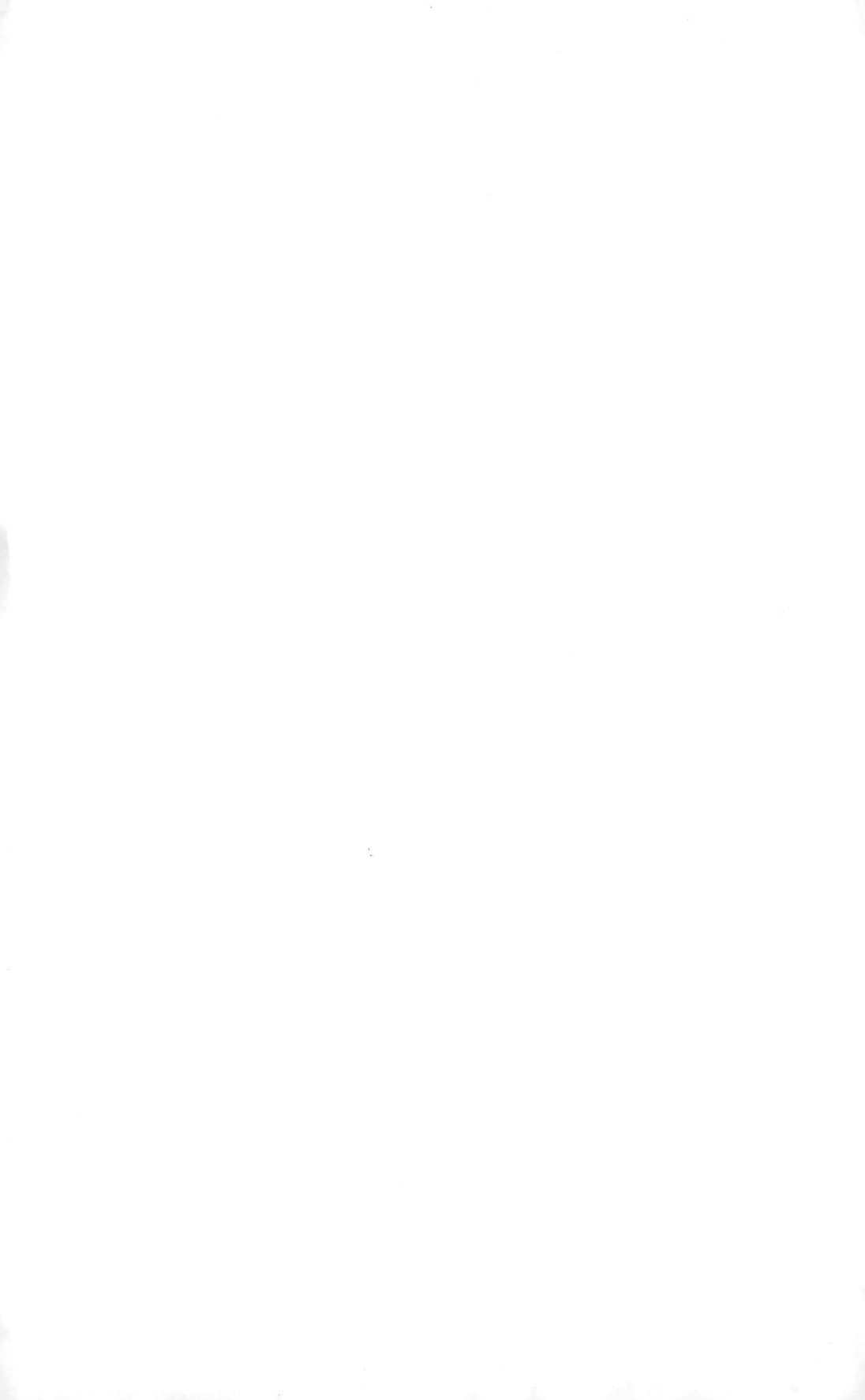

# Mobilizing Knowledge in Physiotherapy

*Mobilizing Knowledge in Physiotherapy: Critical Reflections on Foundations and Practices* is a collection of 15 collaboratively written critical essays by 39 authors from 15 disciplines and seven countries. The book challenges some of the most important contemporary assumptions about physiotherapy knowledge, and makes the case for much more critical theory, practice, and education in physiotherapy health and social care.

The book challenges the kinds of thinking that have traditionally bounded the profession and highlights the ways in which knowledge is now increasingly fluid, complex, and diffuse. The collection engages a range of critical social theories and interdisciplinary perspectives from within and without the profession. It includes sections focusing on evidence, practice, patient perspectives, embodiment, culture, diversity, digital worlds, and research methods. The book makes an important contribution to how we think about mobilizing knowledge, and it speaks to a diverse audience of academics, practitioners, educators, policy-makers, and students – both within physiotherapy and from a range of related health and social care disciplines.

This book will be a useful reference for scholars interested in conceptions of professional knowledge and the theory of professional education and practice in physiotherapy and beyond.

**David A. Nicholls** is Professor in the School of Clinical Sciences at AUT University, New Zealand.

**Karen Synne Groven** is Associate Professor in the Institute of Physiotherapy, Oslo Metropolitan University, Norway. She is also Professor at the Faculty of Health at VID Specialized University, Norway.

**Elizabeth Anne Kinsella** is Professor in the School of Occupational Therapy and the Health Professions Education Graduate Program, Western University, Canada.

**Rani Lill Anjum** is Professor and Co-Director of the Centre for Applied Philosophy of Science at the Norwegian University of Life Sciences, Norway.

# Routledge Advances in Physiotherapy

**Mobilizing Knowledge in Physiotherapy**
Critical Reflections on Foundations and Practices
*Edited by David A. Nicholls, Karen Synne Groven, Elizabeth Anne Kinsella and Rani Lill Anjum*

# Mobilizing Knowledge in Physiotherapy

Critical Reflections on Foundations and Practices

Edited by David A. Nicholls, Karen Synne Groven, Elizabeth Anne Kinsella and Rani Lill Anjum

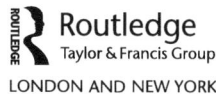

LONDON AND NEW YORK

First published 2021
by Routledge
2 Park Square, Milton Park, Abingdon, Oxon OX14 4RN

and by Routledge
52 Vanderbilt Avenue, New York, NY 10017

*Routledge is an imprint of the Taylor & Francis Group, an informa business*

© 2021 selection and editorial matter, David A. Nicholls, Karen Synne Groven, Elizabeth Anne Kinsella and Rani Lill Anjum; individual chapters, the contributors.

The right of David A. Nicholls, Karen Synne Groven, Elizabeth Anne Kinsella and Rani Lill Anjum to be identified as the authors of the editorial material, and of the authors for their individual chapters, has been asserted in accordance with sections 77 and 78 of the Copyright, Designs and Patents Act 1988.

All rights reserved. No part of this book may be reprinted or reproduced or utilised in any form or by any electronic, mechanical, or other means, now known or hereafter invented, including photocopying and recording, or in any information storage or retrieval system, without permission in writing from the publishers.

*Trademark notice*: Product or corporate names may be trademarks or registered trademarks, and are used only for identification and explanation without intent to infringe.

*British Library Cataloguing-in-Publication Data*
A catalogue record for this book is available from the British Library

*Library of Congress Cataloging-in-Publication Data*
A catalog record for this book has been requested

ISBN: 978-0-367-42818-1 (hbk)
ISBN: 978-0-367-85533-8 (ebk)

Typeset in Times New Roman
by Apex CoVantage, LLC

# Contents

*List of figures* vii
*List of tables* viii
*List of contributors* ix
*Acknowledgements* xvii

1 **Introduction** 1
  DAVID A. NICHOLLS, KAREN SYNNE GROVEN,
  ELIZABETH ANNE KINSELLA, AND RANI LILL ANJUM

2 **Beyond empathy: how physiotherapists and photographers learn to look** 9
  DAVID A. NICHOLLS AND JON NICHOLLS

3 **Bodily ways of knowing: how students learn *about* and *through* bodies during physiotherapy education** 29
  ANNE GUDRUN LANGAAS AND ANNE-LISE MIDDELTHON

4 **Care in physiotherapy – a ghost story** 41
  BIRGITTE AHLSEN, ALETTE OTTESEN, AND CLEMET ASKHEIM

5 **Rethinking recovery** 54
  ANNE MARIT MENGSHOEL AND MARTE FEIRING

6 **Physiotherapy for children and the construction of the disabled child** 70
  KATE WATERWORTH, DAVID A. NICHOLLS, LISETTE BURROWS,
  AND MICHAEL GAFFNEY

7 **Learning from biology, philosophy, and sourdough bread – challenging the evidence-based practice paradigm for community physiotherapy** 83
  SATU REIVONEN, FINLAY SIM, AND CATHY BULLEY

8 Mâmawi-atoskêwin "working together in partnership" – challenging Eurocentric physical therapy practice guided by Indigenous Métis worldview and knowledge    97
LIRIS SMITH, SYLVIA ABONYI, LIZ DUROCHER, TJ ROY, AND SARAH OOSMAN

9 Feeling good about yourself? An exploration of FitBit "new moms community" as an emergent space for online biosociality    113
ALMA VIVIANA SILVA GUERRERO AND WENDY LOWE

10 Disability as expertise: mobilizing a critique of school-based physical therapy for integrating disability studies into physical therapy professionalization    128
DEVORAH SHUBOWITZ

11 A person-centred and collaborative model for understanding chronic pain. Perspectives from a pain patient, a practitioner, and a philosopher    140
CHRISTINE PRICE, MATTHEW LOW, AND RANI LILL ANJUM

12 Finding the right track: embodied reflecting teams for generous physiotherapy    155
PATRICIA THILLE, ARTHUR W. FRANK, AND TOBBA T. SUDMANN

13 Why care about culture? Encountering diversity in a paediatric rehabilitation context: reflections on epiphanies and transformative processes    167
RUNA KALLESON, LINN JULIE SKAGESTAD, AND SOSAN ASGARI MOLLESTAD

14 Using Deleuze: language, dysphasia, and physiotherapy    182
MICHAEL GARD, REBEKAH DEWBERRY, AND JENNY SETCHELL

15 How are we doing? Placing human relationships at the centre of physiotherapy    197
JEAN BRAITHWAITE, TONE DAHL-MICHELSEN, AND KAREN SYNNE GROVEN

*Index*    210

# Figures

| | | |
|---|---|---|
| 2.1 | A patient with cosmetically unacceptable spastic elbow flexion deformity | 14 |
| 2.2 | CJ, aged 16, cystic fibrosis. (A) Relaxed sitting posture (posterior view). (B) Relaxed sitting posture (side view) | 15 |
| 2.3 | Siân Davey, *The Blue Portrait*, 2018 | 16 |
| 2.4 | Thoracic spine: rotation during traction II | 18 |
| 2.5 | Overpressure to the elbow complex. (A) Flexion. (B) Extension. (C) Supination. (D) Pronation | 18 |
| 2.6 and 2.7 | Pauline with Jamie, Endeavour Academy | 20 |
| 2.8 | Students in clinical room | 21 |
| 2.9 | Piermatteo d'Amelia (Italian, about 1450–1508), *The Annunciation*, about 1487 | 22 |
| 2.10 | Therapist and child | 23 |
| 2.11 | Student therapist mobilizing patient's leg | 24 |
| 2.12 | Therapist and kneeling patient | 25 |
| 9.1 | Participant 1 | 121 |
| 9.2 | Participant 5 | 122 |
| 9.3 | Participant 12 | 123 |
| 11.1 | My first four years of healthcare | 142 |
| 11.2 | The vector model of causation | 147 |
| 11.3 | My experience of good, person-centred, evidence-based practice | 150 |
| 11.4 | Causal and dispositional factors contributing to my experience of pain | 151 |
| 11.5 | The main contributors and improvers of my pain | 152 |
| 15.1 | Flourishing around, toward, and beyond recovery | 198 |

# Tables

9.1    Participant characteristics    117

# Contributors

**Sylvia Abonyi** is an associate professor and a medical anthropologist in the Department of Community Health & Epidemiology, University of Saskatchewan. She is a researcher for the Saskatchewan Population Health & Evaluation Research Unit (SPHERU). She has worked closely with First Nation and Métis peoples and communities in Canada for most of her career.

**Birgitte Ahlsen** is an associate professor specialist in Norwegian psychomotor physiotherapy at the Department of Physiotherapy, Oslo Metropolitan University, Oslo, Norway. Birgitte's research interests include critical perspectives on medicine, healthcare, and physiotherapy. Her doctoral research focused on the role of gender in illness narratives of chronic pain. Birgitte's present research project focuses on the first clinical encounter between patients and physiotherapists and relates to issues of knowledge production and translation, as well as how the patient's position is constituted in physiotherapy practice.

**Rani Lill Anjum** is a researcher in philosophy in the School of Economics and Business at the Norwegian University of Life Sciences (NMBU), where she runs the Centre for Applied Philosophy of Science together with Elena Rocca. Rani is the leader of CauseHealth (Causation, Complexity and Evidence in Health Sciences), funded by the Research Council of Norway between 2015 and 2019, which resulted in a spin-off collaborative project, CauseHealth Risk and Safety, funded by Uppsala Centre for International Drug Monitoring and led by Rani and Elena. In her research, Rani primarily works on the philosophical foundations of science with focus on causality, probability, and dispositions and how philosophical assumptions tacitly motivate choice of theory, approach, and practice.

**Clemet Askheim** is a researcher at Centre for Sustainable Health Care Education (SHE), Faculty of Medicine, University of Oslo. He is a philosopher and is currently exploring the history of the concept of sustainability. His research interests include philosophy of science, political philosophy, history of science, environmental history, medical humanities, care, evidence-based medicine, sustainable development, and the Sustainable Development Goals. He occasionally lectures on philosophy of science for master students in physiotherapy at

OsloMet – Oslo Metropolitan University. A recent publication focused on the lost legacy of Archie Cochrane (2017).

**Jean Braithwaite** is a specialist in nonfiction writing, with particular interests in life writing, health, and philosophy. She now teaches nonfiction writing and graphic literature at University of Texas-Rio Grande Valley and heads the faculty Words + Pictures Group. Braithwaite's publishing history is as eclectic as her education, including a literary memoir and artistic essays alongside scholarly research including cultural criticism and narratology. Braithwaite's long-term research-writing partnership with Groven and Dahl-Michelsen is a source of particular satisfaction.

**Cathy Bulley** is Co-Director of the Centre for Health, Activity and Rehabilitation Research. Cathy has interests in scholarship, innovation, and research, as well as the interplay between these. Her research focuses on supporting people with long-term conditions and has led to Cathy co-founding a social enterprise called 'Health Design Collective', which focuses on user-centred, health-related product design.

**Lisette Burrows** is a professor in community health at the University of Waikato, Hamilton, New Zealand. Her research draws on insights from the sociology of education, sociology of youth, curriculum studies, and cultural studies to explore the place and meaning of physical culture and health in young people's lives. She is also interested in the ways health imperatives expressed at policy and government levels are taken up and responded to in community contexts. She has published work on gender, ethnicity, and disability in school-based physical education and young New Zealanders' constructions of health and fitness.

**Tone Dahl-Michelsen** is a physiotherapist and holds a master's in health sciences. She graduated with her PhD in professional studies in 2015 at the Centre of the Study of Professions (OsloMet) with the thesis: *Gender in Physiotherapy Education. A Study of Gender Performance Among Physiotherapy Students and Changes in the Significance of Gender*. Dahl-Michelsen's range of interests is broad, covering higher education, qualitative methods, ethics, and rehabilitation, among other topics. Her main research interest is knowledge and professional practices in healthcare education and in rehabilitation. Her teaching covers the same areas as her research, and she teaches and supervises students at the bachelor, master, and PhD level.

**Rebekah Dewberry** directs the Red Soup Speech Pathology, a well-established private practice, delivering community-based rehabilitation to adults and children who have sustained an acquired brain injury, with a particular interest in traumatic brain injury.

**Liz Durocher** is a third-generation Métis woman with French ancestry on her dad's side of the family. She is a social worker and community developer with a passion for working with young adults in her community.

Marte Feiring is Professor of Public Health and Rehabilitation in the Institute of Physiotherapy, Faculty of Health Science, Oslo Metropolitan University, Norway. She is educated as an occupational therapist and a sociologist and holds a PhD in sociology from the University of Oslo on the history of rehabilitation. Her research interests cover historical and critical perspectives on health policies, welfare services, professional and multiprofessional knowledge, rehabilitation practices, and civil movements, including recovery. She is currently working on research projects focusing on the global travels of ideas of reablement and task shifts in the care for patients with hand osteoarthritis.

Arthur W. Frank received his doctorate in sociology from Yale in 1975 and spent his entire teaching career at the University of Calgary, where he is Professor Emeritus. He is an elected fellow of the Royal Society of Canada and 2008 winner of the Society's medal in bioethics. In 2016, he received the lifetime achievement award of the Canadian Bioethics Society. His current project is vulnerable reading, an approach to literature from the perspective of the needs of people who seek help living with some form of suffering.

Michael Gaffney teaches early childhood education students in the initial teacher education programme at the College of Education University of Otago, with his main responsibilities being inclusive education and teaching practice. Michael has an interest in understanding children's experiences within the theoretical frameworks of sociocultural theory and childhood studies with connections to disability studies, children's rights, and the sociology of childhood. He is also interested in how concepts from new materialism and post-humanism might reframe his theoretical understandings of children and families with respect to agency, relationships, and identity.

Michael Gard holds a master's degree in exercise science and a PhD in the sociology and history of dance. He has written several books on a variety of subjects, including obesity, science, and public health policy. While his primary field of research is in health and physical education, Michael is also a social scientist who has intentionally contributed to broader sociological scholarship of health and the body.

Karen Synne Groven is a physical therapist and holds a PhD in health science from the University of Oslo, Faculty of Medicine. She is a professor of public health and rehabilitation at the Department of Physiotherapy, Faculty of Health Science, Oslo Metropolitan University, Norway. She is also Professor at VID Specialized University, Faculty of Health. Groven's research interests are in the fields of obesity, long-term illness and pain, and rehabilitation from long-term conditions (including chronic fatigue syndrome, vulva pain, and so on). She is also involved in research projects focusing on children with disabilities and their experiences of a meaningful life.

Runa Kalleson is a physiotherapist with a master's degree in rehabilitation and habilitation. Runa has more than ten years of experience working with children with disabilities and their families in the municipal health services in Oslo, Norway. She is a PhD candidate in health sciences at Oslo Metropolitan University (OsloMet) working on a project relating to children with cerebral palsy, family empowerment, and provision of services directed to children with disabilities and their families. She also teaches in the Department of Physiotherapy at OsloMet.

**Elizabeth Anne Kinsella** is a professor at Western University in London, Ontario Canada. Elizabeth Anne's scholarship increases awareness of the impact that epistemological understandings of reflection can have on conceptions of professional knowledge, education, and practice in health and social care. Her work investigates a continuum of reflection that includes reflective practice, embodied reflection, critical reflection, reflexivity, and mindfulness. Her scholarship encompasses reflective approaches oriented toward phronesis, praxis, ethics of care, relational autonomy, disability rights, justice, equity, and inclusion.

**Anne Gudrun Langaas** is an associate professor in the bachelor program in physiotherapy, the master's in rehabilitation, and the master's in physiotherapy, and she is in charge of a PhD course in qualitative methods in the Faculty of Health Sciences at Oslo Metropolitan University. Her research interests are within qualitative methodologies, medical and social anthropology, pedagogy, epistemology, philosophy, and semiotics related to embodiment, bodily ways of knowing, critical reflection on professional encounters in physiotherapy, and social inequality in health.

**Matthew Low** is a consultant physiotherapist in the NHS and is a visiting associate at the Orthopaedic Research Institute at Bournemouth University. He has interests in compassionate person-centred care, the theory of causation within the healthcare setting, philosophy, clinical reasoning, reflective practice, and critical thinking skills.

**Wendy Lowe** is a senior lecturer in medical sociology and medical education and Module Lead for the Human Science Public Health module of the MBBS and GEP at Barts and the London School of Medicine and Dentistry. Her PhD explored how health professionals are educated and some of the consequences of that. Her PhD study arose from her previous training and experience as a physiotherapist, then developed through further biomechanical research and learning on pedagogy, sociology, and the medical humanities.

**Anne Marit Mengshoel** is a professor at the Department of Interdisciplinary Health Sciences, Medical Faculty, at the University of Oslo, a doctor of medical science, and a physiotherapist with postgraduate training in manual therapy. She founded and chaired the research group self-management in her department until last year. Her recent research has mainly focused on patients' experiences of living with long-term illnesses; recovery processes; and currently developing, implementing, and evaluating a new rehabilitation programme for patients with fibromyalgia. Mengshoel is lecturing on theories of disease, health, and illness, academic writing, qualitative analysis, and project planning.

Contributors xiii

**Anne-Lise Middelthon** is a professor at the Section for Medical Anthropology and Medical History at the Faculty of Medicine, University of Oslo, Norway. She is a social anthropologist by training, working mainly within the field of medical anthropology. Anne-Lise's research work focuses on the body and medicalization of food, as well as the cultural and social dimension of infectious diseases. Theoretically, she is particularly interested in semiotics – more specifically, semiotics in the Peircean tradition. Works and thinking of this tradition largely inform her research.

**Sosan Asgari Mollestad** sought safety and protection in Norway after a dramatic escape from Iran in 1985. Her education background is in child protection and welfare; however, her work has largely focused on facilitating the support and integration of newcomers – refugees, asylum seekers, and immigrants – to Norway. Through her company, Ektabana Consulting, she offers courses and training for private and public sectors on topics such as refugees, integration, multicultural understanding, and intercultural communication. She now works as a project manager and integration advisor at the Norwegian Society of Rural Women.

**David A. Nicholls** is a professor in the School of Clinical Sciences at AUT University in Auckland, New Zealand. He is a physiotherapist, lecturer, researcher, and writer, with a passion for critical thinking in and around the physical therapies. David is the founder of the Critical Physiotherapy Network, co-founder and chair of the International Physiotherapy History Association, and founding executive member of the Environmental Physiotherapy Association. David's own research work focuses on the critical history and sociology of physiotherapy.

**Jon Nicholls** is Director of Arts & Creativity at Thomas Tallis School in London, UK, a teacher of photography. Jon has collaborated with Photoworks, the Royal Photographic Society, and the Photographers' Gallery on a number of educational projects and resources. He also leads the school's pioneering work on creative learning and its projects with Tate Exchange, an experiment in public engagement with art at Tate Modern, which explores the role of contemporary arts pedagogy in schools, particularly for young people with special educational needs and disabilities.

**Sarah Oosman** is an associate professor at the University of Saskatchewan and a researcher for the Saskatchewan Population Health & Evaluation Research Unit (SPHERU). Sarah is a first-generation settler Canadian, mother of two children. She has had the honour of working with Métis community members from northern Saskatchewan for over ten years.

**Alette Ottesen** is a physiotherapist and specialist in (Norwegian) psychomotor physiotherapy, with her own practice and long experience (almost 40 years) working as a clinician. She is an assistant in FYSIOPRIM, a research program at the University of Oslo, Norway, which aims to improve research in primary healthcare and to bridge the gap between research and clinical practice. Alette also works as a lecturer at OsloMet – Oslo Metropolitan University – teaching practical skills to students in professional development courses in the area of psychomotor physiotherapy. Alette's interests are related to issues concerning physiotherapy practice and questions about what physiotherapy is and could be.

**Christine Price** is affected by neuropathic pain (sciatica), which she has lived with since an injury in 2008. Recently, she started to write, blog, and talk about her experiences of living well with pain, directed at both clinicians and patients. Christine has been invited to sit on research advisory panels and is the first patient representative on the Executive Board of the UK's Physiotherapy Pain Association. She is involved in the production of learning materials about persistent pain for both patients and clinicians.

**Satu Reivonen** is a paediatric physiotherapist at the Helsinki University Hospital. Satu graduated with an MSc in physiotherapy in 2018 from Queen Margaret University in Edinburgh, Scotland. Before this, she completed a research-oriented master's in psychology at the University of Edinburgh. During her studies, she developed a strong interest in interdisciplinary connections, qualitative research, and critical thinking, which led her to join the Critical Physiotherapy Network. She currently has the long-term aim of combining research with clinical work.

**TJ Roy** is a community developer at the University of Saskatchewan. TJ is a Plains Cree and Métis man, having a bloodline with two rich cultures. His mom was a Cree First Nation woman and a Treaty Indian; his dad was Métis with French and Irish heritage and a strong connection to the land.

**Jenny Setchell** is a senior research fellow in physiotherapy at the School of Health and Rehabilitation Sciences, University of Queensland. Her research interests include post-structuralist critical perspectives on healthcare broadly and physiotherapy specifically. Her PhD was in psychology and focused on weight stigma in physiotherapy. She is experienced in a range of qualitative and post-qualitative research methodologies. Dr Setchell also has 20 years of diverse clinical experience in Australia and internationally, primarily in the musculoskeletal and sports subdisciplines. She is a founding member and past co-chair of the Executive Committee of the International Critical Physiotherapy Network and on the Executive Committee of the International Society for Critical Health Psychology. Dr Setchell has held a number of grants and awards and was the recipient of an NHMRC Fellowship in 2019 and the Margaret Mittelheuser Fellowship in 2015. She has also been an acrobat and a human rights worker.

**Devorah Shubowitz** currently works as a physical therapist for the NYC Department of Education. Her PhD is in social cultural anthropology. She is interested in the integration of disability studies, disability movement expertise, dance, somatic practices, and physical therapy.

Contributors xv

**Alma Viviana Silva Guerrero** is a physiotherapist with 20 years of clinical experience in the fields of musculoskeletal, orthopaedics, and cardiopulmonary care in Bogota, Colombia, and recently in age care and sports in Australia. She has critically explored the sociopolitical and economic forces that impact professional practice in Colombia, as well as sharing her experiences and reflections in relation to recent policy changes in Colombia at the WCPT conference, *The Impact of Neoliberal Ideology on Physiotherapy Practice – A Colombian Physiotherapist's Experience*, and explored the links between physiotherapy in Latin America, changes in healthcare delivery, shifting social values, and the relationship between physiotherapy and medicine. Her work focused particularly on the gendered history of the profession in Latin America and its influence on physiotherapy over the last few decades, *Narrative Histories of Physiotherapy in Colombia, Ecuador, and Argentina*.

**Finlay Sim** is a baker and research assistant in grain technology at the University of Helsinki. Finlay is an MSc graduate in dietetics from Queen Margaret University, Edinburgh, who completed his thesis in the topic of sourdough microbiology and sensory science in artisan baking. Upon graduating, he decided to dive deeper in the craft and philosophy of sourdough baking by working as a baker at a community artisan bakery located in the heart of Scotland. Currently, he continues to work as a baker in Finland, as well as working part-time as a research assistant within the Grain Technology research group at the University of Helsinki.

**Linn Julie Skagestad** is a licensed psychologist and PhD candidate at Oslo Metropolitan University. Her professional experience includes counselling and interprofessional work within the Norwegian Specialist Psychiatric Health Services and the Norwegian Educational and Psychological Counselling Service. Her research interests relate to contextualized and relational approaches to (inter)professional practices with children and adults, disability studies, and childhood/adolescence. Her PhD project addresses collaborations around youth living with disability and their caregivers and professional helpers and is particularly concerned with how youth participation relates to parent/helper involvement and broader cultural-institutional structures.

**Liris Smith** is a mother of two adults and a physical therapist who has worked for almost three decades in rural/remote/northern practice and leadership. She is a first-generation Canadian on her mother's side and third generation on her father's side. She is now a graduate student, working with older Métis adults to understand how they experience physical activity through their life journey. She believes that as physical therapists, it is incumbent on us, when working within Indigenous communities, to use reflective practice within an ethical space of engagement and thereby find transformative ways to support health and wellness.

**Tobba T. Sudmann** is a full-time professor of public health, physiotherapist, and medical sociologist. She is head of the PhD Program in Health, Functioning and Participation at Western Norway University of Applied Sciences in Norway, and she has an adjunct position as an outdoor riding physiotherapist. Her research interests are related to how people use their bodily resources to enhance their well-being and social participation, whether the means are indoor or outdoor physical activity, technology, nature, or animals. Her research is directed towards the person(s)'s agency, barriers for interaction and social participation, and anti-oppressive professional practice, irrespective of empirical field.

**Patricia Thille** is an assistant professor in the Department of Physical Therapy at the University of Manitoba. She is a PhD-trained medical sociologist with a clinical physiotherapy degree. Her research program bridges critical social scientific theories and methodologies into the health services and health professions education fields, focusing on the topics of stigmatization of patients, health behaviour change support, organizational change, and chronic disease management.

**Kate Waterworth** is a PhD student and teacher at the School of Clinical Sciences, AUT University, New Zealand. She enjoys exploring ideas around children, childhood, disability, and rehabilitation. She works at AUT University teaching in the areas of critical disability studies and the undergraduate physiotherapy curriculum. She is particularly interested in thinking with philosophy to critique and challenge conventional thinking and practices. At the moment, she is grappling with concepts from Deleuze, Guattari, and others in post-structural/post-qualitative spaces for a PhD project on rethinking disability for children. She also loves playing in the outdoors with her wee boy Sammy.

# Acknowledgements

David and Jon Nicholls would like to acknowledge Frank Weedon's family for allowing them to reproduce the images from his collection. We also acknowledge the Isabella Stewart Gardner Gallery for permission to reproduce 'The Annunciation'; Polly Braden and Siân Davey for permission to reprint their photographs; and Elsevier for permission to reproduce images from Main and Denehy, Montgomery, Petty and Moore. A recording of Weedon talking about his time at the Otago Physiotherapy School can be found at http://tinyurl.com/uh4njn2, and a full set of Weedon's photographs used in this chapter can be found at http://tinyurl.com/sqczlyc. Anne Langaas and Anne-Lise Middelthon would like to thank all students and colleagues at the physiotherapy program at Oslo Metropolitan University for their participation, patience, and contribution throughout the project period. A special thanks to associate professor Sidsel Byhring for always being available for discussions and reflections and to philosophy professor Vincent Colapietro for his explications of William James' thoughts. We would also like to thank the Centre for the Study of Professions (SPS) at Oslo Metropolitan University for making already collected data available for inclusion in our project. Birgitte Ahlsen, Alette Ottesen, and Clemet Askheim acknowledge the financial support from The Norwegian Fund for Post-Graduate Training in Physiotherapy through the FYSIOPRIM project. Liris Smith and co-authors acknowledge the traditional indigenous territories of Canada that include treaty lands, unceded lands, and Métis homelands on which we, the authors, live, work, teach, and learn. The authors engage in their work together on Treaty 6 and Treaty 10 territory and the Homeland of the Métis and affirm our commitment to respectful relationships with one another and the land. We acknowledge the Métis people and the community of Île-à-la-Crosse and the Sakitiwak Elders Council for being open and patient in guiding our learning journey and for their ongoing support and partnership. Alva Viviana Silva and Wendy Lowe wish to thank Adele Pavlidis at Griffith University for her help in reviewing and editing of some sections of their chapter. Patricia Thille, Arthur Frank, and Tobba Sudmann would like to acknowledge and thank Louise, whose own generosity and reflections added depth to ours, and Emilly Munguía Marshall, for publishing her own reflective story about physiotherapy practice. In a multivoiced dialogue among stories, we hope they find their contributions and reflections on physiotherapy care in good company. And finally, Jean Braithwaite, Tone Dahl-Michelsen, and Karen Synne Groven wish to express their thanks to Stephen Buetow for permission to reproduce the figure illustrating his concept of ultrabilitation.

# 1 Introduction

*David A. Nicholls, Karen Synne Groven,
Elizabeth Anne Kinsella, and Rani Lill Anjum*

This manuscript began its life at a book launch for *Manipulating Practices*, the first-ever edited collection of critical physiotherapy writings. In February 2018, just two months after the book had been released online, some of the authors gathered at the Litteraturhuset, in Oslo, to formally launch the book and celebrate its success. Achieved in part because it was open access and therefore freely available, more than 6,000 people had downloaded the book, and today it has been accessed by more than 20,000 people, making it the most-accessed text in publisher Cappelen Damm's history. Perhaps it was appropriate, then, that at the book launch, four eminent scholars offered critical commentaries. Two of the discussants – Dr Rani Lill Anjum and Professor Per Koren Solvang – commended the book, describing it as an important contribution to critical physiotherapy, but also suggested that because it focused on physiotherapy authors looking critically *at* physiotherapy practice, it was rather *inward looking*. It would be good, they suggested, to also have a text that encouraged physiotherapists to be more *outward looking*. And so, at the end of that meeting, a plan was hatched to begin work on a follow-up to *Manipulating Practices* and to find a way to be more exoteric.

Professors Karen Synne Groven and Dave A. Nicholls met in Sydney in June 2018 for the In Sickness and In Health conference, and while there, decided that we would invite contributions for a second book from physiotherapists on the condition that they collaborate with a non-physiotherapy author. And with the first book focusing on practices, we wanted to focus this book on knowledge. We then invited interdisciplinary scholars Dr Rani Lill Anjum and Professor Elizabeth Anne Kinsella to join us on the editorial team. Both were close to the Critical Physiotherapy Network (CPN), both were established scholars interested in epistemological questions relevant to professional knowledge, and neither was a physiotherapist, so our editorial team reflected our focus on epistemology and honoured our commitment to be more outward looking.

We were somewhat nervous about our call for abstracts because critical physiotherapy studies are still in their infancy, and we had no idea whether we had exhausted our field with the first book. We need not have worried. We received 49 diverse and powerful chapter proposals from all over the world for this (second) book, which gave us the enviable but no less difficult task of selecting for the collection.

Our production schedule began mid-2019, and authors completed their chapters by February 2020. As had been the case with the first book, the response from the authors and the quality and diversity of their work has been breathtaking. This is particularly gratifying given that this is still virgin territory for a lot of physiotherapists.

Although critical writings in medicine, nursing, and psychology have been the norm for nearly half a century now, and medical sociology is a vibrant scholarly field, critical physiotherapy studies really only began in earnest in 2014 with the formation of the CPN. Since then, there has been a dramatic increase in the number of articles, editorials, blog posts, social media posts, conference presentations, and even a handful of long-form manuscripts produced that give voice to critical physiotherapy. There can be little doubt now that critical physiotherapy is a sub-discipline in its own right, and the publication of this book offers evidence of an emerging, vibrant, critical community of scholars, keen to be a positive force for an 'otherwise' physiotherapy.

But the success of critical physiotherapy as a field of study in recent years does not mean anyone can rest on their laurels. No one can have any doubt that we are at the crossroads of one of the most exciting and challenging points in the history of the profession and healthcare generally. Health systems around the world are in flux; we have unprecedented access to health knowledge and information technology that could transform everyone's work. We have healthcare happening in myriad locations, perhaps only a relatively small portion of which is regulated. We have a looming climate catastrophe and the ever-present threat of globalised pandemics. We have a world map that is being reshaped demographically and transformed attitudes towards our bodies, health, movement, relationships, and meaning. Who knows what physiotherapy will look like in 50 years' time. All we can say is that it will be very different from today.

So how does this book make a contribution to this epochal debate? First, as with all of us, we can try in our own modest way to engage in these discussions; to be a part of the *polis* and have our voice heard. Second, we can offer ideas that may never have been articulated before; we can say things that may have been too difficult or disallowed or not visible in the past. Third, we can make our mark, literally in print. We can stand for something. Perhaps that something is greater diversity, tolerance, and inclusion, or perhaps it is a call for greater clarity, precision, and definition. And finally, we can come together and give voice to ideas that we believe *can* and *do* make a difference.

When Donald Schon wrote *The Reflective Practitioner* 35 years ago, he was doing far more than guiding practitioners to engage in reflection on their practices: his insights were far more radical. He was pointing to the limits of technical knowledge as a guiding rationality for the professions and calling for recognition of the epistemological significance of other forms of knowledge, particularly those generated through reflection in and on professional practices.

Many of the chapters in this collection illuminate this seemingly radical proposition, that knowledge generated through various forms of reflection, critical reflection, and critical reflexivity is epistemologically significant. Knowledge generated through critical forms of reflection in and on practice is shown throughout this collection to render important epistemological contributions that expand the borders of our understandings, that radically shift how we think about what it is to mobilize knowledge in physiotherapy education and practice.

Knowledge comes to the fore in this collection, not as something situated in a distant, technical, objectivist, universalist, foundationalist milieu, nor as something to be 'implemented' by practitioners onto service users. Rather knowledge reveals itself here through radically constituted dialogue that brings attention to the practice-based experiences, disjunctures, tensions, ruptures, reflections, and insights of practitioners and service users, in conversation with critical social theoretical and philosophical perspectives, to generate new forms of knowledge that are palpable and compelling in their logic and relevance to professional education and practice.

As a collection, the various perspectives presented here make visible and bring to the centre a number of hidden, or marginalized, yet epistemically significant perspectives. This work mobilizes knowledge by redressing past epistemic imbalances, by reclaiming the space for marginalized perspectives, by re-centring important conversations from the periphery, by 'showing' the significance of practice-based perspectives through exemplars and conversations with philosophy and critical social theory. Through this broad recognition of the knowledge contributions of people, theories, discourses, and concepts at the periphery, this work moves us closer to epistemic justice and to more inclusivity in our quest to generate and mobilize knowledge across divides.

Where *Manipulating Practices* focused on a broad range of philosophical and theoretical questions, broadly applied to physiotherapy practice, *Mobilizing Knowledge* concentrates on some of the epistemological questions now surrounding physiotherapy. These questions were raised by Monika Nerland, writing in Trede and McEwan's *Educating the Deliberate Professional*, who argued that the future for professions like physiotherapy relies on their ability to respond to the transformations now taking place in knowledge production and distribution (Nerland, 2016). Implicit in these arguments is the belief that the epistemological presuppositions that once provided orthodox professions with their social status are in decline, being replaced by a heterodox matrix of complex assemblages and discourses that call into question and open conversations concerning the fabric of professional curricula, codes of conduct, practice theories, and socially validated roles. *Mobilizing Knowledge* steps into this space by bringing together scholars in and around the field of physiotherapy who are challenging the kinds of knowledge that have traditionally bounded the profession.

The book's founding premise is that the world in which physiotherapy now operates is evolving rapidly, and so it is axiomatic that physiotherapists will need to be open to new kinds of knowledge and new ways of thinking. There are works in this volume, then, that explore:

- Historical development of physiotherapy knowledge
- Ways in which physiotherapists have claimed particular kinds of knowledge and marginalised others

- Links between physiotherapy knowledge in theory and in practice
- Emerging knowledges being deployed by educators, practitioners, and researchers
- Rethinking the significance of practice-based knowledges and epistemologies of practice in physiotherapy
- Students' experiences of knowledge acquisition
- Challenges of adapting physiotherapy to new kinds of knowledge
- Alter-, cross-, inter-, meta-, multi-, pluri-, post-, and trans-disciplinary contributions to knowledge generation
- Possibilities for radically rethinking what physiotherapy is or can be
- Synergies, collaborations, and fruitful boundary breaches that may transform physiotherapy thinking and practice
- Ruptures, disruptions, interruptions, disjunctures, and disorientations that invite reflection on the boundaries of physiotherapy knowledge
- Cultural, economic, philosophical, political, social, or spiritual challenges to physiotherapy's traditional biomedical worldview
- Radical and critical emancipatory challenges to western, androcentric, heteronormative, colonial, sanist, and ableist hegemonies
- Methods for developing, evaluating, implementing, and critiquing physiotherapy knowledge
- Knowledge and physiotherapy curriculum
- Knowledge as a limiting factor in transforming future practice
- Emerging research methodologies that challenge bio-scientific and interpretivist modes of knowledge production
- Consideration of epistemic justice in relation to whose testimonies are privileged and legitimated and whose testimonies may be silenced or excluded in physiotherapy practice

Overall, we hope to provoke, prompt, and prime the profession, however modestly, for a transformation that may exceed anything we could have imagined even six years ago when the CPN was formed. To that end, we have brought together 39 authors across 15 chapters, from seven countries and more than 14 disciplines. As well as physiotherapy academics, clinicians, researchers, and doctoral students, the collection includes authors who are health service users and authors from medical anthropology, philosophy, non-fiction, community health, speech and language therapy, social work, occupational therapy, sociology, education, child protection, photography, dietetics, and psychology.

We see that, although all the chapters start from the perspective of physiotherapy, each chapter actually tackles some deeper, more general issues that have relevance far beyond physiotherapy. The book is thus an example of how one can use critical reflection as a methodology to mobilize a profession, contribute to the transformation of epistemic insights, and broaden conceptualizations of knowledge and thus avoid becoming locked into a dogmatic mindset where the epistemic premises, such as concepts, approaches, and methods, are simply decided by the dominating paradigm. In this sense, this book is as much a contribution to the philosophy of science and ethics as it is a contribution to critical scholarship in physiotherapy.

The book opens with Dave and Jon Nicholls' chapter 'Beyond Empathy: How Physiotherapists and Photographers Learn to Look', which explores physiotherapists' traditional biomedical and normative ways of looking at bodies. Drawing inspiration from contemporary photography, especially the work of amateur photographer Frank Weedon, they argue for a change of focus – a focus in which an empathic and relational approach is acknowledged. Such a shift in focus is paramount, they argue, in order for the profession to develop in a more reciprocal relationship with their patients.

In the next chapter, 'Bodily Ways of Knowing: How Students Learn *About* and *Through* Bodies During Physiotherapy Education', Anne Gudrun Langaas and Anne-Lise Middelthon argue for the centrality of bodily knowledge in physiotherapy education. The authors argue that education must move beyond technical, theoretical, biomedical, and communicative domains to also focus on the cultivation of physiotherapists' bodily knowledge. Theoretical constructs such as Polanyi's tacit knowledge, Sheets-Johnstone's primacy of movement, and Despret's insights that having a body entails being affected by other entities are used to draw attention to the relationship between embodiment and knowledge generation. The authors examine how students learn both *about* and *through* bodies – how bodies are shaped and what bodies *do* – in physiotherapy education. This chapter calls for educational approaches that make the centrality of bodily knowledge and its importance to competent physiotherapy practice more explicit.

Next, in 'Care in Physiotherapy – A Ghost Story', Birgitte Ahlsen, Alette Ottesen, and Clemet Askheim make a compelling case for re-centring 'care' in physiotherapy practice. The authors draw on practice-based vignettes from a physiotherapist's encounters with a patient; in dialogue with the Roman myth of Cura (or Care); and theoretical insights from Freud, Heidegger, and Mol to show how 'care' is latent and repressed in physiotherapy practice. They argue that this is a result of a predominant emphasis on biomedical perspectives and a focus on the body that excludes mind and soul. The authors contend that the logic of choice and the logic of care frequently come into collision and that this results in the suppression of care and a failure to acknowledge its importance. The chapter makes visible the ways in which care is central to what it means to be human and consequently to the practice of physiotherapy and to the recovery of the profession. This work opens an important dialogue concerning the need to make space for care in physiotherapy practice.

'Rethinking Recovery' by Anne Marit Mengshoel and Marte Feiring explores two different understandings of recovery: disease- and outcome-oriented, compared with process- and experience-oriented. While recovery as an outcome motivates current evidence-based practice, where the goal of therapy is its curative effect, the same cannot apply to many chronic conditions. Here, recovery is seen as the process of coming to terms with and adapting to the new situation, which would motivate a more person-centred and individualized approach to therapy. The authors discuss how the two understandings may be integrated or co-produced.

They use examples from physiotherapy, but the insights apply generally to all health professions.

Kate Waterworth, Dave A. Nicholls, Lisette Burrows, and Michael Gaffney's chapter 'Physiotherapy for Children and the Construction of the Disabled Child' embarks on a historical examination of the physiotherapy profession. Exploring the construction of particular forms of knowledge, the authors explore how notions of normality and otherness gained ground following World War II, inspiring physiotherapists to give priority to children's rehabilitation potential. In this era, two discourses emerged shaping contemporary physiotherapy: the disabled child as having 'potential' and the disabled child as not normal. These discourses are, however, problematic, as they create what the authors term a particular social identity for disabled children – that of the 'other'. In order to change this emphasis, the authors argue for the need to expand physiotherapists' knowledge base through a number of post-critical perspectives.

The chapter 'Learning From Biology, Philosophy, and Sourdough Bread: Challenging the Evidence-Based Practice Paradigm for Community Physiotherapy', written by Satu Reivonen, Finlay Sim, and Cathy Bulley, invites us to critically review the philosophical foundations of the current paradigm of evidence-based practice. More specifically, the authors show that whether one thinks of knowledge and evidence in terms of controllable, context-independent static entities (things, substances) or as highly complex, context-dependent, dynamic, and non-linear processes, one's choice will affect the way evidence is understood, generated, and used to inform complex care plans for individuals with multiple long-term conditions.

Guided by indigenous Métis worldview and knowledge, Liris Smith, Sylvia Abonyi, Liz Durocher, TJ Roy, and Sarah Oosman challenge what they term a predominant 'Eurocentric focus' in physical therapy. In their chapter, 'Mâmawi-Atoskêwin, "Working Together in Partnership" – Challenging Eurocentric Physical Therapy Practice Guided by Indigenous Métis Worldview and Knowledge', Smith and co-authors argue that contemporary physiotherapy has grown within western paradigms of thought and epistemology. In this process, however, the profession has failed to acknowledge alternative knowledge systems, such as those practised by Indigenous populations. In this chapter, the authors propose possibilities for innovatively rethinking the practice of physical therapy in partnership with Indigenous communities. In particular, they suggest applying an 'ethical space' approach to collaboratively working within a northern Canadian Métis community to co-create research and practice. Bridging the strengths of Western and Indigenous worldviews, they pinpoint what is paramount in meeting the needs and priorities of healthy ageing in the Métis community while acquiring new perspectives that transform contemporary physical therapy practice.

In 'Feeling Good About Yourself? An Exploration of FitBit "New Moms Community" as an Emergent Space for Online Biosociality', Alma Viviana Silva Guerrero and Wendy Lowe explore the competitive self-policing, physical accomplishments, and existential tensions experienced by women post-partum. Analysing a community of women engaging in a FitBit community site, the authors draw on feminist post-structural praxiographic research to examine the motivations, frustrations, self-imposed judgements, and aspirations of women as they engage with their bodies through a variety of contemporary health practices. The authors see new roles for physiotherapists emerging at a time when many people are turning to online communities for health advice and support.

In Devorah Shubowitz's chapter, 'Disability as Expertise: Mobilizing a Critique of School-Based Physical Therapy for Integrating Disability Studies into Physiotherapy Professionalization', Shubowitz applies a socially progressive approach to encounters with children with disabilities in New York schools. The author argues how such an emphasis narrows the field of physiotherapy practice, including school physiotherapists' sensitivity as to how to adjust their approaches to each 'disabled' child's needs and desires. Rather than narrowing the scope of practice, there is a need to open up, drawing inspiration from critical disability studies. This entails acknowledging the expertise of the child as well as acknowledging the need for physiotherapists to broaden and somewhat rethink their notion of expertise.

Christine Price, Matthew Low, and Rani Lill Anjum explore dispositionalism as a viable alternative to Humean accounts of causation. Co-authoring the chapter from the perspective of a service user, a physiotherapist, and philosopher of health, 'A Person-Centred and Collaborative Model for Understanding Chronic Pain. Perspectives from a Pain Patient, a Practitioner, and a Philosopher', asks how it might be possible to derive a more complex, nuanced, context-sensitive, and reflexive approach to causation than is currently available. An approach that moves beyond assessment, diagnosis, and the reconciliation of research evidence is needed because we have become over-reliant on descriptive and categorical diagnoses, which leave little room for the patient's voice. Instead, Price, Low, and Anjum make a case for an approach that honours and respects the person at the centre of clinical decision-making.

In 'Finding the Right Track: Embodied Reflecting Teams for Generous Physiotherapy', Patricia Thille, Arthur W. Frank, and Tobba T. Sudmann explore the embodied, situated nature of knowledge. Drawing on the idea of 'mindlines', the authors explore the role of reflective teams in the co-construction of health and healthcare. Creating a reflective team among themselves, the authors think through their own and others' stories of healthcare and reflect on how physiotherapy mindlines can sometimes limit generous, recuperative relations with patients, particularly when facing sadness that exceeds intervention. Calling, instead, for generosity in practice, the authors open a space for dialogue with the profession that reaches beyond the boundaries of current practice.

In the next chapter, 'Why Care About Culture? Encountering Diversity in a Paediatric Rehabilitation Context: Reflections on Epiphanies and Transformative Processes', Runa Kalleson, Linn Julie Skagestad, and Sosan Asgari Mollestad examine a physiotherapist's transformation toward increased cultural awareness. This chapter draws on autoethnographic reflections and epiphanies arising through a physiotherapist's practice-based encounters with a newcomer family from a different country. These reflections are brought into dialogue with a social worker who served as a cultural liaison, a psychologist, and a range of sociocultural and philosophical perspectives. The discussion raises awareness of how assumptions, biases, values, and positioning may unintentionally shape practice. The chapter advances knowledge about approaches that counter ethnocentric perspectives and move to more relational and collaborative practices. The authors argue that cultural humility, and recognition of how two cultures come to meet, are central to culturally relevant healthcare services.

"Using Deleuze: Language, Dysphasia, and Physiotherapy', by Michael Gard, Rebekah Dewberry, and Jenny Setchell, draws on an extensive account of one of the author's experiences of recovering from a traumatic brain injury. Using both the 'patient' narrative, accounts of clinical management, and a novel 'dysphasanalysis' – inspired by Gilles Deleuze – the authors engage in a creative exploration of the intersection between the previously contested world and explore methodological possibilities for boundary breaches. Celebrating the lyrical, poetic, and musical possibility of lost words and the ability to find new avenues of engagement, the authors radically disrupt conventional approaches to therapy, embodiment, health, and the body.

In the final chapter in the collection, Jean Braithwaite, Tone Dahl-Michelsen, and Karen Synne Groven ask a question whose theme runs through the whole book: 'How Are We Doing? Placing Human Relationships at the Centre of Physiotherapy'. The authors call for a critical self-reflection over the aims and practice of physiotherapy. They argue that since the ultimate goal of treatment should be to help the patient flourish, there can be no normal, best, or one-size-fits-all form of therapy that does not take into account the patients' individual values and goals. By reflecting over two contrasting cases of young Scandinavians born with cerebral palsy with very different relationships to their own rehabilitation process and physiotherapy, the authors argue that a more individualized and relationship-centred approach to physiotherapy is needed to help promote bodily pleasure and wellbeing for their patients.

## Reference

Nerland, M. (2016). Learning to master profession-specific knowledge practices: A prerequisite for the deliberate practitioner. In F. Trede & C. McEwan (Eds.), *Educating the deliberate professional* (pp. 127–140). Amsterdam: Springer.

## 2 Beyond empathy

How physiotherapists and photographers learn to look

*David A. Nicholls and Jon Nicholls*

### Background

The inspiration for this chapter came during a family holiday in New Zealand in early 2018. During a week-long road trip, we (Jon, the older brother of Dave) talked a lot about art and photography and its intersection with physiotherapy practice. Jon is a photography teacher at a high-school in London, United Kingdom, and a practiced photographer, and Dave is a professor of physiotherapy in Auckland, New Zealand. As we talked about images, the techniques of photography, and the ways skilled photographers looked at subjects, we began to talk about the kinds of images seen by physiotherapists. Since then, we have met regularly online to discuss images and talk about how physiotherapists can look different(ly).

It seems an obvious thing to say, but looking is a key part of physiotherapy practice (with the notable exception of our visually impaired colleagues). Physiotherapy students are taught how to look at the body and develop their observation skills so that they can identify patterns of movement, bodily reactions, expressions of pain or relief, tension, skin changes, muscle atrophy, and so on. So one might imagine that the skills of looking would be a specific subject in university curricula or that it would be a subject of considerable academic scholarship. But this is not the case. In fact, in the history of the physiotherapy profession, our particular ways of looking have passed almost unnoticed.

And yet without specific images showing specific techniques, performed by expert practitioners, it would be impossible to imagine how physiotherapy techniques could have been developed, learned, and disseminated. Images have also been used heavily to promote physiotherapy in particular ways, especially through marketing images, and these say something distinctive about practice, particularly today in the age of image-saturated social media. Images are important and ubiquitous because they say something particular about their subject, in this case about physiotherapy practice, the profession, its ideals, and distinctive philosophy. So some very powerful things are being said in these images, and the people using them are on some level aware of this, cognisant, perhaps, that they are saying some important things whilst denying others. But what it is that these images convey about physiotherapy remains elusive.

During our road trip, we talked a lot about the shift that had occurred in photography after the 1960s, as photographers began to ask challenging questions about their presumed objectivity and value-neutrality. Was it okay for photographers to simply document a war zone, a humanitarian disaster, or an anorexic model, for example, or should photographers consider their own ethics and responsibilities? Drawing direct parallels with photography, we became interested in the parallels to physiotherapy, which also has a strong culture of technical rationalism (Schön, 1983), and has, for much of its history, privileged the skilled competence of the practitioner over aesthetic considerations. But physiotherapists are now being asked to reflect on the culture and nature of their practice, and there are increasing calls for an otherwise physiotherapy (Setchell, Nicholls, & Gibson, 2018; Nicholls, 2017). So our belief is that there are lessons to be learned by physiotherapists studying the ways that photographers learned to look at bodies and people and that there is merit in us looking more critically at the taken-for-granted gaze of the therapist that predominates in our textbooks and practice manuals.

## How did photography arrive at its critical moment?

Photography is a democratic and diverse medium with a number of competing histories. Any visit to the photography section of a large bookshop shows that photography can be understood as a technical craft, an art form, and the subject of philosophical debate. 'How To' manuals compete for shelf space with artist monographs, gallery catalogues, and theoretical treatises. Thanks largely to Kodak, the picture magazines, and the smartphone, photography has shaped our everyday lives for good and ill since its 'invention' in 1839. The hybrid identity of photography has its roots in the origins of the medium, and debate about its aesthetic, empirical, and technical qualities has been lively.

Photographs, unlike drawings, engravings, or paintings, contain the indexical trace of their subjects. A photograph implies a degree of objectivity, hence its swift acceptance by members of the medical and judicial professions. Prized for its seemingly 'natural and neutral vision', scientists quickly embraced the potential of photographic ways of seeing. And yet a photograph is an abstraction. No matter how lifelike a photograph appears, the world is not flat and does not have an edge. The choices made by a photographer – where to stand, what angle to point the camera, when to open the shutter – have a profound impact on the resulting image: 'Every single choice made by the photographer influences the manner in which the abstraction from reality, which is the final product, will be rendered' (Goldblatt, Haworth-Booth, & Danelzik-Bruggemann, 2005, p. 94).

From the outset, photographers pointed their cameras at bodies: from illicit, erotic images for buttoned-up Victorians to nude studies for painters; from scientific and ethnographic illustrations to modernist abstractions of the human form. Today, the body remains a primary subject for photographers as they tackle issues of identity politics and representation. In the early years, photographers relied on supplementary devices designed to control and constrain the body. Contraptions were invented to keep the heads of portrait sitters still for lengthy daguerreotype exposures. Metal stands, used to support the upright bodies of medical patients, like those of Dr H.W. Berend in the early 1860s, were disguised with neo-classical drapery. And ethnologists devised measurement systems to better compare the body types of various racial groups. Photographs of French neurologist Guillaume-Benjamin Duchenne show him applying electrical currents to facial muscles to better understand human emotion. Bodies have been the subject of violence, have been disfigured by war and famine, have been symbols of health and wellbeing, and have been used to sell all sorts of products, and photographers have been on hand to make images of them.

By the early 20th century, photography had become an independent art form with its own aesthetic criteria: sharp focus, good contrast, and a full range of tones. As the century progressed, photographers experimented with the full range of possibilities for the camera, and questions of the veracity and proper use of visual images as a tool for representing the truth began to emerge. By the late 1960s and early 1970s, photographers (many of whom considered themselves artists who used a camera) began to ask difficult but important questions about the ethics of their trade. Photographers asked about their role in the racist colonialism of early ethnographers and the institutional sexism of advertising and fashion photography. The violent, voyeuristic, fetishising tendencies of photography were summarized by Susan Sontag:

> there is something predatory in the act of taking a picture. To photograph people is to violate them, by seeing them as they never see themselves, by having knowledge of them that they can never have; it turns people into objects that can be symbolically possessed.
>
> (1978, p. 14)

Other critics wrote about the complicity of photography in the process of 'othering', in the creation of capitalist and totalitarian propaganda, of mirroring power inequalities and reinforcing the machinery of oppression. Photographers responded in various ways. Some embraced the critiques and responded with more ethical approaches that acknowledged their inherent privilege as image makers. Many ignored these challenges, seeking refuge in postmodern pluralism and a burgeoning market for fine art photography. But it was impossible to avoid the realisation that something significant had changed. A naïve faith in the objective 'truth' of photography, and its legitimacy as a form of incontestable 'evidence', had been replaced by a sense of documentary uncertainty and the realisation that photographs could exacerbate the pain of others.

Contemporary photographers are consequently having to confront the ethical complexities of seeing bodies through a camera lens. As fast as photography is changing, so are our attitudes to the human body. As curator, author, and museum director William A. Ewing notes: 'What puts the body squarely in the centre of debate is not fashion, but urgency. The body is being rethought and reconsidered by artists and writers because it is being restructured and reconstituted by scientists and engineers' (2009, p. 9).

## Visual methods emerging in healthcare

Physiotherapists are not the first practitioners in healthcare to consider the ethics of visual methods. Research into the use of photographs as a medium and practice has increased dramatically in the health literature in recent years. This is due, in part, to the availability of mobile devices with high-quality cameras; the ability to edit, store, and distribute billions of digital images; and a growing interest in the psychology of imagery (vis à vis the 'selfie') (Tembeck, 2016; Charles & Felton, 2019).

As King, Miller, and Donoghue recently explained:

> As a culture, we are now visually literate – from childhood we are exposed to photographs in a wide variety of contexts and arrangements. This enables us to develop the techniques required to draw meaning and social value from images and to situate the images themselves as historical artefacts in both individual and collective social memories.
>
> (2019, p. 35)

Such has been the growing interest in imagery that visual sociology has become its own specialized field of academic inquiry (Harper, 2012; Nathansohn, 2013; Pink, 2007), with visual methodologies extending from (auto)ethnography to narrative, phenomenology to new materialism. Feminists and postmodernists especially have embraced the possibilities of this emerging field, seeing it as a vehicle to change the ways that social scientists conduct research, opening up 'new possibilities for participatory approaches that appeal to diverse audiences and reposition participants and co-producers of knowledge and potentially co-researchers' (Gubrium, 2016, p. 13).

Other authors have sought to use visual research methods to interrogate 'sociological factors such as class, gender, ethno-racial power relations and institutionalization' (Nathansohn, 2013, pp. 1–2). And approaches like photo-elicitation and visual participatory inquiry are emerging as new visual methods for theorizing complex issues relating to health, particularly among traditionally marginalized communities (Charles & Felton, 2019; Yellowlees, Dingemans, Veldhuis, & Bij de Vaate, 2019; Ortega-Alcázar & Dyck, 2012).

The use of visual methods in healthcare has mostly centred on public health, nursing, and mental health, but little focus has been given to physiotherapy practice. Törnbom and colleagues' recent photo-voice study of stroke recovery (Törnbom, Lundälv, Palstam, & Sunnerhagen, 2019) echoed others' beliefs that visual methods offered new ways to understand people's lived experience of physical disability and disorder (Maratos, Huynh, Tan, Lui, & Jarus, 2016; Dassah, Aldersey, & Norman, 2017), although no studies to date, that we are aware of, focus specifically on physiotherapists' own ways of looking (Wimpenny, Gouzouasis, & Benthall, 2018; Gardner, 2018).

And while images are certainly important in some aspects of physiotherapy practice (for example, Arifa, Thangadurai, & Ebrahim, 2019), we were interested here in exploring a very specific, yet ubiquitous set of images that are central to the way that physiotherapists learn to see. These images are the basis for the way physiotherapists develop their skills of looking and how they learn a particular way to be a therapist. It may be that there is something in the way that physiotherapists learn to define themselves as physiotherapists that is learnt through the way they are taught to look, and if practitioners want to broaden their horizons, this could begin with a different approach to the way we regard ourselves and our patients.

## How we sampled the images

For much of the first half of the 20th century, line drawings were the main method used to convey physiotherapy techniques to the reader. Most likely, this was because of the cost of producing and reproducing photographs of sufficient quality for a small readership. Some of the most widely reproduced texts in physiotherapy used no images at all and relied on textual descriptions to convey proper technique. The first physiotherapy books to make extensive use of photography were produced by doctors and focused on tissue mobilization and manipulation techniques. Only in the second half of the twentieth century, as image reproduction become easier, did physiotherapists begin to use photographs to convey different techniques and modalities of assessment and treatment.

We are most interested, therefore, in the way images have been used to communicate proper practice and professional conduct to readers, especially physiotherapy students, because beyond the specifics of particular technique, images of practicing physiotherapists serve to socialize the student to proper physiotherapy conduct; they define how one should be a good, effective, and proficient practitioner.

We examined photographs of physiotherapists performing assessment or treatment techniques. We concentrated on images in textbooks of physiotherapy practice because these had an overt focus on conveying expertise, and we assumed that the images used were part of a conscious design decision by the authors. We excluded images of microscopic pathology and images of physiotherapists used in advertising. We also excluded images used to convey social status, as in the common 19th-century portrayal of the doctor and 'his' staff. Finally, we excluded line drawings and other non-photographic means for conveying techniques, patients, and therapists.

## Three types of physiotherapy image

### *Style 1: the typical presentation*

The first style of image used in the physiotherapy literature are images that illustrate the typical presentation of a normal physiological or abnormal pathological presentation. Here there are two parties involved: the photographer, whose 'eye' acts as a proxy for the practitioner, and the subject of the image (see Figure 2.1).

14  *David A. Nicholls and Jon Nicholls*

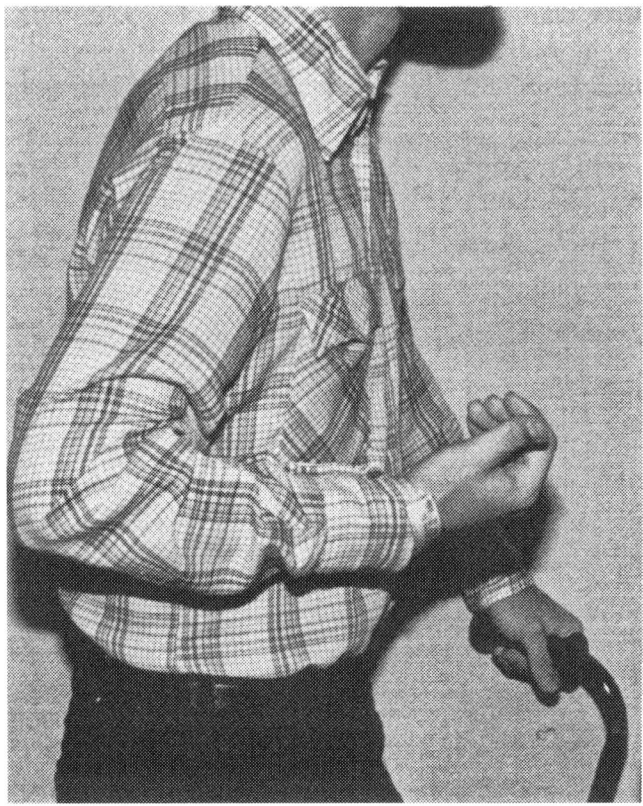

*Figure 2.1* A patient with cosmetically unacceptable spastic elbow flexion deformity.
Source: Montgomery (1995, p. 184).

What is striking about this type of image is how consistently it situates both parties. The camera hovers over the subject. The lighting is stark and revealing, and the subject is exposed entirely to our gaze. There is little empathy here, because the purpose of the image is to convey to the viewer what they might see in practice if they encounter an asymmetrical tonic neck reflex or a subluxed acromio-clavicular joint.

These images resemble Victorian taxonomies of plants, or mannequins in a clothing catalogue. The subject is merely a specimen, akin to the way that medical photographers represent clinical pathologies. The role of the photographer is to catalogue variations and differences as clearly as possible, so that you, the therapist, will translate the resemblance to your own practice.

The text accompanying the image is always intended to be non-judgemental, decontextualized, and ahistorical (see the caption for Figure 2.2 subsequently), but it is the image that dramatically amplifies the idea of the detached, value-neutral

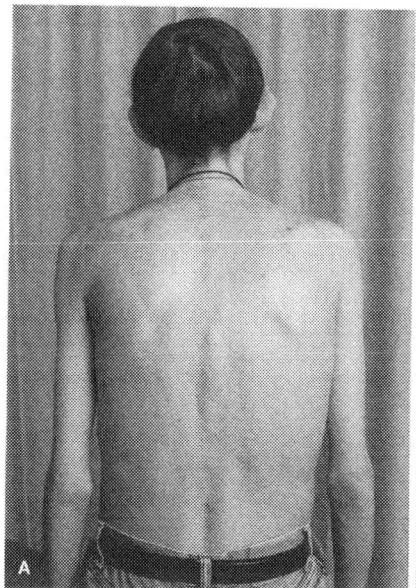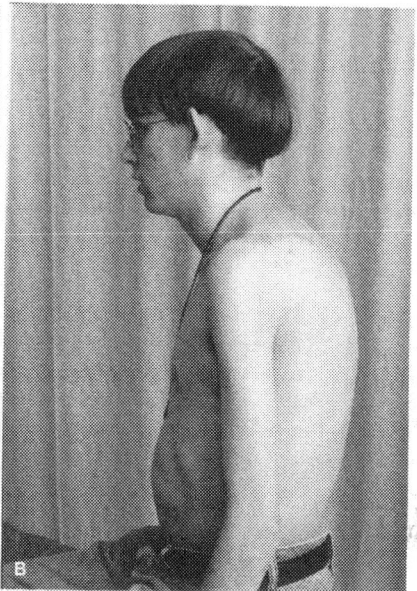

*Figure 2.2* CJ, aged 16, cystic fibrosis. (A) Relaxed sitting posture (posterior view). Note forward head position, tight suboccipital and mid-cervical extensors, tight upper and middle fibres of trapezius, asymmetry and abducted and protracted position of the scapulae, increased thoracic kyphosis, reduced upper lumbar lordosis, and posterior rotation of pelvis. (B) Relaxed sitting posture (side view). Note forward head position, increased sternocleidomastoid activity, increased low cervical lordosis and thoracic kyphosis, abducted and protracted scapulae, anterior position of humerus in glenoid fossa, internal rotation of humerus, and lax abdominal muscles.

Source: Main and Denehy (2016, p. 357).

gaze of the objective clinician. This is the optimal two-dimensional representation of the proper attitude towards the body-as-machine.

Photographs, like Figures 2.1 and 2.2, are useful for presenting bodies in this way because of their perceived indexicality and therefore reliability. This is a superficial but powerfully persuasive feature of photography. As many commentators have noted, photographs are far from value neutral, and their lifelikeness masks a range of ideological, technological, and iconographic meanings. In Figure 2.1, for example, we are not really looking at a portrait of a person but rather an illustration of a medical phenomenon.

Consider the contrast between the previous images – cold, clinical, and impersonal – with the work of contemporary photographer Siân Davey (Figure 2.3). Davey is similarly concerned with the ethics of looking, but, in her case, her role as both mother and photographer complicates the process. Her work is informed by her family and community, and she draws on her experiences as a psychotherapist and mother to make portraits which explore the charged space between photographer and subject. Davey, in common with many contemporary women portrait photographers, is interested in being fully present in the moment when a photograph is made and in exploring how it might be possible to be more responsive and vulnerable in the face of the other:

> I am always there as the photographer, as [Martha's] step-mother, as mentor and friend, but where I am and where I place myself become a more questioning issue as she grows and moves further away from her childhood. The exchange of looks between us, that complex reflected gaze, begins to shift as she tries to define her own sense of self, to decide who she is becoming.
> (Davey, 2018)

In Figure 2.3, Martha looks directly back at us with an enigmatic expression. Her eyeline is level with ours. The implied viewer's gaze is that of a mother, encountering her daughter in a domestic space and wondering about her growing independence. The lighting is key here. The bright light from a window falls across the girl's body, leaving her face in partial shadow. Martha is emerging into the light, but her face occupies a liminal zone, a threshold, between full sun and deep shade. Davey evokes the blossoming of her step-daughter and the complex, confusing, disorientating experience of growing up, both through the exchange

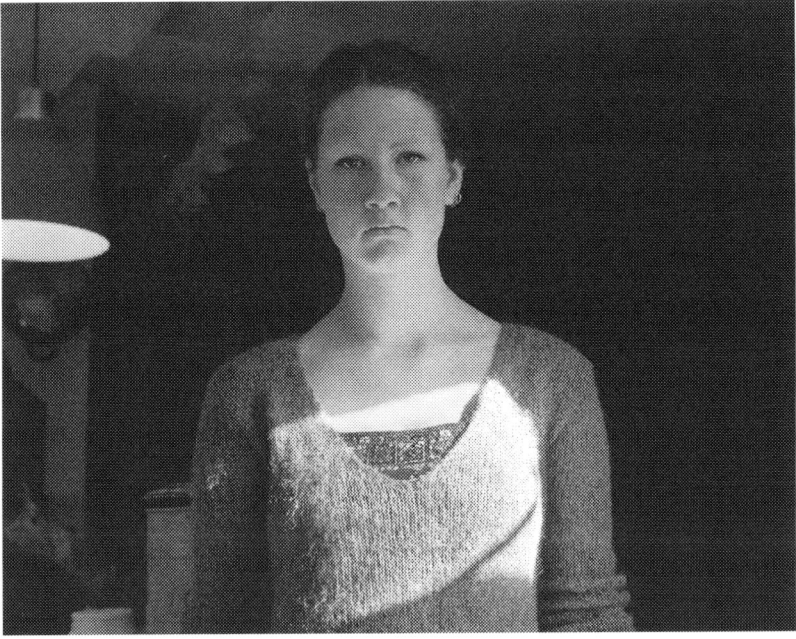

*Figure 2.3* Siân Davey, *The Blue Portrait*, 2018.
Source: From the series 'Martha'.

*Beyond empathy* 17

of a knowing but ambiguous gaze and through the symbolism of light. Davey's portraits function as part of a longer conversation with her children. They traverse a psychological landscape of charged emotions in which the photographer is working on instinct. The resulting images suggest a deep connection, something beyond empathy, in which the vulnerabilities of being present are made manifest. As curator Kate Bush notices:

> For Sian, photography involves reciprocity: it is a 'dance' between photographer and subject, a quest for simultaneous, self-understanding and mutual recognition. . . . Martha returns the gaze of the photographer, her mother, on equal terms, with a frankness than can be both affecting and disarming for the viewer, who becomes bound up in their intimate exchange.
>
> (2018)

If we now look back at Figures 2.1 and 2.2, it seems clear that this type of photography makes no overt attempt to engage with the subject as person. Images like this succeed only in communicating detached, disembodied attitudes to the viewer. We are asked to think of the other as a medical problem to be recognized and catalogued, not an individual person with a life, a future, and a set of emotions. The viewer is conceived of as the powerful agent in this dynamic, the potential fixer, whereas the subject is the docile recipient of the observer's skill and expertise. Photography reinforces this power imbalance through its rhetoric of viewpoint, lighting, focus, and composition.

## *Style 2: Proper treatment*

The second set of images we encountered differ from the first group for a seemingly trivial reason, but they serve a very different purpose for the viewer. Where images of 'the typical presentation' involve only a viewer/photographer and subject, in this group, we have the addition of a therapist.

In images like Figure 2.4, much more attention is given to the therapeutic space, which is often designed to convey the idea of an abstracted clinical setting. Equipment and aids to the practitioner are kept to a minimum, and the focus is on the expert's technique.

Attention is given to the performative aspect of the expert: how he stands, how he positions his hands, the direction of push or pull, and the ability to visualize the 'effective neutrality' of the therapist. As Hughes explains:

> During the process of professional socialisation the health professional learns to objectify the patient. This probably helps the professional to internalise the unwritten rules of physical engagement, so that in the actual medical encounter the definition of touch brooks no dubiety.
>
> (2000, p. 24)

To some degree, all of the people in Figure 2.4 are meant to recede into the background, to allow us to focus on the skill being demonstrated. We see this especially in images where only part of the practitioner performing the technique is shown (see Figure 2.5).

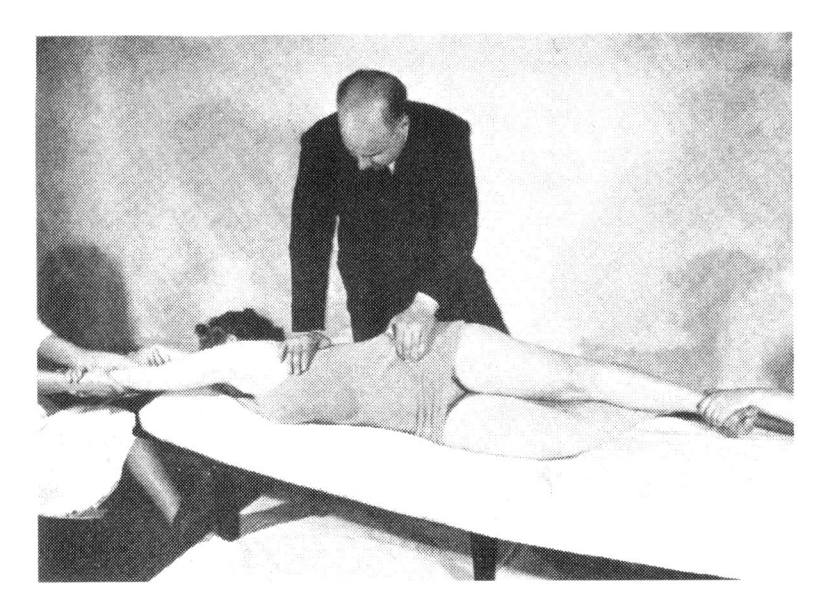

*Figure 2.4* Thoracic spine: rotation during traction II.
Source: Cyriax (1955, p. 241).

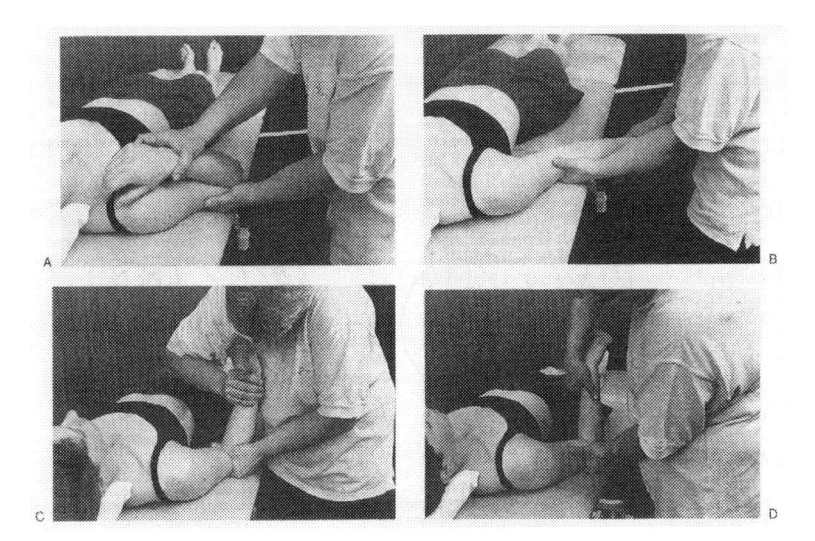

*Figure 2.5* Overpressure to the elbow complex. (A) Flexion. Note that the left hand supports underneath the elbow, while the right hand flexes the elbow. (B) Extension. The left hand supports underneath the elbow, while the right hand extends the elbow. (C) Supination. The left hand supports underneath the elbow, while the right hand supinates the forearm. (D) Pronation. The left hand supports underneath the elbow, while the right hand pronates the forearm.
Source: Petty and Moore (2011, p. 220).

Because the centre of the frame frequently focuses on the expert's hands, one cannot help but see a hierarchy at work in which the (male) expert is the dynamic agent of restoration and recovery – the true artist – and the patient is a mere dupe, a living 'cadaver' of sorts (Nicholls, 2017), a Body-*with*-Organs (Deleuze & Guattari, 1983). The camera angle positions the viewer as if you are privy to a live demonstration, and the message is clear: 'This is an important technique to learn. Let me show you how it should be done'.

Contemporary photographer Polly Braden employs a different approach when photographing young people and adults with autism and learning difficulties (see Figures 2.6 and 2.7). In her project, 'Great Interactions: Life with Learning Disabilities and Autism' (Braden, 2016), Braden employs sequences of portraits rather than snapshots. She explains:

> Single photographs often present a person as a final statement . . . [a]ll of us are in ongoing states of being and becoming. With two images you can at least see the next movement, the next gesture, the ongoing moment, not the definitive moment.
>
> (2016)

It is often difficult to tell in Braden's portraits who is the support worker and who is being supported. Braden acknowledges the importance of hands as indicators of emotion and that it was important to her to capture the flow of empathy and support through the hands from one person to another.

Rather than interpose herself in the dynamics of the places where she photographs, Braden has become adept at watching and waiting for moments where she can capture the subtle language of gestures. In order to allow us to concentrate on these gestures, she manoeuvres backdrops and lights into place, careful not to disturb the activity. In Figures 2.6 and 2.7, Pauline encourages Jamie to taste and smell the chocolate bits in the cookie dough; 'Jamie is completely absorbed in all the sensations he is feeling. We can't actually feel that through the photographs but we can empathise, and we can see that Pauline is feeling great empathy for Jamie' (ibid).

In these situations, we are reminded that we are not seeing someone manipulate an inanimate object, like we might see in a cookery or carpentry demonstration, but a person in touch with another. The images in the physiotherapy literature are interesting photographically, then, because it seems that in an effort to show us the part of the therapeutic encounter that can be reduced to physical technique, the photographer and author have made a conscious effort to strip away the human dimensions of practice and convey a dispassionate image of physiotherapy practice to the viewer.

### *Style 3: Real physiotherapy*

Frank Weedon was a physiotherapist, teacher, and amateur photographer in Dunedin, New Zealand. Qualifying in 1949, he followed his parents and grandfather into physiotherapy (Shaw, 2013, p. 87). Weedon taught at the Otago Physiotherapy School from 1966 until 1990 and during that time also practiced amateur

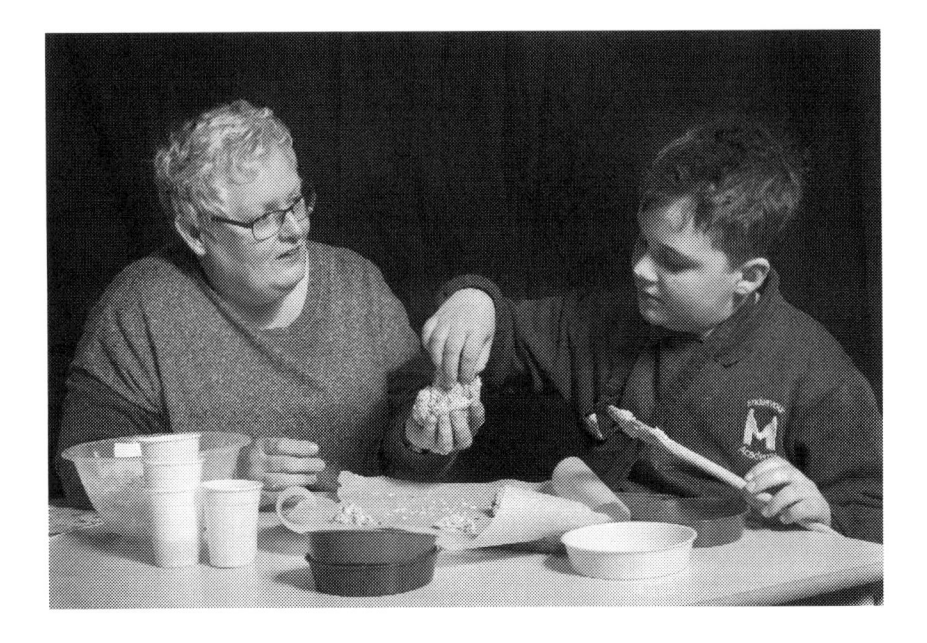

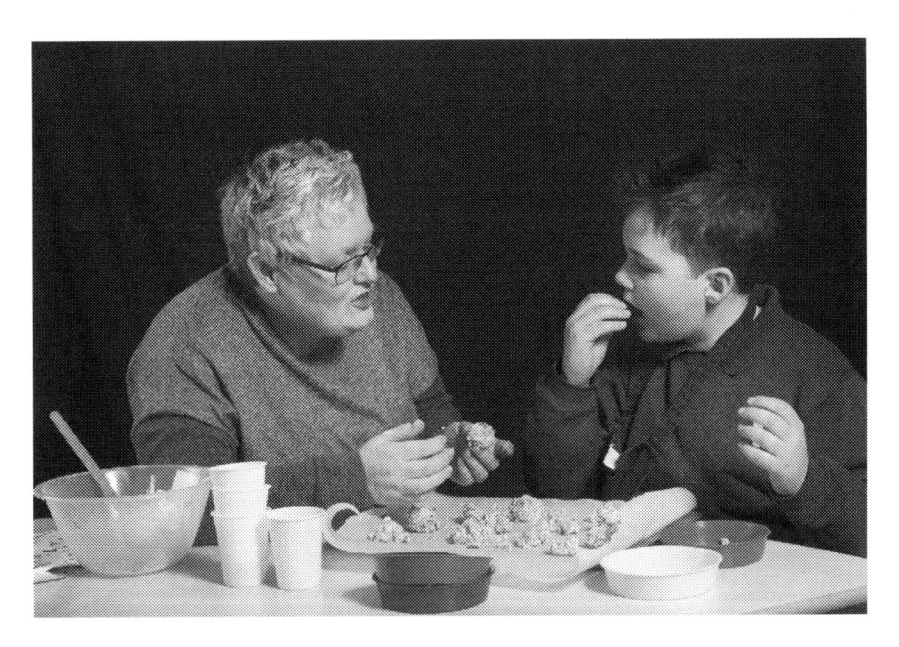

*Figures 2.6* and *2.7* Pauline with Jamie, Endeavour Academy.
Source: From Braden (2016, pp. 48–49).

photography, bequeathing a set of prints to the New Zealand physiotherapy centenary celebrations in 2013.

Weedon's images are striking because they convey a different aesthetic about physiotherapy practice to those found elsewhere in the literature. Never used for any academic or professional purpose, they show that it is possible to present a different image about physiotherapy to students and therapists.

First, Weedon's images are beautifully shot and composed. The images are carefully lit. He creates detailed negatives with a wide range of tones and lots of detail and clearly understands something about the development and printing process. More than this, though, he has a photographer's sense for the aesthetics of the image and a portraitist's sensitivity for gesture. His subjects are 'present'. The therapeutic encounters are full of latent emotion and empathy. The compositions make us part of the experience rather than forcing us into a paternalistic, detached, judging, clinical gaze. Weedon shows a more humanistic, nuanced appreciation for the artistry of physiotherapy. These pictures reveal something of people's vulnerability and the sensitivity and quality of touch.

Since the early Renaissance, artists have concentrated on the representation of hands in order to convey deep-seated emotion. The 'master' would often complete the painting, taking over from the apprentices in order to paint the faces and hands of the figures (see Figure 2.9 subsequently). Weedon has a sense of this, too. Although his images don't aspire to be works of art, great care has been taken to produce images that, for him, convey the physical subtleties and emotional dimension of physiotherapy.

Despite the medical equipment in the background, the robed figure, cloistered setting, and sombre encounter in Weedon's photograph of students in a clinical room (Figure 2.8) are reminiscent of images of d'Amelia's 15th-century painting

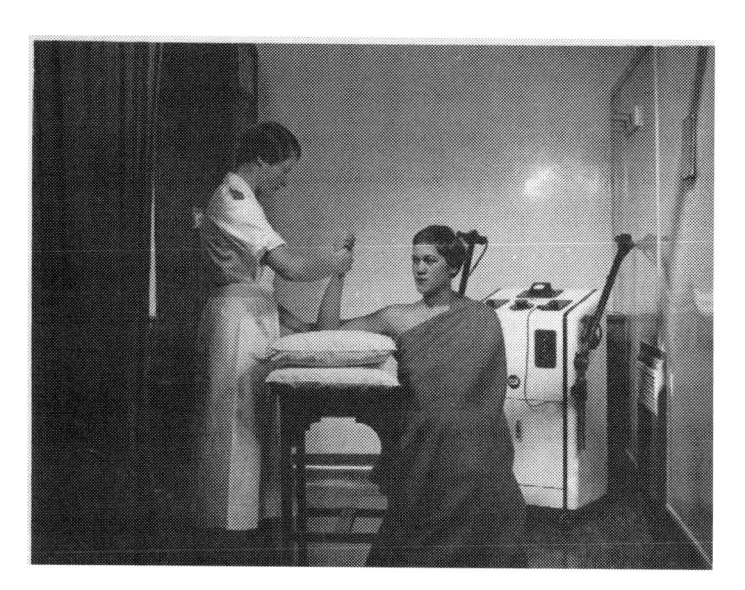

*Figure 2.8* Students in clinical room.
Source: From Frank Weedon collection. Author's personal copy.

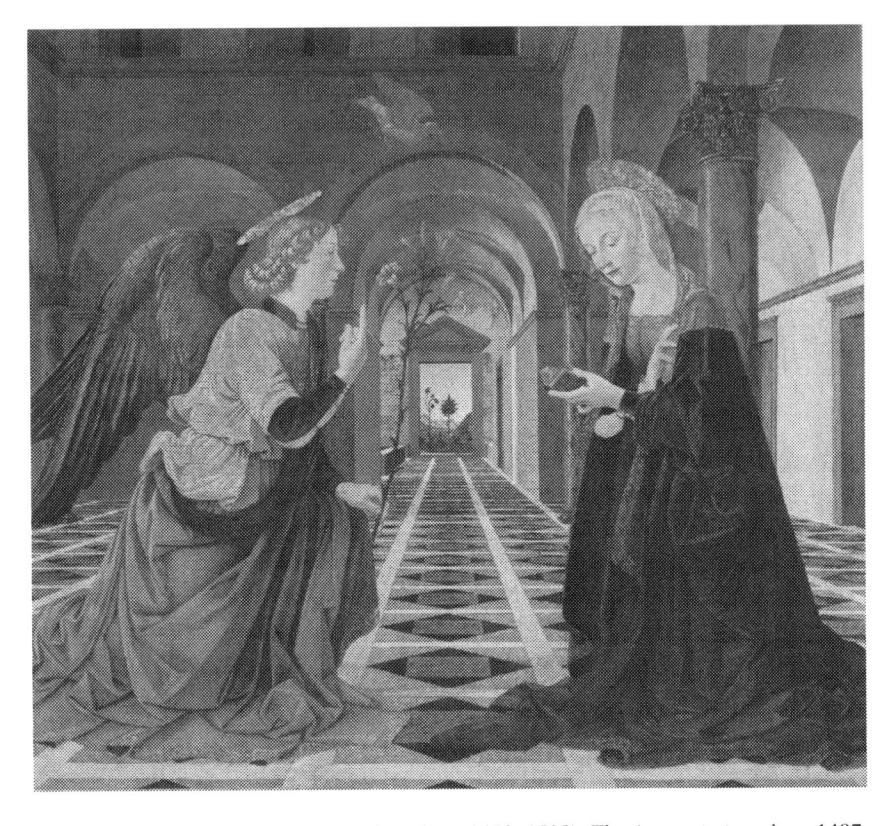

*Figure 2.9* Piermatteo d'Amelia (Italian, about 1450–1508), *The Annunciation*, about 1487. Tempera on panel, 102.4 × 114.8 cm (40 5/16 × 45 3/16 in.).
Source: Isabella Stewart Gardner Museum, Boston (P16w4).

of *The Annunciation*. Consider the harmonious composition and respect for both figures, their postures, and facial expressions. Weedon seems repeatedly drawn to crepuscular light, folded drapery, and eloquent gestures.

Weedon often captures a remarkable sense of the intrapersonal dynamics at play in a therapeutic encounter. In Figure 2.10, for example, the photographer is witness to a familiar bedside scene in which a female therapist holds a young boy's leg. But here the composition is beautifully balanced, pivoting on the fulcrum of the lamp in which we see the whole scene reflected. The lamp arm also functions as a leading line, linking the boy's gaze to that of the therapist. Weedon has captured the therapist's reassuring, kindly look, and the boy's ambivalence. More remarkable still is the inclusion of the toys, especially the tank, which reinforces the boy's need to be brave (because this will hurt). His gestures and facial expression suggest the tank offers him little comfort. Weedon seems at pains to assert the human dimension of this encounter, in which the empathy of the

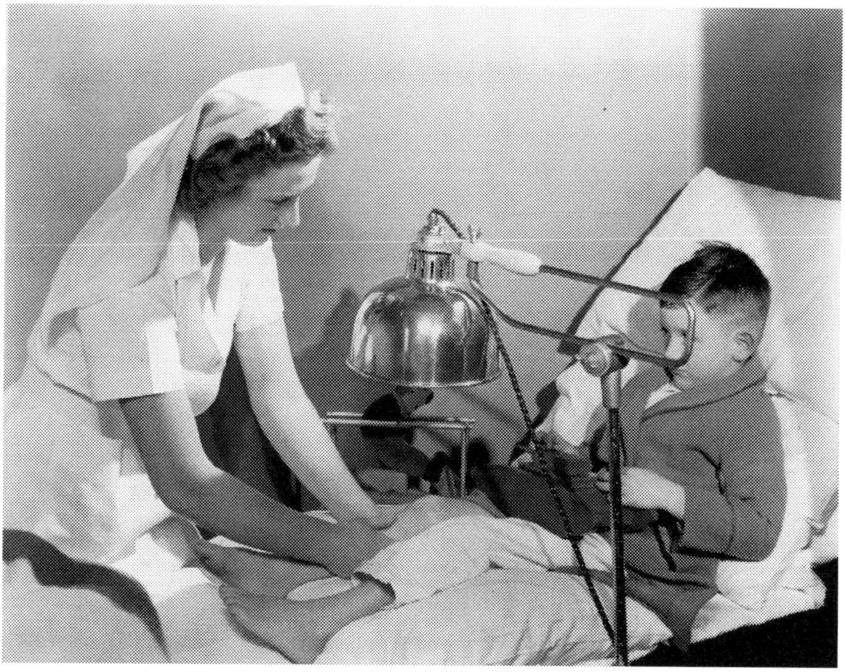

*Figure 2.10* Therapist and child.
Source: Frank Weedon collection. Author's personal copy.

therapist is at least as significant as her skill or technique. We can admire the balance and grace of the image, the subtlety of the gestures, not unlike the perfectly poised toy acrobat beneath the lamp, a play on the patient regaining mobility in parallel bars perhaps? Weedon may not have intended this symbolic reading, but it is present nonetheless.

In many of the images, we see the faces of the patient and the backs of the practitioner. Many of the faces are themselves 'looking'. The focus of the image is reversed from the standard textbook photograph where the main interest is in the practitioner and the model/patient is barely present. In Figure 2.11, Weedon seems far more interested in the gaze of the patient than in illustrating the therapist's technique, since the blanket obscures the hands mobilizing the lower leg. It is as if Weedon is distracted by the light falling on the blanket and the patient's face. One might ask whether an image like this would be useful in a 'clinical' textbook, but then should clinical textbooks only show dispassionate technique and not also convey a story about person-centred care?

It seems important to Weedon that we see how the patient feels. He seems eager to represent the participants in the images as people who happen to be having physiotherapy. He is respectful of the space they take up, and through these images,

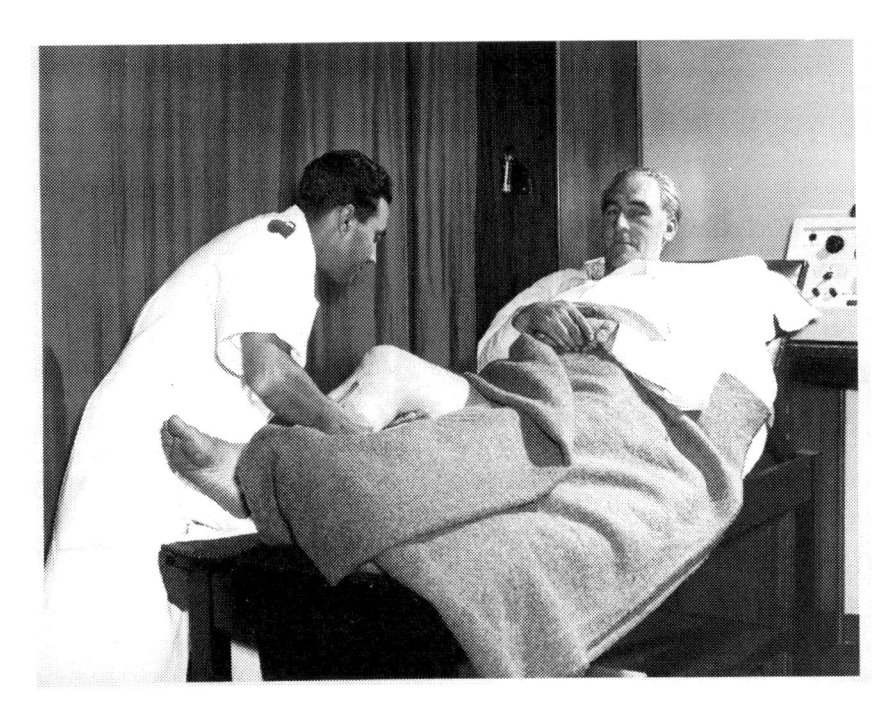

*Figure 2.11* Student therapist mobilizing patient's leg.
Source: Frank Weedon collection.

you, the viewer, are tacitly asked to respect them, too. There is a gentleness to the work that is almost never seen in physiotherapy textbooks.

In Figure 2.12, Weedon has chosen an unusually low angle in order to capture this balance training. We look up at the therapist and patient, who create a beautifully balanced bridge shape, echoed by the chair in the background. The therapist is faintly, reassuringly smiling, and the patient returns her gaze with what appears to be an expression of confidence, determination, and trust. Here we not only see a procedure being carried out but also a human transaction, a meeting of two individuals, who, although figuratively at 'arm's length', are depicted in a mutual exchange of energies. The choices made by the photographer, in this case, help to communicate a particularly humane impression of the physiotherapist's professionalism and competence.

Contemporary photographers are interested in the same kinds of energy between the photographer and subject as physiotherapists are in practice. This goes beyond empathy and is more about reciprocity. Although we are provided with unambiguous cues to recognize this as a therapeutic encounter, in which there is a characteristic power asymmetry between the therapist and patient – through the therapist's uniform and the clinical setting, for example – Weedon appeared to want to enrich

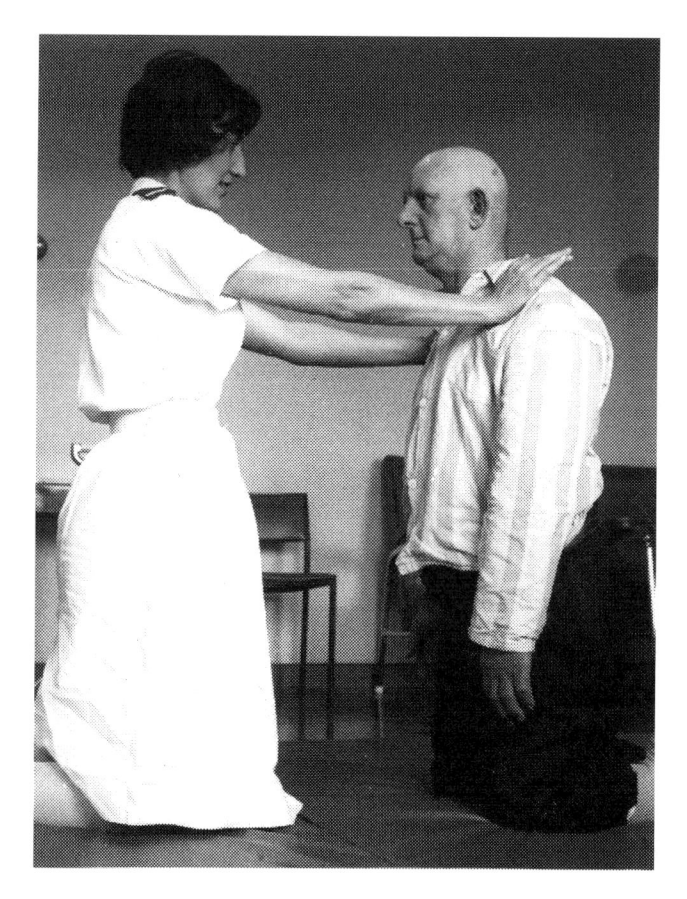

*Figure 2.12* Therapist and kneeling patient.
Source: Frank Weedon collection.

this with a deeper, more authentic appreciation for the full richness of real physiotherapy practice. Weedon had a deep connection with the world of physiotherapy. He was embedded in it, felt comfortable with it, and respected his profession. And his images celebrated the modest pleasures of everyday practice.

## Can the lessons of photography help us to be more empathic?

A recent study by Sullivan, Hebron, and Vuoskoski (Sullivan, Hebron, & Vuoskoski, 2019) looking at the way clinicians 'sell' their own understanding of chronic nonspecific low back pain to patients, suggests that physiotherapists often try to be patient centred but feel uncomfortable dealing with uncertainty, patient counter-narratives, and the ensuing conflict. The therapists' response in the study betrayed 'an underlying paternalistic wish to get patients "on board"' (ibid) – a finding that has been echoed elsewhere in recent years (Dierckx, Deveugele, Roosen, & Devisch, 2013; Stenner, Swinkels, Mitchell, & Palmer, 2016; Mudge, Stretton, & Kayes, 2013). Much of the anxiety experienced by clinicians relates to patients' experiential and sociocultural understandings that can differ markedly from the therapists' biomedical orientation. Practitioners report being ill equipped to manage skills like rapport-building (Sullivan et al., 2019). Perhaps this is a function of the way physiotherapists are taught to see their purpose?

One of the problems with the biomechanical approach to health is that it promotes the perception of illness and injury as 'a physical reality independent of time, space and changing moral evaluation' (Freidson, 1970, p. 208). In doing so, it accentuates the idea that physical illness resides within the body, regardless of the persons culture, psyche, location, personal history, spirituality, values, and beliefs.

We found a strong message of detachment, objectivity, and paternalism in the way physiotherapy practice was conveyed in images we viewed for this chapter. And we felt a distinct lack of empathy or reciprocity being conveyed in the myriad images used convey proper physiotherapy conduct to students and peers. This must surely have an effect on the attitudes, values, and beliefs of practitioners learning how to relate to the clients/patients they serve.

Toye, Seers, Hannink, and Barker (2017) have recently show that clinicians are finding it hard to move beyond their biomedical heritage to embrace the complex reality of health and healthcare for people today (ibid). We would suggest that one way to help this process might be to consider closely how ideas about physiotherapy practice are conveyed through images. More than 40 years ago, Ivan Illich suggested that 'the age of disabling professions . . . when people had "problems", experts had "solutions" and scientists measured imponderables such as "abilities" and "needs"', is at an end (Illich, 1977, p. 6). What Frank Weedon's images remind us is that if we want practitioners to engage with clients/patients empathically and embrace the kinds of reciprocity that is at the heart of person-centred care, then we might look to the lessons of photography to show us some ways to do this.

## References

Arifa, M., Thangadurai, C., & Ebrahim, S. A. R. (2019). Effectiveness of gaze stability and conventional exercises on balance in vestibular hypofunction patients. *Indian Journal of Physiotherapy and Occupational Therapy: An International Journal, 13*(2), 95. doi:10.5958/0973-5674.2019.00053.4

Braden, P. (2016). *Great interactions: Life with learning disabilities and autism*. Stockport, UK: Dewi Lewis.

Bush, K. (2018). *Review of Siân Davey's "Martha" series*. Retrieved from www.siandavey.com/portraiture/eng4qpa5lz22i6kwhsw6ginae0xeup

Charles, A., & Felton, A. (2019). Exploring young people's experiences and perceptions of mental health and well-being using photography. *Child and Adolescent Mental Health*. doi:10.1111/camh.12351

Cyriax, J. (1955). *Textbook of orthopaedic medicine: Treatment by manipulation and massage* (Vol. 2). London, UK: Cassell and Company.

Dassah, E., Aldersey, H. M., & Norman, K. E. (2017). Photovoice and persons with physical disabilities: A scoping review of the literature. *Qualitative Health Research, 27*(9), 1412–1422. doi:10.1177/1049732316687731

Davey, S. (2018). *Martha*. Retrieved from www.siandavey.com/portraiture/71c0nm6dosdbvwx6n09axju37d65tv

Deleuze, G., & Guattari, F. (1983). *Anti-Oedipus: Capitalism and schizophrenia*. Minneapolis, MN: University of Minnesota Press.

Dierckx, K., Deveugele, M., Roosen, P., & Devisch, I. (2013). Implementation of shared decision making in physical therapy: Observed level of involvement and patient preference. *Physical Therapy, 93*(10), 1321–1330. doi:10.2522/ptj.20120286

Ewing, W. (2009). *The body: Photoworks of the human form*. London, UK: Thames & Hudson.

Freidson, E. (1970). *The profession of medicine: A study of the sociology of applied knowledge*. New York, NY: Dodd Mead.

Gardner, J. (2018). *Rethinking the clinical gaze: Patient-centred innovation in paediatric neurology*. Basingstoke, UK: Palgrave Macmillan.

Goldblatt, D., Haworth-Booth, M., & Danelzik-Bruggemann, C. (2005). *South African intersections*. Munich, Germany: Prestel.

Gubrium, A. (2016). *Participatory visual and digital methods*. Abingdon, UK: Routledge.

Harper, D. (2012). *Visual sociology*. Abingdon, UK: Routledge.

Hughes, B. (2000). Medicalized bodies. In P. Hancock, B. Hughes, E. Jagger, K. Peterson, R. Russell, E. Tulle-Winton, & M. Tyler (Eds.), *The body, culture and society* (pp. 12–28). Buckingham, UK: Open University Press.

Illich, I. (1977). *Disabling professions*. London, UK: Marion Boyars.

King, T., Miller, E., & Donoghue, G. (2019). Spaces, sauce and schedules: A photographic journey of aged care. *Social Alternatives, 38*(1), 35–44.

Main, E., & Denehy, L. (2016). *Cardiorespiratory physiotherapy: Adults and paediatrics* (5th ed.). Edinburgh, Scotland: Elsevier.

Maratos, M., Huynh, L., Tan, J., Lui, J., & Jarus, T. (2016). Picture this: Exploring the lived experience of high-functioning stroke survivors using photovoice. *Qualitative Health Research, 26*(8), 1055–1066. doi:10.1177/1049732316648114

Montgomery, J. (1995). *Physical therapy for traumatic brain injury*. New York, NY: Churchill Livingstone.

Mudge, S., Stretton, C., & Kayes, N. (2013). Are physiotherapists comfortable with person-centred practice? An autoethnographic insight. *Disability and Rehabilitation*. doi:10.3109/09638288.2013.797515

Nathansohn, R. (2013). *Sociology of the visual sphere*. Abingdon, UK: Routledge.

Nicholls, D. A. (2017). *The end of physiotherapy*. Abingdon, UK: Routledge.

Ortega-Alcázar, I., & Dyck, I. (2012). Migrant narratives of health and well-being: Challenging "othering" processes through photo-elicitation interviews. *Critical Social Policy, 32*(1), 106–125. doi:10.1177/0261018311425981

Petty, N. J., & Moore, A. (2011). *Neuromusculoskeletal examination and assessment: A handbook for therapists* (4th ed.). Edinburgh, Scotland: Elsevier.

Pink, S. (2007). *Doing visual ethnography*. London, UK: Sage Publications.

Schön, D. A. (1983). *The reflective practitioner: How professionals think in action*. New York, NY: Basic Books.

Setchell, J., Nicholls, D. A., & Gibson, B. E. (2018). Objecting: Multiplicity and the practice of physiotherapy. *Health* (London), *22*(2), 165–184. doi:10.1177/1363459316688519

Shaw, L. (2013). *In our hands: 100 years of the school of physiotherapy in Otago 1913–2013*. Dunedin, New Zealand: University of Otago.

Sontag, S. (1978). *On photography*. London, UK: Allen Lane.

Stenner, R., Swinkels, A., Mitchell, T., & Palmer, S. (2016). Exercise prescription for patients with non-specific chronic low back pain: A qualitative exploration of decision making in physiotherapy practice. *Physiotherapy*, *102*(4), 332–338. doi:10.1016/j.physio.2015.05.004

Sullivan, N., Hebron, C., & Vuoskoski, P. (2019). "Selling" chronic pain: Physiotherapists' lived experiences of communicating the diagnosis of chronic nonspecific lower back pain to their patients. *Physiotherapy Theory & Practice*, 1–20. doi:10.1080/09593985.2019.1672227

Tembeck, T. (2016). Selfies of ill health: Online autopathographic photography and the dramaturgy of the everyday. *Social Media + Society*, *2*(1), 205630511664134. doi:10.1177/2056305116641343

Törnbom, K., Lundälv, J., Palstam, A., & Sunnerhagen, K. S. (2019). "My life after stroke through a camera lens": A photovoice study on participation in Sweden. *PLOS ONE*, *14*(9), e0222099. doi:10.1371/journal.pone.0222099

Toye, F., Seers, K., Hannink, E., & Barker, K. (2017). A mega-ethnography of eleven qualitative evidence syntheses exploring the experience of living with chronic non-malignant pain. *BMC Medical Research Methodology*, *17*(1), 116. doi:10.1186/s12874-017-0392-7

Wimpenny, K., Gouzouasis, P., & Benthall, K. (2018). Remembering, reflecting, returning: A return to professional practice journey through poetry, music and images. *Media Practice and Education*, *19*(1), 98–115. doi:10.1080/14682753.2017.1362179

Yellowlees, R., Dingemans, A. E., Veldhuis, J., & Bij de Vaate, A. J. D. (2019). Face yourself(ie): Investigating selfie-behavior in females with severe eating disorder symptoms. *Computers in Human Behavior*, *101*, 77–83. doi:10.1016/j.chb.2019.07.018

# 3 Bodily ways of knowing

How students learn *about* and *through* bodies during physiotherapy education

*Anne Gudrun Langaas and
Anne-Lise Middelthon*

### Introduction: the body in physiotherapy education

We take Olav's reflections in his third year of physiotherapy education as our point of departure in order to explore the phenomenon that one can acknowledge having achieved bodily capacities without knowing how this development came about. In itself, this phenomenon signifies a challenge to the teaching and learning of physiotherapy, as neither professional physiotherapists nor lecturers may be fully aware of the ways in which bodily knowledge is articulated, enacted, or produced through interaction.

> As a result of what I've been doing during my three years of physiotherapy training, I have become more aware of my own body and have developed more body control, thus I'm more in tune with my body, in a way. This has been very positive for me. From previously being unaware of different parts of the body, I am now more aware of my whole body, but I am unsure why and how it has come about. Whether it is movement classes or simply anatomy lessons or other elements. . . . Surely many things may come into play, but anyhow – during the past three years – I have developed in a positive way in terms of my body awareness and I have more connection with all of me.
> 
> (Olav, physiotherapy student)

In physiotherapy – as in many everyday corporal practices – we might find that knowledge acquired *through* the body may not necessarily be exhaustively or satisfactorily articulated through verbal language. Rather, we articulate this way of knowing through what we *do* – it is performed. Thus, the tacit dimensions of knowing in physiotherapy incorporate not only non-verbalized but in some cases perhaps also non-verbalizable knowledge. This is similar to everyday bodily ways of knowing, which we physically acquire through dwelling in different situations rather than through theorization. Once one grants that the education of physiotherapists is not – and cannot solely be – about learning theory, technical, biomedical, and communicative skills but that it is also about educating students' *bodies*, a concomitant need for theorizations and explorations of this very phenomenon arises.

In setting out to study how students learn to become more embodied, how they learn to acquire a competent body that knows in ways specific to physiotherapy, a central challenge was how to scientifically approach, get at, or grasp embodied phenomena that we may not be able to be fully articulate verbally. 'Observation' offers one approach; however, not everything is observable that is felt or experienced by the body. Despite the challenge, we contend nonetheless that it is useful to try to make bodily knowledge explicit by attempting to express verbally what is observed, felt, and experienced in the body. In this chapter, we explore and describe tacit ways of knowing in physiotherapy and also attempt to make more explicit that which cannot be exhaustively articulated through words. More specifically, we have set out to explore and describe how students learn both *about* and *through* bodies – how bodies are being shaped and what bodies *do* – in physiotherapy education. Another aim is to introduce a conceptual framework that we have found enlightening and helpful when seeking to explore dimensions of bodily ways of knowing in physiotherapy. Conceptual frameworks and concepts focused on bodily knowledge are, to our understanding, less frequently used in physiotherapy research.

This chapter answers a call from Nicholls and Gibson (2010, p. 506) to produce more studies that theoretically explore 'the way physiotherapists engage with the body'. There is currently an emerging field within physiotherapy research that seeks to explore the practice of physiotherapy in multiple ways, which include economic, philosophical, political, and sociological perspectives (Nicholls, 2018). This shift attempts to embrace broader epistemological perspectives and to encourage new ways of exploring, understanding and developing physiotherapeutic approaches and encounters, including attention to embodiment. Krieger (2005) writes of 'embodiment' as a concept that highlights that 'our living bodies tell stories about our lives, whether or not these are ever consciously expressed' (p. 350). For Krieger (2005), taking embodiment into account may add nuance to our understandings of how both the physical and psychosocial environments shape health and healthcare.

Macdonald and Nicholls (2017) argue that health workers often need to function alongside the patient, especially when patients need to adapt to a new way of living, and that this includes taking into account the illness, the lived experiences, and the sociocultural context of the patient. They refer to these dimensions as a framework for constituting an embodied view of health and illness. Furthermore, they suggest that many physiotherapists work with an embodied approach towards 'health and illness despite their training not because of it' (Macdonald & Nicholls, 2017, p. 504). Our focus is particularly on how students acquire competent bodies, understood as bodies capable of initiating, participating, and contributing in interaction with patients, in order to establish therapeutic intercorporealities specific to physiotherapy.

Before we proceed to an account of the theoretical conceptual framework applied in this work, we offer a brief description of a study which constitutes the empirical base for the work presented in this chapter. Empirical material, produced through a set of complementary qualitative methods including interviews, participant observation, and analysis of education-related texts, serves as a foundation and is drawn upon for illustrative exemplars within the current chapter. The material consists of interviews with 31 physiotherapy students – 24 of the students engaged in repeat dialogical interviews – for a total of 61 interviews. In addition, participant observations – which included focused conversations – were carried out over an eight-week period at the physiotherapy out-patient department at Oslo University College (now Oslo Metropolitan University) where students worked in clinical practice. Participant observations/conversations also took place in six physiotherapy treatment skill classes and three movement analysis classes at the same university.

## Theoretical framework

Polanyi's (1966) seminal writing which inquired into and theorized 'tacit knowing' is central to this work. We particularly emphasize his much-cited insight that 'we can know more than we can tell' (p. 4). An often-used example is found in the way we learn to walk or to ride a bike and the manner in which these competencies thereafter operate tacitly throughout most of our life. Tacit ways of knowing are a fundamental dimension of human existence and a necessary and inescapable part of everyday life. If injured or ill, however, we might experience a disruption in our abilities to perform our corporeal skills, including those that are operating in a tacit manner.

To illustrate how Polanyi conceptualizes and theorizes activities of daily living, we start by conveying some core insights on tacit knowing from Polanyi's example of hitting a nail with a hammer (Polanyi, 1962 [1958]) as it seems particularly relevant to physiotherapists who work with body and movement. Polanyi operates with two types of attention: focal and subliminal. In order to be able to hit a nail with a hammer, our focal attention will be on the nail. At the same time, we will be subliminally attentive to the pressure the hammer exerts against the palm of our hand and how our grip is exerting a pressure against the shaft of the hammer. When we focus on a whole – an action or a situation – we are at the same time subliminally attentive to its parts. The parts will maintain the 'gestalt' and can in some instances be seen as the meaning of the 'gestalt' (Polanyi, 1962 [1958], p. 58). In this way, the two modes of attention operate together, constituting a whole; indeed, rather than being mutually exclusive, these are mutually dependent modes of attention. To hit a nail with a hammer successfully (at least most of the time) will be the outcome of a process of acquiring a particular bodily habit, just like walking and riding a bike. Habits typically include elements of tacit knowing, as outlined by Polanyi (1966), and although tacit ways of knowing cannot be exhaustively accounted for verbally, tacit knowledge nevertheless plays an active role in creating meaning, and guiding and controlling action. As ways of bodily knowing are articulated mainly through what we do, as already mentioned, it follows that the development of tacit ways of bodily knowing is an ongoing process.

The insights of dancer, philosopher, and evolutionary biologist Maxine Sheets-Johnstone (2002) illustrate how we may come to understand the primacy of movement in all human beings:

> We knew neither that we were coming into the world nor that there was such a thing as a world to begin with. As adults, we tend to think that our primary job as infants was to learn this world. What we tend not to realize is that we had to learn something prior to – or at least something fundamentally essential to, and coincident with – that learning. We had to learn to move ourselves. We had to learn our bodies. . . . We were apprentices of our bodies. By listening to them, by staying attuned kinesthetically, we learned complex details about our kinesthetic aliveness – about bending, stretching, blinking, turning, lifting, opening, closing, and much more. We learned about eyes and ears, not as *things* or as *linguistic labels of things*, but as sites of felt bodily happenings. We learned that we modify our senses by moving, and correlatively, that when we move we take all our senses with us.
>
> (p. 138)

To further explore ways in which bodies may acquire knowledge, we find Sheets-Johnstone's (2002) concept of 'staying attuned kinesthetically' – understood as learning about our own body and also attuning to other peoples' bodies – helpful (p. 138). She also refers to what she conceptualizes as 'thinking in movement' and attending to 'bodily happenings' when she analyzes dance improvisation and describes it as an 'ongoing present' when she explores how movement develops here and now (Sheets-Johnstone, 1999, p. 485). Her theoretical framework resonates with philosopher Vinciane Despret's (2004) insights that having a body means to learn to be affected by other entities, humans or non-humans. Despret emphasizes the dialogical and dialectical elements of both being affected and to affect others when she calls for 'a theory of affected and affecting bodies' (p. 125).

Inspired by Despret, anthropologist Bruno Latour (2004) elaborates on what learning to be affected means, as he relates this to an example of a person who is learning to develop a nose for different scents of perfume. According to Latour, it is all about giving something that previously did not exist for you, for example, a certain smell, attention and meaning. When 'something' both becomes the subject of attention and is attributed meaning, it will affect the person in question. It will make the person more sensitive to, and more knowledgeable about, what the world has to offer. You will also be a more attentive, sensitive, and affected body as you develop a nose able to smell different scents in various perfumes – a nose sensitive to differences. This will require a lot of exposure and training, as one finds cues to increase the ability to differentiate smells through sensory input. This means that the body is sensitized in relation to what the world has to offer by way of the scents of perfume. Sensitization in general occurs through a dynamic learning process and results in a person becoming 'a more embodied body', as Latour (2004, p. 212) phrases it.

Despret's (2004, p. 131) concept of 'with-ness' or 'being with' sheds light on ways bodies and worlds articulate with each other (and are akin to each other). According to Despret, 'with-ness' presupposes interest and immersion in the multitude of problems, pleasures, and functioning of another person, creature, organism, or object. Based on affects or emotions as they are involved in tensions and attention, desires, embodied interests, and bodies learning to feel like another body, Despret (2004, p. 125) draws particular attention to what the body (or bodies) makes us or others do.

The body at the fore of this framework is the body understood *not* as something we have once and for all but rather a body we may acquire more and more through ceaseless interaction with ourselves, objects, other persons, and our surroundings. (Not to forget that the same body may also fail us, as in illness and disease, but this is less relevant when it comes to students of physiotherapy and their development of knowledgeable bodies). The body moves around and dwells in a multitude of situations and settings; as it explores ways of doing things, the body will be challenged, acknowledged, resisted, encouraged, or discouraged. The endeavour of indwelling and moving back and forth between focal and subliminal attention (Polanyi, 1966) or shifting between foreground and background (Merleau-Ponty, 2006 [1945]) is central. Visual illusions like the duck-rabbit are often used as examples of two possible 'readings'. While in the duck-rabbit illusion, there may be only two readings, in other more open exploratory interactions or sensitizing processes, we might find an infinite number of intangible nuances made possible through the movement between focal and subliminal attention. The restrictions and potentials of human experience are also addressed by James, here as 'habits of attention' [square brackets in quotation added by authors]:

> A man's [woman's] empirical thought depends on the things he [she] has experienced, but what these shall be is to a large extent determined by his [her] habits of attention. A thing may be presented to him [her] a thousand times, but if he [she] persistently fails to notice it, it cannot be said to enter into his [her] experience. . . . On the other hand, a thing met only once in a lifetime may leave an indelible experience in the memory.
>
> (James, 1950a [1890], p. 286)

The quote also illustrates how we tend to see and experience what we are looking for and that this can be conceptualized as habits of attention.

With this brief theoretical framing of possible ways bodies learn and what they might be capable of knowing, we now describe, analyze, and discuss insights arising from our study about how students of physiotherapy learn through their bodies during professional education.

## Discussion of emerging insights: tacit and bodily knowing in physiotherapy education

### *Recognizing the relevance of tacit knowing*

Olav's comments about his experiences, as presented at the beginning of this chapter, show his uncertainty as to how he has acquired an increased bodily awareness; he links this increased body awareness as relevant to the combat sport he practices yet not to his learning to become a physiotherapist. He explicitly expresses that this new kind of bodily awareness has contributed to him becoming more skilled in his sport, and he is puzzled about this, since he has not been practicing these skills specifically. His coach has also observed that Olav has acquired an increased bodily presence. While Olav identifies and reflects on an increased bodily awareness, he does not identify this growth of bodily ways of knowing as a specific physiotherapeutic corporeal way of knowing – nor does he even make mention of its relevance to his professional life.

During the interviews and conversations in the participant observations, many of the students were challenged by Olav's example, which was sometimes presented to them as a way to initiate a conversation on the topic. Most of the students expressed uncertainty, interest, and wonder about what might have brought about Olav's increase in bodily awareness during physiotherapy education.

Although not widely recognized by students and educators, we argue that tacit ways of bodily knowing are not only relevant to physiotherapy but are also inescapable if one is to develop the competent body of a physiotherapist, that is, a body that holds ways of knowing specific to physiotherapy. Furthermore, we identify some particular processes that we contend are needed to acquire such knowledge.

In the following section, we present examples to discuss how students might be seen to *do* bodies and learn *about* and *through* bodies in order to elaborate how learning seemed to take place.

### *Attending to the generalized body*

Students meet a multitude of bodies during training: the anatomical, physiological, and biomechanical body – that is, the generalized body from books and anatomical atlases – and a myriad of particular and individual, sensing, and meaning-making bodies – for example, their own body, other students' bodies, and the patients' bodies. The first is 'the anatomical body' operating as a norm. The latter refers to living, individual bodies with particular histories and memories. When student bodies enter into dialogue with a non-perceiving generalized body norm, the norm could operate as a horizon of comparison and thus influence the meaning making of the individual.

Nina, a first-year student, elaborates on her experience of what has contributed to an aspect of her increased bodily awareness: 'one knows where the hip joint and the pelvis are, thus, it is easier to be conscious about it'. She adds that this is a new kind of attentiveness and that she generally has become 'attentive to a lot more' in relation to what she has learned about the generalized body. Thus, we find that a generalized body norm – an image of what is common in all human bodies – may be conceptualized as a horizon for the comparison of living bodies, thus playing an important role in sensitizing and meaning-making processes. Anatomical visualizations may operate as cues in sensitizing processes, implicitly or explicitly, and in the case of Nina, she made this explicit through retrospective verbal reflection.

### *Attending to bodily happenings during basic activities of daily living*

We also inquired into how students analyze movements, with emphasis on how it feels in the body and how using cues and visualizations might nourish the experience. At the time of the study, the physiotherapy students participated in movement sessions in the gym during the first semester of training. We chose to observe and have conversations within these movement sessions, as the sessions had the explicit aim of exposing students to a variety of movement experiences and thus had the potential to open up to new experiences and ways of understanding. These sessions were designed to constitute a breach with everyday habitual movements. A variety of metaphors and other tropes were introduced, which many of the students found unfamiliar. Most of the students described these movement sessions as 'strange' and some added 'strange but fun'. A few described them as a 'waste of time'. We present an example from a movement session where students were asked to register what was happening in their own body when they performed the daily activity of standing and shifting bodyweight. This specific activity was selected as it was known to the students and operates in a tacit and taken-for-granted manner at all times in everyday activities. While standing, they were asked to shift their weight forward and backward and from side to side, and they were asked to draw attention to how this felt in their bodies by accentuating the pressure under their feet. Visualization was then introduced to the exercise as the teacher asked them to imagine that there was a weight attached to a string and the string was hanging from an axis inside their heads. This string with the weight was a visualization of the gravitational force. When this image had been introduced, they were asked again to register how this shift of weight *now* felt in their bodies. The teacher continued to construct new images, toward the base of support, described as the area covered by the feet and the area in between the feet. By focusing on the relation between the gravitational force and the base of support, the students were again asked to register how this felt in their bodies and to explore how the body will be brought out of balance if the force of gravity falls outside the base of support.

This activity can be understood in multiple ways, and we highlight two: 1) the ways in which students commonly understood the activity and 2) the intention of the teacher. The students commonly understood this activity as a way of living or doing biomechanics practically, as opposed to doing it on paper with biomechanical calculations with weight-arms and fulcrums, that is, to experience *in* your body how the interaction between the force of gravity and the base of support affects your balance. Understood in this way, it will suffice to do it once. Another purpose of this activity, from the teacher's point of view, was for it to operate as a *sensitizing process* by providing tools with the potential to make the experience of shifting the bodyweight more nuanced and multifaceted. This way of understanding the activity is akin to the dynamic way in which Despret's (2004) concept of 'learning to become affected' operates or how Schön's (1987) conceptions of 'learning by doing' and 'reflection-in-action' are understood. Polanyi's concept of 'indwelling' – a concept also used by Despret – is actualized in this example, as the strategy of the teacher was to provide possibilities for the students to immerse themselves in the situation and mobilize interest in exploring this simple, everyday activity in the way intended by the teacher. This way of engaging *bodily* awareness while *doing* brings into focus something which normally operates tacitly or subliminally and may perhaps most fruitfully be described as a dialogic and dynamic way of *experimenting* with and *exploring* bodies. In sensitizing processes, such as the one under scrutiny here, the students learn to identify, register, and differentiate nuances and details in what their bodies sense and perceive, while clearly recognizing that this endeavour can never be exhaustive. For such a learning situation to work as a sensitizing process which will be known to the person, what is *felt* in the body must be given *focal* attention; it will not suffice, as in everyday life, for it to exist in subliminal spheres; rather, it must be brought to the fore. By learning to shift attention to phenomena between a foreground and a background position, there is a potential that students will learn and acknowledge this as a process in which bodily awareness, as a way of bodily knowing, is established and constructed in a rich and skilled way. Moreover, the aim is for the students to acquire this new capacity, such that they will be able to dwell in this new knowledge, and apply this conceptual framework, in the same way that they dwell in their bodies (Polanyi, 1962 [1958], pp. 59–60). In the shifting-of-weight example, the students recognize – with immediacy – the gravitational force as something that exists and affects them, and although it usually operates in subliminal spheres, it holds the potential to become more 'alive' when brought to the fore by visualizations of a string with a weight (as a metaphor).

The teacher provides this sensitizing cue, the string with the weight, together with verbal suggestions to direct focal attention also to the pressure felt under the sole of the foot where the heel and the forefoot will be activated as sites of bodily felt happenings. Other sites of bodily felt happenings may also surface – which might be different bodily or muscular responses to being brought out of balance or emotional responses of anxiety or fear, as the body recalls earlier occurrences of maybe falling and hurting oneself. Going through these kinds of educational practices seem to have the potential to establish tacitly operating (bodily) habits in the students – 'habits' here are understood as a disposition to act (including thinking) in certain ways under certain conditions or circumstances (Colapietro, 1993).

Unlike Olav, quoted previously, Kjetil, a second-year student with a background as a dancer, states in an interview that moving can be understood as the body's way of reflecting in its own non-verbal way. Kjetil says, 'it is the activity which is the experience when it comes to the body, not the talking'. Kjetil has previous bodily experiences that appear more compatible to the understanding of movement as a sensitizing process. He conceives the body as reflecting in or through movement and that movement is a bodily form of wordless reflection, something we also find elaborated by Sheets-Johnstone (1981, 1999), through her concept of 'thinking in movement', and also by Schön (1987) and his 'reflection-in-action'. When it comes to 'thinking in movement', Sheets-Johnstone (1981, p. 402) describes how she experiences reflection-in-movement when she improvises in dance, in a process characterized as an 'ongoing or prolonged present': 'As one may wonder about the world in words, I am wondering the world directly, in movement; I am actively exploring its possibilities and what I perceive in the course of that wondering or exploration is enfolded in the very process of moving' (p. 405).

Kjetil's insights align with those of Sheets-Johnstone (1981, 1999), who elaborates that tacit ways of bodily knowing are articulated through performativity but still not exhaustively, as 'thinking in movement' is an open, ongoing process where the body is enacted and intertwined with that which appears in the environment and in the person moving. Kjetil is critical of physiotherapy education and says he had expected more emphasis on exploration of and experimentation in movement, which he thought would have been central in physiotherapy education.

## *Attending to bodily happenings in relation to one another and to patients*

In addition to what students do, more or less within their own bodies, there are also situations where they practice with each other, where their bodies are in relation. As the execution of physiotherapy is both relational and intercorporeal (Sheets-Johnstone, 1994), the student's practical training of palpation and massage can illuminate how touch gives both the therapist and the patient direct and subjectively experienced access to the other person's body and how touch exceeds and goes beyond verbal communication. What you are doing and how you are doing it is incorporated knowledge; it is the tactile-kinaesthetic (Sheets-Johnstone, 2002) and bodily-emotional (James, 1950b [1890]) knowledge that the act of palpating and giving a massage is articulating. This kind of knowledge is articulated in and through bodily practices. Examples of the tactile-kinaesthetic and the bodily-emotional are the adjustment of firmness in the grip, the assessment of the degree of stiffness in a patient's muscles, the sensitively performed transfer of weight when giving a massage, and the way the massage is adjusted to emotional reactions of the person being massaged. The corporeal knowledge we are dealing with here is articulated through performing the palpation and massage in a good way. But it is not only the corporeal skills that are at work here; such skills operate in a dynamic and dialogical relationship with other kinds of theoretical knowledge, such as, for example, anatomy, physiology, mechanics, relational ethics, and other – more or less – tacitly operating relational ways of knowing. You have to practice in order to acquire the necessary bodily knowledge or competence to be able to master a skill as complex as this.

The body has its own tactile-kinaesthetic and bodily-emotional knowledge and processes of making meaning, which cannot always be verbalized fully and directly, but one can nevertheless make efforts to raise awareness about these processes and experiences through dialogue.

Anne was educated and practiced as a massage therapist prior to starting her physiotherapy education. In this section, we present her reflections on what she learned from putting herself into the position of the patient. The aim is for students to learn by putting themselves in the position of both the therapist and the patient. As Anne explores the experiences of being touched, she is also attempting to make meaning of the tactile-kinaesthetic and bodily-emotional processes. She says she learned a lot from being massaged by a fellow student; her words exemplify how shifting between the subject positions of student and therapist opens the potential for a pedagogical opportunity for differential learning:

> You notice that she cares about the one she is massaging. She is attentive to the breathing of the one she is massaging. It feels very different from a person who is just massaging to massage somehow. . . . She is very precise in where she touches. . . . There are some students whose hands move a little all over the place without any particular rhythm, and then you become a little confused as a patient as well, I think.
>
> (Anne, first year)

When physiotherapists interact with patients in what would be considered a good practice, we suggest that this is an expression of what Sheets-Johnstone is alluding to through her concepts of – 'kinesthetically and kinetically attuned' – they attend both to bodily happenings in their own body and in that of the patients. This can also be conceptualized as bodily intentionality (Merleau-Ponty, 2006 [1945]) or a habitual way of being in the world (James, 1950b [1890], Polanyi, 1962 [1958], Polanyi, 1966). From Anne's experiences of being massaged/touched, we see that reflections on felt bodily happenings can, at least in part, be expressed through verbal language, movements, touch, or other non-verbal signs and cues. Indeed, she reads along many lines, accentuating different qualities, multiple signs, and sign languages.

To further elaborate upon ways in which physiotherapy may operate as an interactive and intercorporeal endeavour, we present an example from a clinical setting where a physiotherapist is cooperating with a patient in moving the patient's arm while supervising a student in how to do it. The example illustrates how bodily phenomena may surface and start to exist in awareness and thus become experiences and new gestalts when patients and therapists interact. We do not attempt to identify all elements in such an intercorporeal experience, to use Sheets-Johnstone's term, but rather to acknowledge that several elements may be intertwined and operate in a complex and inseparable manner.

The physiotherapist experiences resistance to passive movement of the arm of a patient, and the physiotherapist asks if the patient is aware that there is increased tension. The patient responds that she did not realize this up until now and neither does she know why it is occurring. The same situation might also spur the physiotherapist to consider the way she is supporting the arm – is it sufficient for the patient to trust that the arm will be adequately supported? Thus, the physiotherapist will also, by questioning what is felt in her own body, learn to adjust to and be affected by the patient. By experiencing this increased tension through bodily sensation, it is acknowledged as a phenomenon that exists. It becomes or emerges as a corporal (bodily) reality – what Sheets-Johnstone refers to as 'corporeality'. The interaction between the patient and the physiotherapist has brought a phenomenon into focal attention, thus establishing a new gestalt or 'reality' – as an 'intercorporeality'. In the situation of moving the arm, the physiotherapist may ask the patient to 'let go of your arm' or 'rest your arm in my hands' in order for the patient to experience the release of tension and thus accentuate and acknowledge that the tension actually was there in the first place. The situation demands an adequate verbalization, which may be explorative, as the physiotherapist tries out different metaphors or words in order to achieve a bodily response or a changed bodily awareness in the patient. The bodily signs and cues performed by the physiotherapist in order to articulate sufficient support to the patient's arm to encourage the patient to trust the physiotherapist enough to let go of the arm are also an important dimension of the intercorporeal exchange between therapist and patient. Thus, this gestalt or intercorporeality will be enacted and explored within both tactile-kinaesthetic and bodily-emotional domains.

## Concluding remarks

We have explored and theorized ways in which the body of the physiotherapist – as an instrument of treatment – is at work in physiotherapeutic intercorporeal encounters. In doing so, we have applied conceptual frameworks that are both familiar and unfamiliar to mainstream physiotherapy research.

We have sought to bring to the fore and analyze how students of physiotherapy learn *about* and *through* a myriad of bodies. Moreover, we discuss how students acquire a competent body that knows in ways specific to physiotherapy. We hence argue that there is such a thing as a competent physiotherapeutic body and that there are distinctive ways of acquiring this body. By providing – and indeed introducing – our discussion with Olav, we aim to draw attention to elements of physiotherapy education that, despite being effective in bringing about such a body, are frequently not recognized by students as doing so; something which suggests that some elements of their education are not necessarily accompanied by explicit theorization, exploration, clarification, and questioning of bodily ways of knowing and intercorporeality.

Acknowledging that some core elements of the profession's knowledge base operate tacitly is of importance, as this kind of knowledge is among the inescapable elements at work in the intercorporeal practice of physiotherapy. It seems imperative that teaching instituions elaborate and make explicit the existence of tacit aspects of physiotherapy in order to gain a deeper understanding of *if, when, how*, and *why* physiotherapy works.

## References

Colapietro, V. M. (1993). *Glossary of semiotics*. New York: Paragon House.
Despret, V. (2004). The body we care for: Figures of anthropo-zoo-genesis. *Body & Society, 10*(2–3), 111–134.
James, W. (1950a [1890]). *The principles of psychology* (Vol. 1). New York: Dover.
James, W. (1950b [1890]). *The principles of psychology* (Vol. 2). New York: Dover.
Krieger, N. (2005). Embodiment: A conceptual glossary for epidemiology. *Journal of Epidemiology and Community Health, 59*(5), 350.
Latour, B. (2004). How to talk about the body? The normative dimension of science studies. *Body & Society, 10*(2–3), 205–229.

Macdonald, H., & Nicholls, D. A. (2017). Teaching physiotherapy students to "be content with a body that refuses to hold still". *Physiotherapy Theory & Practice*, *33*(4), 303–315.

Merleau-Ponty, M. (2006 [1945]). *Phenomenology of perception*. New York: Routledge & Kegan Paul.

Nicholls, D. A. (2018). *The end of physiotherapy*. Abingdon, UK: Routledge.

Nicholls, D. A., & Gibson, B. E. (2010). The body and physiotherapy. *Physiotherapy Theory and Practice*, *26*, 497–509.

Polanyi, M. (1962 [1958]). *Personal knowledge: Towards a post-critical philosophy*. Chicago, IL: The University of Chicago Press.

Polanyi, M. (1966). *The tacit dimension*. New York: Doubleday & Company.

Schön, D. A. (1987). *Educating the reflective practitioner*. San Francisco, CA: Jossey-Bass.

Sheets-Johnstone, M. (1981). Thinking in movement. *The Journal of Aesthetics and Art Criticism*, *39* (4), 399–407.

Sheets-Johnstone, M. (1994). *The roots of power: Animate form and gendered bodies*. Chicago: Open Court.

Sheets-Johnstone, M. (1999). *The primacy of movement*. Amsterdam: John Benjamins.

Sheets-Johnstone, M. (2002). Rationality and caring: An ontogenetic and phylogenetic perspective. *Journal of the Philosophy of Sport*, *29*, 136–148.

# 4 Care in physiotherapy – a ghost story

*Birgitte Ahlsen, Alette Ottesen, and Clemet Askheim*

## Introducing care

During the early days of imperial Rome, the writer and grammarian Gaius Julius Hyginus (64 BC–17 AD) collected and wrote down ancient myths and fables. Among them was the myth of the goddess Cura (in Latin, *cura* means 'care' or 'concern'). In the translation provided by Mary Grant, the story runs thus:

> When Cura (Care) was crossing a certain river, she saw some clayey mud. She took it up thoughtfully and began to fashion a man. While she was pondering on what she had done, Jove (Jupiter) came up; Cura asked him to give the image life, and Jove (Jupiter) readily granted this. When Cura wanted to give it her name, Jove forbade her, and said that his name should be given it. But while they were disputing about the name, Tellus (Mother Earth) arose and said that it should have her name, since she had given her own body. They took it to Saturn to judge; he seems to have decided for them: Jove, since you gave him life take his soul after death; since Tellus offered her body let her receive his body; since Cura first fashioned him, let her possess him as long as he lives, but since there is controversy about his name, let him be called homo [human being], since he seems to be made from humus [earth].
>
> (Hyginus, 1960)

A central function of myths is to tell us something about 'the human condition' and presumably give some meaning to it. The creation myth of Cura, which involves at least three different deities (Cura, Jupiter, and Tellus), tells of the manifold nature of our origin as human beings. The myth also speaks of our being created in such a way as to be somewhat out of tune with our own elements, putting us constantly at risk of dissolving. The primordial role of Cura, or Care, is to keep our body and our soul temporarily together, as a whole, throughout our life. This makes the myth a suitable inspiration for dealing with dualisms and an interesting starting point for rethinking care, both in the health sector as a whole (Kristeva, Moro, Odemark, & Engebretsen, 2018) and more specifically within physiotherapy (Nicholls, 2018a; Nicholls & Cheek, 2006).

While there has been an ongoing conversation about the role of care within nursing (Martinsen & Kjerland, 2006), this has been largely absent within physiotherapy (Nicholls & Gibson, 2010; Nicholls & Holmes, 2012). Could this silence derive from the profession's tendency to focus primarily on *curing* patients, rather than offering them care? Does this emphasis on 'cure' have something to do with the invisibility of care in both clinical practice and research?

In an attempt to answer such questions and begin a wider reflection on the role of care within physiotherapy, we want to tell a story: a complex ghost story inspired by the philosopher Jacques Derrida's writing on 'hauntology' (Derrida, 2006). Our story comprises several seemingly unrelated episodes and elements, which will be woven back together as the story unfolds. Some parts of it are stories in their own right, as in the case of the ancient creation myth involving Cura. There is also a case narrative drawn from clinical practice, starring a patient and a physiotherapist. Finally, there are episodes from the history of physiotherapy as a profession, including the fateful liaison between physiotherapy and medical science.

Sara, the patient in the case narrative, is a real individual who has actually been treated by one of the authors (AO). Sara's name and some details have been changed to preserve her confidentiality. In *our* story, however, the 'patient' is the physiotherapy profession itself. For the purposes of this chapter, we place the entire profession on the psychoanalyst's couch. Our story can thus be read as itself a symptomatic reading of physiotherapy (Althusser & Balibar, 2009). As is the case in Freudian psychoanalysis, the ambition is to make latent and repressed content manifest and visible and by that means open it up to being consciously interpreted and dealt with. We argue that *care constitutes the latent content in our analysis*. By making it manifest, we hope to start a conversation on the role of care in physiotherapy.

Towards the end of the article, we return to the myth of Cura (Care). Inspired by the philosophers Martin Heidegger and Annemarie Mol, we seek to identify some fundamental aspects of care in physiotherapy: aspects that could contribute to a revaluation of the role of care in our profession.

## The case history

> Sara is an elderly woman well into her eighties, with children and grandchildren. She is a widow and lives alone in an assisted living facility. A sociable individual, she leaves the house almost every day, supported by two crutches and with her knee well bandaged. In-home nursing care is provided to her daily. After a couple of falls, she now has a safety alarm in her living space. Sara feels dizzy at times and worries that she is becoming forgetful. She has received several diagnoses, including one of osteoarthritis in her hips and knees. When she walks, her hips and knees are slightly bent, and she suffers from stiffness with kyphosis in her back. She sleeps badly. Her body is very tense, and she experiences chronic pain in various parts of her body, particularly her knees. Because of this she was referred to physiotherapy by her general practitioner (GP). AO has treated Sara periodically for several years. Sara comes for treatment only once or twice a month.

To justify the need for physiotherapy, the treatment offered should yield some measurable effect (Jamtvedt, Dahm, Holm, & Flottorp, 2008; Mikhail, Korner-Bitensky, Rossignol, & Dumas, 2005). Such evaluations are often made through assessments of the patient's pain experiences, functionality, working capacity, independence, and quality of life (Jamtvedt et al., 2008; Pencharz & MacLean, 2004). In other words, physiotherapy, like other healthcare practices, is required to work from an evidence-based perspective (Herbert, Jamtvedt, Hagen, & Mead, 2011). In general terms, physiotherapy is associated with short-term, goal-oriented interventions aimed at alleviating physical impairment and restoring mobility to the patient (Ahlsen, Engebretsen, Nicholls, & Mengshoel, 2019).

In Sara's case, however, her health issues make it difficult for treatment to fulfil these objectives. She is elderly and her illness is complex. She is probably not going to recover in the sense of having less pain and increased body function. She will probably not become more active or less dependent on help from others in her daily living. Her condition will most likely not improve significantly. Instead, Sara needs ongoing care and support in order to manage her daily life. The best that can be expected of treatment is that it may prevent her from falling, slow down her rate of decline, and mitigate the need for her to seek a greater measure of (expensive) help from the healthcare system.

## The treatment

> Sara is often very tired when she arrives for her physiotherapy and will ask to lie down on the plinth. The session usually begins with Sara talking about the pain she's been experiencing, along with her health problems in general. "I don't like complaining," she says, "But it's very good for me to come here and talk about it. I can't always be bothering others with my problems." An average session with Sara begins with AO helping her find a good resting position to allow her to relax. Then AO massages Sara's legs and gives assisted movements to her hips and knees. Together they work on knee extensions to help Sara maintain her walking function. Sara states that she feels whole-body relief during the session. Towards the end of the treatment, Sara is allowed to rest for a while on the plinth, during which she often falls asleep. When she is woken, she describes the fact that she has slept as 'fantastic'.

Touch is one of the defining characteristics of physiotherapy (Bjorbaekmo & Mengshoel, 2016; Moffatt & Kerry, 2018; Nicholls & Holmes, 2012; Roger et al., 2002). Physiotherapists utilize different forms of touch through massage, assisted movements, mobilization, and manipulation. However, the profession tends to frown upon passive forms of therapy that do not require an active effort on the patient's part and where the purpose is simply to create relief and increase the patient's well-being (Nicholls, 2018b; Nicholls & Holmes, 2012).

The origins of physiotherapy as a profession date back to the late 19th century, when a controversy related to massage treatment surfaced in London (Nicholls & Cheek, 2006). Massage institutes were flourishing at that time, but the business was unregulated, and practices were subject to considerable variation. Then, in

1894, it was alleged by an editorial in the *British Medical Journal* that many of the massage institutes were actually brothels in disguise. In order to legitimize massage as a health-related practice, its practitioners entered into an alliance with medicine by which it was agreed that massage would only be administered under medical direction. Consequently, the biomedical model was adopted as the basis for massage practices. Through the application of this model, massage was rendered a legitimate part of healthcare practice and the body was stripped of its sensuality (Nicholls & Cheek, 2006).

Subsequent events, particularly polio epidemics and the multiplicity of injuries generated by the First World War, contributed to the further development of physiotherapy as a profession (Nicholls, 2018a). Along with dramatically increasing the demand for massage services, these events also reinforced the search for treatments that required fewer resources – while being capable of returning soldiers speedily to the front and rehabilitating polio patients. In this context, massage was seen as excessively comfortable and passive, even as something that might discourage patients from making the effort necessary for recovery (Nicholls, 2018a). Overall, these events tended to reinforce the focus on cure and recovery. Repairing injuries and restoring loss of function became the watchwords of the profession. The aim was to restore the patient to leading a productive and useful life.

In Norway (and Sweden), the history of the profession came to be dominated by a struggle for position and power between the various health professions, a struggle which had a pronounced gender inflection (Ottosson, 2016). In both countries, physiotherapy practice was closely affiliated with medicine. Recovery was seen to result from physical exercises (gymnastics), discipline, and the individual's own motivation to make an effort (Nicholls, 2018a; Nicholls & Holmes, 2012; Ottosson, 2016; Thornquist, 2014). This tended to involve a conscious demarcation, a reconfiguring of both the ends (recovery) and the means (exercise) to enable both to conform with clear categories and measurable standards – drawn largely from a biomedical vocabulary.

It is evident, however, that Sara does not easily fit into such a treatment regime. Her enjoyment of physiotherapy can neither be properly measured nor legitimized, and it certainly has no place in professional journals (Mattingly & Lawlor, 2001). Sara does not have the strength and energy for physical exercises outside her routine daily activities. She is tired, sleeps poorly, and needs rest, something she experiences during the treatment session with AO. Sara describes her physiotherapy sessions as 'fantastic'. But her therapist is experiencing growing unease and uncertainty about the treatment of Sara.

## That which must not be named

> Sara truly enjoys her physiotherapy treatment; she always shows up on time and never misses a session. She always tells AO how important it is for her to come to physiotherapy, every time adding: 'It is such good care. You don't know how much it means to me'. 'Care!?' The very word makes AO feel a bit irritated but also a little ashamed. 'Yes, care is what it is,' she tells herself. 'I can hardly call it physiotherapy!'

While its alliance with medicine has endowed physiotherapy with respect as well as recognition as an indispensable part of healthcare and the healthcare system (Nicholls, 2018a; Thornquist, 2014), it has also created a circumscribed understanding of what physiotherapy is and can be. This has reached the point at which offering care is seen to be beyond the frontiers of professional practice (Nicholls, 2018b; Nicholls & Gibson, 2010; Nicholls & Holmes, 2012). In effect, care is out of bounds.

There is a necessary reductionism within the biomedical paradigm, where the patient is primarily conceived as a body to be treated, and the body is likened to a machine (Nicholls & Gibson, 2010). Related to this is the seemingly inescapable separation between soul and body, mind and matter. This dualism, often framed in terms of 'Cartesianism', is reproduced in specific ways in the biomedical worldview (Nicholls & Gibson, 2010). Even when medical practice draws on psychological and social insights, holistic interpretations or other alternative viewpoints, the hierarchy remains in place, with the body and the physical/biological firmly at the summit.

The imagery of the body as a machine fits well with the notion of physiotherapy as a curative enterprise (Nicholls & Gibson, 2010; Thornquist, 2006). When a functional body is broken, it can be brought to the physiotherapist, who is then supposed to diagnose the problem and find a solution to it. Ideally the patient will regain their previous functional abilities, return to work, and move on (Ahlsen et al., 2019). Such is the way the biomedical model, with its Cartesian tendency to separate mind and body and prioritize the latter, creates a situation where cure is emphasized at the expense of care (Askheim, Sandset, & Engebretsen, 2017). Within the physiotherapy profession, the dualism and the focus on the body has led to an unconscious blindness towards other dimensions of human experience, such as the soul or the mind. The resulting inattention to care can be seen as a result of subconscious processes of repression.

In physiotherapy research, there is little mention of care as a component of practice (although there are indications of a growing interest in the issue) (Dahl-Michelsen, 2015; Nicholls & Holmes, 2012). And while care may find its way into clinical settings, it will not be named as such. Viewing themselves through the lens of biomedicine, where cure eclipses care, physiotherapists are unable to recognize themselves as providers of care, as we shall argue.

This situation threatens to create real problems in clinical practice. Conflict can arise between what is actually happening (the reality of everyday practice) and what has been instilled in practitioners by prevailing discourses, theory, guidelines, and norms (including evidence-based practice). As a result of this clash, offering care becomes something 'one should not do' – or, if it does happen, 'one should not talk about it'. It becomes a kind of taboo, something ineffable or beyond comment (Freud, 2001).

## Clinical consequences

> To make a long story short, AO subsequently finds an opportunity to terminate her work with Sara. As AO explains to Sara, it's difficult to find reasons that would justify further physiotherapy treatment for her. 'Perhaps there are other treatment alternatives?' suggests AO. 'How about trying a balance group for older adults?'

What happens to the patient in this context? When Sara walks in the door, she does so as a person, a complex individual. However, for the purposes of physiotherapy, she must be stripped of her soul. She must become her 'body', pure and simple. Sara's osteoarthritis diagnosis (degeneration of joints), balance issues, and physical pain provide her with a legitimate claim to physiotherapy, since she has problems with her body. In order to maintain the legitimacy of treatment, AO and Sara must collaborate on Sara's osteoarthritis, her knees, the tenseness of her body, and problems with her balance and her mobility – always towards the goal of improving bodily function. In Sara's case, however, such improvement can take place only within very narrow limits. Treatment may help prevent falls or slow down Sara's loss of physical function or possibly help her cope with the pain. When Sara goes for physiotherapy, she seeks respite for her inner being, perhaps nourishment for her soul. But this does not lie within the accepted boundaries of physiotherapy as presently constituted. It is not what physiotherapists 'do'. Care is not a legitimate wish. The patient must under no circumstances utter the word 'care'. The physiotherapist is there to treat the body, full stop.

But what of the rest? Is Sara simply an 'illegitimate' form of patient? And what happens to the physiotherapist? AO must turn a blind eye to Sara's need for care. She must prioritize her work in accordance with current guidelines (Øyehaug, Paulsen, Vøllestad, & Robinson, 2019). In her journal, she must justify her clinical decisions with reference to effect and goal attainment. After all, Sara is not going back to work, her condition is not improving, and there will be no significant recovery, no future horizon where things change for the better. There is no room for care, since AO must reduce her patients to bodies, to machine-like objects. But in the process, she risks being turned into a machine herself.

If a physiotherapist is reduced to the status of a body-treating machine, this may lead to a sense of powerlessness (Mattingly & Lawlor, 2001). To care too much becomes a transgression. It is not a legitimate option within the prevailing conception of physiotherapy. It is impossible to argue for continued treatment based on care and well-being. As a result, the physiotherapist confronts the same dilemma as that experienced by every other health practitioner: whether to give primacy to the patient and their needs and preferences or to remain 'loyal' to the guidelines, rules, and regulations laid down by the healthcare system.

## The uncanny

In his essay on the uncanny ('Das Unheimliche' [1919]), Freud defines something as uncanny when it borders on the well-known and homelike ('heimlich' in German) but in a twisted way that feels threatening or uncomfortable. The uncanny is too close for comfort, 'that class of the frightening which leads back to what is known of old and long familiar' (Freud, 1955, p. 220). Freud continues thus:

> In the first place, if psycho-analytic theory is correct in maintaining that every affect belonging to an emotional impulse, whatever its kind, is transformed, if it is repressed, into anxiety, then among instances of frightening things

there must be one class in which the frightening element can be shown to be something repressed which recurs. This class of frightening things would then constitute the uncanny; and it must be a matter of indifference whether what is uncanny was itself originally frightening or whether it carried some other affect. In the second place if this is indeed the secret nature of the uncanny, we can understand why linguistic usage has extended das Heimliche ['homely'] into its opposite, das Unheimliche; for this uncanny is in reality nothing new or alien, but something which is familiar and old-established in the mind and which has become alienated from it only through the process of repression.

(Freud, 1955, p. 241)

Following Freud, if an affect associated with care, such as shame, is repressed, it may turn into anxiety. When care comes up on the agenda again, it is likely to be seen or felt as something uncanny. An additional meaning of 'uncanny' (unheimlich) is something that ought to remain hidden (Svenaeus, 2000a). In German, there is both a phonetic and an etymological similarity between 'heimlich' and 'heimisch', the latter deriving from 'geheim': 'that which is hidden or secret'. In the context of physiotherapy, this sense of something that 'ought to remain hidden' appears applicable to care.

It can be argued that physiotherapy's adoption of the biomedical paradigm, along with its reliance on 'hard facts', is what gives it status and potency. But this requires the repression of the sensual, 'softer' aspects of the profession, both in its theoretical formulations and in its everyday practice (Nicholls & Holmes, 2012). A Freudian interpretation might link this with a 'castration complex' or a fear of castration (Freud, 1955). Here, physiotherapy's tendency to clutch on to 'hard' elements (cure), while repressing softer ones (care) is seen to result from its fear of being rendered impotent as a practice and profession: metaphorical castration, in Freudian terms.

## Return of the repressed

> One day a few weeks later, well after treatment has ended, AO sees Sara walking along the other side of the street, supported by her crutches. 'What a brave woman', AO says to herself with a pang of conscience. 'If physiotherapy means that much to her, why can't she come and see me every now and again'?

This 'pang of conscience' can be likened to an experience of the uncanny. In this scene, the patient becomes a phantom-like presence haunting the physiotherapist in broad daylight. But the spectre at the centre of *our* story is not the patient – it is care itself.

In a reappraisal of Freud's metapsychological theory of the unconscious, Svenaeus asks whether it might not be;

> precisely a sophisticated model for explaining how various phenomena make the individual aware of not being at home in him- or herself? Something that

belongs to the person, but which is still not known by him or her, presents itself in dreams and slips of the tongue.

(Svenaeus, 1999, p. 244)

Or perhaps this 'something' presents itself in phantom form. In our story, the physiotherapy profession comes face to face with care: a repressed element of its being that continues to haunt it. Sara here becomes symbolic or representative of the illegitimacy and repression of care within physiotherapy. By virtue of its repression, care has turned into something uncanny: a ghost. Upholding the scientific basis, effectiveness and purity of physiotherapy requires the continuous exorcism of the ghost of care, with its blurry boundaries and unclear status. But the spectral presence of care keeps coming back.

## The spectre of care

As with the Latin term 'cura', considerable ambiguity is attached to the English word 'care'. On the one hand, it denotes thoughtfulness, attentiveness, concern. On the other, it can mean sorrow, anxiety, and solicitude (Hamilton, 2013). In the myth that began our story, Care personifies all these meanings, thereby rendering herself more complex than the stock figure of the caring mother. What Care creates is human life (homo) – in all its complexity.

Jupiter is the god of the sky, associated with light and lightning (enlightenment). He is also the son of Saturn. Tellus or Terra is 'Mother Earth', associated with both agriculture, ground, and fertility. She is also the mother of Saturn. Saturn is, among other things, the god of time and the old king of the gods. In the myth, humans are both earthbound, grounded creatures and spirit-infused beings who look upwards towards the sky. What unites them, what holds them together in time – temporarily – is Care. When she thoughtfully picks up some clay, she is at the threshold of change (as symbolized by the river). Humans are born into time with the ability to think and to respond to Care's solicitude. This involves the knowledge of our mortality and the sorrow and anxiety that come with it. Rather than representing something that is soft and pleasurable, Care is often dark and painful. As long as we live, Care is something we cannot escape.

## The ghost in the machine

The myth of care has featured in European philosophy and literature for many centuries (Reich, 1995). In modern times, the most influential engagement with it remains the reinterpretation offered by Martin Heidegger in *Being and Time* (Heidegger, 1996). Here, Heidegger gives the myth an existential twist. He sees it as conveying the centrality of Care to what it means to be human and to live a human life. In addition, the myth reveals how humankind as a social totality is brought into the world by Care and then sustained by it. Just as it binds humans together, Care binds us to our environments – out of necessity rather than as part of a quest for harmony. Finally, the myth expresses the temporal dimension of human existence, its quality of being 'always already' thrown into the world, and the reality that every human life has an end.

Heidegger's interpretation of the myth, together with his more comprehensive concept of care, have inspired considerable debate, including within the health sciences (Kleinman & Van Der Geest, 2009). In the field of nursing in particular, the ethics of care has been a central topic of research since the 1970s (Martinsen & Kjerland, 2006). But while several authors have written about Heidegger in relation to physiotherapy, they have largely avoided the topic of care (Shaw & Connelly, 2012).

## In the company of ghosts

One reason for this silence could be the 'uncanniness' of care in physiotherapy, a profession which has always focused on the curative dimension of clinical practice. While every physiotherapist is aware of the presence of care, there is a reluctance to acknowledge it or bring it into the discussion. Care is uncomfortable yet strangely familiar: a monster from the 'id' (for Freud, the basic level of our subconscious) which 'ought to have remained hidden' (Freud, 1961, p. 241). And if it does happen to be revealed, then it must be quickly repressed. However, there is also the possibility that this spectral presence could be confronted, embraced, and brought into the light of day.

For Heidegger, care is the constitutive element of our humanness. We *are* care! We constantly take care of different issues; we care for others and ourselves. We cannot *not* care, since we exist at the mercy of care. We have never been, and will never be, completely autonomous, self-contained, or independent individuals. Instead, we are dependent on others, and this makes us vulnerable, worried, anxious, and solicitous. At the moment of birth, we are already in a web of relationships. We are victims of circumstance, surrounded by expectations and obligations. This goes for patients and physiotherapists as much as for anyone else. Yet within physiotherapy, these basic truths appear to go unrecognized. Or worse: they become subjected to a form of denial.

Taking Heidegger's perspective on the human condition as our starting point, we can state that physiotherapy necessarily includes care. Indeed, it is impossible to practice physiotherapy *without* care, given that care is integral to human interaction with the world. The problem is that the preeminence of the biomedical model in physiotherapy makes it difficult for the profession to recognize care or acknowledge its centrality.

In the health sciences, care tends to be viewed as separate from cure. While cure is associated with interventions geared to healing an injury or combating a disease, care is associated with add-on activities: 'friendly extras' (Mol, 2008). While cure is associated with evidence-based practice, technology, science, and facts, care is seen as something vague and indistinct – an optional 'soft supplement' (Askheim et al., 2017; Kristeva et al., 2018).

While there is now some recognition that care-related activities (such as communication) can usefully supplement physical exercises in physiotherapy practice, traditionally, the profession has tended to view care, and caring, almost as obstacles, as impediments to recovery (Nicholls & Holmes, 2012). If treatment seems too comfortable, not including active effort from the patient, then there's something suspect about it. Something is not quite right; something is just a touch uncanny.

## The logic of care

The Dutch ethnographer and philosopher Annemarie Mol argues that care has its own logic: the logic of care (Mol, 2008). In contrast, physiotherapy, with its historical alliance with medicine, is still rooted in what Mol calls the logic of choice. Although resting on different ideological foundations, these two types of logic can coexist and blend in concrete situations (Mol, 2008).

Care is not recognized, Mol contends, when there is not enough time to listen to the patient. Care is not recognized when physical parameters are isolated from their context, when the patient's daily life and values are not taken into consideration, or when measurement of a few discrete parameters diverts attention from the sometimes-painful intricacies of day-to-day life with disease. Care is not recognized when the patient is not recognized as such (Mol, 2008).

Mol argues that the logic of choice derives from a specific ideological standpoint: the view that human beings are autonomous, independent, choice-making individuals. This ideology permeates the dominant discourse of medicine and other health sciences, emerging in concepts such as 'shared decision-making', 'empowerment', and 'self-management' (Kristeva et al., 2018). The body, according to the logic of choice, is an object (a machine) to be controlled, kept in order, and subjected to treatment. In the case of physiotherapy, treatment is seen as a pre-defined product about which patients can exercise their own free choice. 'You could join a balance group for older adults – it's entirely up to you'. According to the logic of choice, treatment has a beginning and an end; evaluations are made once it is over.

In contrast, the logic of care derives from an understanding of humans as interdependent, vulnerable, and profoundly social beings who exist within a network of relationships and require the support of others. From this perspective, care has neither a beginning nor an end. As with the ancient myth and Heidegger's existential exploration, care is 'always already': an ongoing and open process. In Sara's story, care manifests itself in relation to the open-endedness of her treatment. From Sara's viewpoint, there is no predetermined end to the treatment she is receiving, and she finds comfort in the fact that she can come for her physiotherapy every now and then.

For Mol, care is not a transaction where something is exchanged (Mol, 2008). Nor is it simply a matter of offering treatment or giving the patient a sheet of paper with descriptions and diagrams of different physical exercises. Instead, care is all about interaction and recognition. Care includes listening to the patient's problems and worries. Care is when the therapist attunes to the patient's body and acknowledges the patient's needs (Svenaeus, 2000a, 2000b). Care is the therapist and patient working together, perhaps exploring various resting positions and movements. In the logic of care, the patient's body is not separated from that patient's self and approached as something to be fixed. Rather, self and body form a totality that must be acknowledged and nourished. Care is an interactive, open-ended process that constantly evolves and shifts. Rather than existing as pre-fixed entities that are independent of treatment, goals are integral to its practice and evolution.

While it remains possible for the logic of care and the logic of choice to function well together in daily healthcare practice, Mol argues that very often, they come into collision. In the case of physiotherapy, we argue that this clash has resulted in the suppression of care and a failure to acknowledge its centrality.

## Coda

Our story presents care in physiotherapy as something uncanny or 'unheimlich': something familiar and well known, yet repressed and hidden. By explicitly acknowledging care as an integral part of physiotherapy, we want to open up more space for the logic of care in clinical practice. It concerns making our profession a place where the patient's pain and problems are recognized, a place of cooperative endeavour where therapist and patient together explore movements and bodily habits and gain new bodily experiences. We foresee the opening up of new paths and possibilities: ones which enable the patient to feel 'at home' while making it possible for the physiotherapist to be recognized and acknowledged as one who cares.

Not everyone in need of care is entitled to physiotherapy; physiotherapists will have to continue making difficult choices. But as our evolving profession seeks to improve its practice, we argue that it needs to confront the ghosts from the past that haunt it still. Above all, it needs to embrace the centrality of care, to draw it into the light and welcome its life-enhancing possibilities.

## References

Ahlsen, B., Engebretsen, E., Nicholls, D., & Mengshoel, A. M. (2019). The singular patient in patient-centred care: Physiotherapists' accounts of treatment of patients with chronic muscle pain. *Medical Humanities*, On-line early. doi:10.1136/medhum-2018-011603

Althusser, L., & Balibar, É. (2009). *Reading capital*. London, UK: Verso.

Askheim, C., Sandset, T., & Engebretsen, E. (2017). Who cares? The lost legacy of Archie Cochrane. *Medical Humanities*, *43*(1), 41–46. doi:10.1136/medhum-2016-011037

Bjorbaekmo, W. S., & Mengshoel, A. M. (2016). "A touch of physiotherapy": The significance and meaning of touch in the practice of physiotherapy. *Physiotherapy Theory and Practice*, *32*(1), 10–19. doi:10.3109/09593985.2015.1071449

Dahl-Michelsen, T. (2015). Curing and caring competences in the skills training of physiotherapy students. *Physiotherapy Theory and Practice*, *31*(1), 8–16. doi:10.3109/09593985.2014.949946

Derrida, J. (2006). *Specters of Marx: The state of the debt, the work of mourning and the new international*. New York: Routledge Classics.

Freud, S. (1955). The uncanny. In J. Strachey & A. Freud (Eds.), *The standard edition of the complete psychological works of Sigmund Freud: Vol. 17: An infantile neurosis, and other works (1917–1919)*. London, UK: Hogarth Press and the Institute of Psycho-Analysis.

Freud, S. (1961). The ego and the id. In J. Strachey & A. Freud (Eds.), *The standard edition of the complete psychological works of Sigmund Freud: Vol. 19: The ego and the id, and other works (1923–1925)*. London, UK: Hogarth Press and the Institute of Psycho-Analysis.

Freud, S. (2001). Totem and taboo. In S. James & A. Freud (Eds.), *The standard edition of the complete psychological works of Sigmund Freud: Vol. 13: Totem and taboo, and other works (1913–1914)*. London, UK: Vintage.

Hamilton, J. T. (2013). *Security: Politics, humanity, and the philology of care*. Princeton and Oxford: Princeton University Press.

Heidegger, M. (1996). *Being and time: A translation of Sein Und Zeit*. Albany, NY: State University of New York Press.

Herbert, R., Jamtvedt, G., Hagen, K. B., & Mead, J. (2011). *Practical evidence-based physiotherapy* (2nd ed.). Edinburgh: Elsevier.

Hyginus, G. J. (1960). *The myths of Hyginus* (M. Grant, Trans., Vol. 34). Lawrence: University of Kansas Publications.

Jamtvedt, G., Dahm, K. T., Holm, I., & Flottorp, S. (2008). Measuring physiotherapy performance in patients with osteoarthritis of the knee: A prospective study. *BMC Health Services Research*, 8(145). doi:10.1186/1472-6963-8-145

Kleinman, A., & Van Der Geest, S. (2009). "Care" in health care: Remaking the moral world of medicine. *Medische Antropologie*, 21(1), 159–168.

Kristeva, J., Moro, M. R., Odemark, J., & Engebretsen, E. (2018). Cultural crossings of care: An appeal to the medical humanities. *Medical Humanities*, 44(1), 55–58. doi:10.1136/medhum-2017-011263

Martinsen, K., & Kjerland, L. E. (2006). *Care and vulnerability*. Oslo, NO: Akribe.

Mattingly, C., & Lawlor, M. (2001). The fragility of healing. *American Anthropologist*, 29(1), 30–57. doi:10.1525/eth.2001.29.1.30

Mikhail, C., Korner-Bitensky, N., Rossignol, M., & Dumas, J. P. (2005). Physical therapists' use of interventions with high evidence of effectiveness in the management of a hypothetical typical patient with acute low back pain. *Physical Therapy*, 85(11), 1151–1167.

Moffatt, F., & Kerry, R. (2018). The desire for "hands-on" therapy: A critical analysis of the phenomenon of touch. In B. E. Gibson, D. A. Nicholls, J. Setchell, & K. S. Groven (Eds.), *Manipulating practices: A critical physiotherapy reader* (pp. 174–190). Oslo, NO: Cappelen Damm Akademisk.

Mol, A. (2008). *The logic of care: Health and the problem of patient choice*. Abington, UK: Routledge.

Nicholls, D. A. (2018a). *The end of physiotherapy*. Abington, UK and New York: Routledge.

Nicholls, D. A. (2018b). Aged care as a bellwether of future physiotherapy. *Physiotherapy Theory and Practice*, 1–13. doi:10.1080/09593985.2018.1513105

Nicholls, D. A., & Cheek, J. (2006). Physiotherapy and the shadow of prostitution: The society of trained masseuses and the massage scandals of 1894. *Social Science and Medicine*, 62(9), 2336–2348. doi:10.1016/j.socscimed.2005.09.010

Nicholls, D. A., & Gibson, B. E. (2010). The body and physiotherapy. *Physiotherapy Theory and Practice*, 26(8), 497–509. doi:10.3109/09593981003710316

Nicholls, D. A., & Holmes, D. (2012). Discipline, desire, and transgression in physiotherapy practice. *Physiotherapy Theory and Practice*, 28(6), 454–465. doi:10.3109/09593985.2012.676940

Ottosson, A. (2016). One history or many herstories? Gender politics and the history of physiotherapy's origins in the nineteenth and early twentieth century. *Women's History Review, 25*(2), 296–319.

Øyehaug, G. A., Paulsen, A. K., Vøllestad, N. K., & Robinson, H. S. (2019). Prioritering og venteliste hos avtalefysioterapeuter – en tverrsnittstudie [Prioritization and waiting times for physiotherapy in private practice: A cross-sectional study]. *Fysioterapeuten, 7*, 22–27.

Pencharz, J. N., & MacLean, C. H. (2004). Measuring quality in arthritis care: The Arthritis Foundation's quality indicator set for osteoarthritis. *Arthritis and Rheumatism, 51*(4), 538–548. doi:10.1002/art.20521

Reich, W. T. (1995). History of the nation of "care". In W. T. Reich (Ed.), *Encyclopedia of bioethics* (Revised ed., Vol. 5, pp. 319–331). New York: Simon & Schuster Macmillan.

Roger, J., Darfour, D., Dham, A., Hickman, O., Shaubach, L., & Shepard, K. (2002). Physiotherapists' use of touch in inpatient settings. *Physiotherapy Research International, 7*(3), 170–186.

Shaw, J. A., & Connelly, D. M. (2012). Phenomenology and physiotherapy: Meaning in research and practice. *Physical Therapy Reviews, 17*(6), 398–408.

Svenaeus, F. (1999). Freud's philosophy of the uncanny. *The Scandinavian Psychoanalytic Review, 22*(2), 239–254.

Svenaeus, F. (2000a). Das unheimliche: Towards a phenomenology of illness. *Medicine, Health Care, and Philosophy, 3*(1), 3–16. doi:10.1023/a:1009943524301

Svenaeus, F. (2000b). The body uncanny: Further steps towards a phenomenology of illness. *Medicine, Health Care, and Philosophy, 3*(2), 125–137.

Thornquist, E. (2006). Face-to-face and hands-on: Assumptions and assessments in the physiotherapy clinic. *Medical Anthropology, 25*(1), 65–97. doi:10.1080/01459740500514489

Thornquist, E. (2014). Fysioterapeutene: Fra kosmologi til fagpolitikk. In R. Slagstad & J. Messel (Eds.), *Profesjonshistorier* (pp. 138–176). Oslo, NO: Pax forlag A/S.

# 5 Rethinking recovery

*Anne Marit Mengshoel and Marte Feiring*

## Introduction

The term 'recovery' frequently occurs in medical and in public settings. For example, in medical care, people can recover from a disease, such as bronchitis or cancer, and are said to be in recovery when they learn how to cope with symptoms and manage practical everyday tasks despite limitations set by chronic illness. While laypeople often say they have recovered from a cold, mental illness, or cancer, drug addicts will describe themselves as being in recovery when they become sober or abstinent. Recovery may encompass becoming better or being cured, returning to, or arriving at a healthy state or life as it used to be, regaining something that was lost, or recreating a meaningful or well life.

Inspired by Jacobson (2004), we refer to different meanings and uses of the term recovery. These include *recovery as outcome* (evidence), which was first used in mental hospital services in the mid-19th century, and *recovery as experience* (personal healing process), an understanding that was constituted as a response to the former by the voices of mental health survivors and ex-patients during the 1930s. In addition, *recovery as co-production* covers the new public emphasis on partnerships as well as people's accountability for their own health and the reduction of health costs (Jasanoff, 2004; Jacobson, 2004). In the sociology of science, the concept 'co-production of knowledge' is applied on a new combined approach, analysing the social structure and cultural meanings, integrating theory and practice, macro and micro, and objects and subjects, as well as historical and contemporary studies (Jasanoff, 2004). In our society today, in both mental and somatic healthcare systems and in research, political documents emphasize evidence-based practice and consumers' or users' expertise. In these contexts, recovery is an umbrella term with various interpretations and meanings.

A search of scientific databases, using the term recovery alone or in combination with health professions including physiotherapy, results in thousands of hits. Often, studies by health professionals refer to treatment outcomes in terms of their effectiveness in minimizing symptoms and disease-related limitations in functioning. Less frequently, studies address how people experience illness or, even less commonly, illuminate people's recovery experiences. However, since the 1980s, the disease-oriented quantitative studies on recovery outcome have been complemented by qualitative studies of ill people's experiences (Jacobson, 2004). We characterize the quantitative studies as disease-oriented, outcome-based research, defining recovery as a dimension of pathology or disease-related deficits and a real event represented by the nonappearance of certain disease indicators. On the other hand, the qualitative studies focus on personal experiential processes where recovery is constructed in the process of learning how to live a safe, dignified, and self-determined life.

The disease-oriented recovery outcome is informed by evidence from quantitative studies aiming to produce knowledge that can be valid for groups of patients across contexts and cultures, and the qualitative and mixed studies consider recovery experiences as contextual and occurring in an interplay between individuals, their clinical treatment, and their social surroundings. We refer to the first approaches as a disease-oriented recovery outcome and the second as a personal experiential recovery process. Our aim is to unpack these two applications of the term 'recovery', analysed as different ways of producing knowledge, first in terms of curing disease and second in the language of a person's process of overcoming or coming to terms with disruptions from illness. Third, we discuss how it is possible to critically integrate recovery as outcome and recovery as experience in professional health practices into what Jasanoff (2004) has referred to as co-production of knowledge.

## Disease-oriented recovery outcome

For centuries, physicians were committed to understanding people's suffering based on information from interviews of individuals and their own observations through gaze, smell, and taste (Johannisson, 2004). Treatment was a product of the physician's skill at interpreting what people told them, as well as the meanings of their conversations with patients and their own observations. But when the nature of disease and the idea of specific disease aetiology emerged, the physician's task became to translate what ill persons told them into a classification of symptoms to be used to further trace the cause of disease (Bury, 2005, Chap. 1). Accordingly, the focus of medical practice shifted from subjective experiences to objective measures of pathology and from personalized and symptom-oriented logics to disease-oriented ones.

The disease-oriented perspective is based on a biomedical understanding wherein disease is defined in terms of deviance from statistical norms of organ functioning in healthy populations (Boorse, 1977). The deviances or signs of disease that are hidden inside the body become visible through technological measures, for example, radiological imaging and blood tests. The aim of treatment becomes to 'normalize' what is wrong by targeting abnormal organ structures and functioning with appropriate treatment. In order to make decisions concerning treatment or therapy, health professionals translate patients' illness experiences into symptoms, which in turn serve as clues to guide further testing for plausible diseases (Eriksen & Risør, 2014). In the International Classification of Diseases (ICD), clusters of typical symptoms and bodily malfunctioning create criteria for diagnosis, and if clinical findings match these criteria, a disease is named by a diagnostic label (Jutel, 2011). In other words, a person's perceptions and bodily changes are translated into nomenclature and disease taxonomy that constitutes an objective 'it' that exists beyond the particular patient (Kleinman, 1988). From this point, the disease becomes a real 'thing' that justifies a person's suffering and legitimizes a need for help (Lian, 2007). A similar logic can be found in physiotherapy, for example, in physiotherapists' attempts to develop a pathokinaesiological classification system of limitations in physical functioning (Rose, 1988), as well as in the importance they place on arriving at a functioning diagnosis and connecting treatment to this diagnosis (Rose, 1989; Sahrman, 1988).

## What is similar should be treated similarly

At the beginning of the 1900s, medicine became enchanted by the idea that the nature of diseases could be discovered and their specific causes and treatment found, and the hunt for precision in diagnosis and treatment continues to this day (Cassell, 2004). According to this view, each disease is believed to have a particular cause that can be revealed by observing changes in inner organs' function and structure, and in turn, treatment should target such disease-specific changes and normalize them to recover health. Physicians should act upon a particular disease with specific treatments; for example, a targeting drug should destroy bacteria that cause disease. During the last couple of decades, medical treatment has become even more specific by targeting specific disease mechanisms within a diagnostic category. For example, patients with prostate cancer receive various medical therapies specifically designed to target different pathological patterns. Thus, in some areas of medicine, personalized medicine has become an alternative. In this context, personalization means that each person's specific disease pathology within a diagnostic category should be acted on, and those with similar pathology should be treated similarly in order to become better or be cured.

The idea of classification and using targeted therapy to help patients recover their health can be traced to early in the history of physiotherapy. At the beginning of the 1800s, Per Henrik Ling, the founder of physiotherapy in Scandinavia, developed an exercise system tailored to promote healing of musculoskeletal pain (Haugen, 1997). This was carried further; for example, during the poliomyelitis epidemic in the 1950s, physiotherapists developed a method for assessing the strength of specific muscles (Kendall, 1983). The aim was to identify which muscles were affected by poliomyelitis and tailor specific exercises to revitalize the affected muscles. Treatment modalities have also been developed to normalize the functioning of other organs; for example, joint mobilization techniques aim to reduce stiffness in joint capsules (Kaltenborn, 2003). The idea that similar problems should be treated similarly can also be seen in the model of evidence-based practice (EBP), in which treatment recommendations are grouped according to diagnosis (Herbert, Jamtvedt, Mead, & Hagen, 2005).

## Recovery as absence of disease, deficits, or dysfunctions

Within biomedicine, health is defined as the absence of disease (Hofmann, 2001). Health and disease are understood as dichotomous phenomena, and recovery is usually understood as an endpoint or a treatment outcome where the disease is absent and a cure is reached. Recovery results from either a natural biological healing process or an effective curative treatment. In addition to cures, recovery outcomes can also be expressed as partial recovery (fewer disease-related deficits and dysfunctions) or remission (normalized biology but not the absence of disease).

In 1948, the World Health Organization (WHO) expanded the biomedical definition of health to include not merely absence of disease or infirmity but also a state of complete physical, mental, and social well-being (Larson, 1996). Later, Engel (1977) argued that disease should be understood as complex, dynamic, interacting processes between biological, psychological, and social phenomena. He coined the concept 'biopsychosocial' and expanded the biomedical understanding of disease (White, 2005). This was followed up by the WHO's (1980) introduction of a supplement to the biomedical classification of disease (the ICD), launching the International Classification of Impairments, Disabilities and Handicaps (ICIDH), which included a theoretical model describing that disease-related bodily impairments could lead to disabilities and handicaps and, second, a classification of multiple factors under the terms impairments, disabilities, and handicaps. In the years that followed, the ICIDH was criticized, first for its biomedical understanding by indicating a causal chain from biological impairments to disability and handicap and second for labelling people with impairment as disabled and handicapped.

The ICIDH was revised several times, leading to the present International Classification of Health and Functioning (ICF; WHO, 2001). The ICF model shows reciprocal interrelationships between body function (previously impairment) and personal limitations in functioning under activities and participation (previously disability and handicap). Accordingly, the ICF model now reflects a biopsychosocial understanding of disease, and it still includes a classification system. However, in contrast to the biomedical understanding of disease, the present ICF model of reciprocal interactions suggests that a person's health can be targeted in multiple ways. The ICF has been embraced within the field of rehabilitation, including among physiotherapists. In clinical practice and research, the ICF and the biopsychosocial model are presented as a more comprehensive and complex understanding of disease and health than the biomedical model. But the ICF can still be criticized for having an individualistic perspective and not taking into account social and political barriers to a person's health, functioning, or well-being. Also, the ICF follows the biomedical principle of objectivity and value-neutrality. Thus, Hammell (2006) argues that the application of this classification tool does not have any benefit for the persons being objectified and coded; rather, classification systems are tools for health professionals. The use of classification tools, such as the ICF, is also criticized in physiotherapy, for example by Leplège et al. (2015) and by Gibson (2016).

## Recovery determined by measured treatment outcomes

Recovery outcomes, in terms of treatment effects, are determined by evaluating the extent to which disease-related measures approximate statistically based or socially determined norms, as well as by the disappearance of symptoms. In physiotherapy, body function is assessed by objective measures such as aerobic capacity, muscle strength, and range of motion. Limitations in activities and participation are assessed by patient self-report questionnaires. Questionnaires can be generic instruments developed to assess what is normal in a general population, such as quality of life and presence at work. Alternatively, in physiotherapy research, disease-specific questionnaires are often used to assess the reduction of typical disease-related symptoms and limitations in daily functioning. In both cases, recovery is determined by external criteria for what is considered normal among healthy people or within a society. However, norms determined by statistics or social values of functioning do not always match what is important in the treatment of an individual patient. In particular, occupational therapists and physiotherapists within the field of rehabilitation have expressed concerns that generic and disease-specific instruments do not capture the effects of therapies tailored to patients' specific activity problems. To address this, they have developed patient-specific instruments that allow clinicians, in collaboration with their patients, to specify the problem to be approached by treatment. The severity of a problem is assessed by scales, and recovery outcome is measured in terms of the amelioration of the problem. Accordingly, improvements are evaluated with respect to self-defined treatment goals and norms for success (Stevens, Beurskens, & Köke, 2013; Stratford, Gill, Westaway, & Binkley, 1995).

## A personal experiential recovery process

### A social movement promoting personal recovery

As a critical response to disease-oriented approaches, consumer communities in the 1930s showed how recovery was related to individuals' experiences of illness (Jacobson, 2004). Alcoholics Anonymous (AA) is an early example of recovery as experience (Feiring, 2013), and Ralph and Corrigan (2005) consider these communities 'historical backdrops' to modern mental health services. In the 1970s and 1980s, people experiencing mental health problems started to oppose the focus within psychiatry on diagnosis, psychopathology, and biological treatments and claimed that it was possible to achieve a life of personal value by focusing on personal experiences and resources. According to Roberts and Boardman (2013), the recovery movement in psychiatry arose as a product of critique, emerging from the writings of survivors and ex-patients.

During the 1980s and 1990s, a social movement also emerged among people with physical disabilities who objected to the 'normalization' of functioning within the field of rehabilitation and claimed their human right to participate in society alongside able-bodied people on equal terms (Oliver, 1990). For example, constructions of public transport and buildings excluded access for people with physical disabilities. Instead, a society accepting and adjusting to diversity among citizens was envisaged as a means to achieving a more inclusive society.

Jacobson (2004) associates recovery as experience with this type of social rights movement. Publicly driven campaigns challenged medical views on people with mental illnesses and physical disabilities, resulting in health reforms highlighting human rights and individuals' possession of the expertise and resources necessary to live well despite illness or disability, as well as changes within health services, including the introduction of patient- or person-centred practice. Over the last couple of decades, a personal resource-oriented approach to recovery in mental healthcare has gradually gained ground with the aim of empowering individuals to act and create a life worth living despite mental illness (Roberts & Wolfson, 2006).

Following Deegan (1997, 2003), who was diagnosed with schizophrenia during adolescence, it is possible for people to actively bring wellness into their lives, but a disease-oriented practice may hamper such a process. For example, Deegan (2003) was told by physicians that schizophrenia was chronic and non-responsive to treatment. This type of message, she argues, sentences patients to a life-long disease and leaves little hope for the future. Ralph and Corrigan (2005, Chap. 2) argue that hope is crucial to motivate personal recovery processes as a way of living, an attitude, and a way of approaching daily challenges. For a person in recovery, making life meaningful is a complex process that includes healing personally and socially by developing new ways of living, adopting new social roles, and rebuilding a life around changed priorities and a new sense of self (Jacobson, 2004). A person in recovery engages in self-discovery, self-renewal, and transformation (Ralph & Corrigan, 2005); being in recovery is a personal process that cannot be separated from life itself (Kleinman, 1988). This process involves learning and personal growth and lacks a definite endpoint; the subject is in constant change, with various transformations occurring over time.

## *Studies on personal recovery experiences*

Scientific studies on personal accounts of recovery see illness as a subjective experience of how disease and its consequences are perceived (Bury, 2005; Nettleton, 2006). According to Bury (2005), health is a taken-for-granted form of wellness, which, paradoxically, is first detected through its absence. When a person is incapacitated by illness or disability, they can experience alienation from their own body; be removed from social roles and obligations; or lose connections to family, colleagues, and friends (Lupton, 2012). Personal recovery implies a process of discovering how to bring wellness back into life – in terms of either overcoming illness or reclaiming wellness despite illness (Davidson, Drake, Schmutte, Dinzeo, & Andres-Hyman, 2009).

Kleinman (1988) has long urged that health professionals and researchers must address not only symptoms and diseases but also the meaning of illness and the practical problems illness creates in a person's life. Since the 1990s, inspired by theories from the social, cultural, and humanistic sciences based on interpretative logics, researchers have been increasingly interested in examining people's illness experiences and what they do to cope and self-manage. To explore recovery as a personal experience, based on qualitative empirical studies, we address the following themes: the meaning of wellness, developing self-knowledge, recovery as an ongoing process, and recovery identified in people's storytelling.

## *Wellness and meaning*

The meaning of wellness is seen in relation to the concept of illness and what illness entails. In accordance with Lupton (2012, Chap. 4), several studies describe falling ill as a process whereby people either suddenly or gradually perceive changes in an otherwise 'silent body' or disturbances in the taken-for-granted performance of daily activities. Thus, illness separates a person from his or her own body and also disrupts ordinary daily routines and social relationships and roles (Njølstad, Mengshoel, & Sveen, 2019). Changes in the social self (Charmaz, 1991) and disruption of a person's biography (Bury, 1982) can also occur, particularly in long-term illnesses. The future may become uncertain, and, according to Mattingly (2010, p. 161), a person may 'lack a hopeful picture of her future self'. In this way, illness disturbs a person's lifeworld (Kleinman, 1988).

Studies of personal recovery illuminate how people replace illness with wellness by accepting and adapting to their changed situation, adjusting their life situation, and adopting alternative social roles while still living a meaningful life (Kearney, 1999). For example, people with schizophrenia, an incurable mental illness from a disease perspective, may feel recovered when they have secured a safe, meaningful social life (Ralph & Corrigan, 2005). Alternatively, for women who had previously suffered from fibromyalgia (a contested, medically incurable musculoskeletal illness), recovery or wellness may mean being free from symptoms or having tolerable, manageable symptoms (Grape, Solbrække, Kirkevold, & Mengshoel, 2015). These two examples illuminate that wellness can imply living well despite being ill and struggling, as well as overcoming an illness and at the same time including new meaning for life.

Kleinman (1988) argues that it is important for people to make sense of their symptoms and suffering, as well as to figure out how to manage the implications of their illness. This means that a type of self-knowledge is considered crucial to recovery. Ill people want answers to many questions, such as, 'What is causing my illness?', 'What does the illness do to my body?', 'What can I expect from treatment?', 'What can I do to manage the illness, its exacerbations and consequences?', and 'What can be expected in the future?' (Kleinman, 1988, p. 43). Many people with chronic illnesses strive to make sense of their illness experiences (Aronowitz, 1998). For example, women who had recovered from fibromyalgia reported that they made sense of their experiences through a mundane, daily exploration of the relationship between their symptoms and their way of living (Grape, Solbrække, Kirkevold, & Mengshoel, 2017).

## *Developing personal expertise*

According to Kearney (1999), a recovery trajectory includes learning to endure the altered situation and grieving over experienced losses, accepting the situation as it presently is, creating hope for a better future, reckoning one's own resources, and the possibility of overcoming losses and making choices about how to adapt and adjust to a new situation. The process of learning how to come to terms with an illness is not linear, and it includes possible setbacks. However, relapses are not necessarily considered a failure but rather events from which a person can learn. Personal knowledge and engagement also include the capacity to build relationships with other people and take part in meaningful activities that create a feeling of connectedness and social belonging (Halding, Wahl, & Heggdal, 2010) that may lead to new, valued social identities (Lau & van Niekerk, 2011). Thus, the personal recovery process includes expanding competence by developing practical skills; adjusting activities, identities, and social roles; and creating new meaning and purpose in life.

People with chronic illnesses are often engaged in an ongoing recovery process to maintain what they have achieved and continue to adjust and adapt to their illness, which can fluctuate or progress. Arthritis, for example, often has a fluctuating course, and for people with arthritis, this means that in addition to reclaiming a life despite illness, they have to act to prevent exacerbations (Tollefsrud & Mengshoel, 2019). A person diagnosed with ankylosing spondylitis portrayed this through the following allegory: Life with arthritis is like living in a spider's web; it is impossible to escape, but there are still many roads to follow to live well. But if strings in the web break, they have to be knit together, and this limits the space (Mengshoel, 2008).

The fluctuations of experiences illustrate that illness and wellness are coexisting rather than dichotomous phenomena, shifting positions between the fore- and background (Paterson et al., 2003). Hope serves as fuel for not giving up, motivating the ongoing recovery process and taking action, and the hope is nurtured by success and belief in further progress (Mengshoel, Bjorbaekmo, Sallinen, & Wahl, 2019). Accordingly, hope is not merely a feeling but an incorporated part of a recovery practice (Mattingly, 2010).

## *Noticing a personal recovery process*

A person's recovery process is an integrated part of their daily life and can be identified in personal stories. Mattingly (1998) and Garro and Mattingly (2000) argues that ill persons' recovery narratives include moments that make a difference, turning points that display a break-through where new insight and activities make new recovery routes possible. Such narratives may portray a shift from withdrawal to active engagement; from loneliness to reconnection with others; from passive adaptation to active coping; from low self-esteem to a positive sense of self; or from alienation to a sense of meaning, purpose, and belonging, as well as the awakening of hope.

Recovering is mirrored by moments or events but can also become evident through the storyline in a person's narrative (Squire et al., 2014). Storylines can be interpreted according to the narrative typologies developed by Frank (1995). A restitution narrative describes falling ill, getting a diagnosis, receiving appropriate treatment, and being cured. In contrast, a chaos narrative is an illness storyline that portrays a lack of understanding of what is happening in which everyday life is chaotic and there is no obvious prospect for the future. Such stories are often fragmented, broken, hesitant, and difficult to listen to and understand (Bülow, 2008). A quest storyline, Frank claims, captures a personal recovery process in which a person trusts their own experiences, arrives at new insights and moments that affect the situation positively, and expresses hope for an optimistic future. Frank's typology thus shows that storylines, like the personal recovery process, display complex interactions between impairment, illness, experience, contexts, and culture.

## Co-production of recovery

### *Standardization and differentiation in clinical practice*

Nowotny, Scott, and Gibbons (2001) characterize knowledge production based on a 'cool' rational logic which is technically rather than culturally determined. This corresponds to knowledge production in a disease-oriented recovery outcome perspective that aims to *explain reality*, and it is essential to operationalize and classify deviances, 'normalize' them through treatment, and evaluate whether treatment produced successful outcomes. This orthodoxy is seen in clinical practices following classification schemes, standardized tools, and treatments. Thus, clinical practice is determined by what Rose (2006) calls political technologies, in forms of protocols, EBP guidelines, and standardized reporting tools, which separate professionals and ill persons from their treatment and healing practices.

Ill persons criticize disease- and deficit-oriented practice for depersonalizing them by reducing them to a disease or failure (Deegan, 2003) or reducing their illness experiences into scores on questionnaires (Gibson et al., 2019). Physiotherapists can devalue a person's illness experiences by asking closed, factual questions when taking patient histories (Ahlsen et al., 2019) or by stereotyping the delivery of physiotherapy according to 'cookbook recipes' (Mengshoel et al., 2019). Studies show that ill persons wish to be at the centre of physiotherapists' concern, preferring the latter to shift their focus away from techniques to providing information they find meaningful (Wijma et al., 2017). To reduce depersonalization in clinical practice, policy documents, as well as users of health services and health professionals, have spoken of person-centred practice that is characterized by clinicians' valuing the autonomy of ill persons and treating people in a respectful way, as well as meeting individuals' particular needs (Gluyas, 2015; Sacristan, 2013). We argue that human rights-based, person-centred practice demands a non-standardized, differentiated clinical approach that has the potential to enhance more than human rights by backing a person's healing practice. However, attending to individuals' needs, personal experiences, and wishes is not straightforward, and complex negotiations between the persons involved and what is possible in a particular context may take place (Gibson et al., 2019). We will, however, argue that knowledge production of personal and sociocultural issues, aligning with a personal experiential recovery process, is helpful for *understanding* what is at stake for an ill person.

Disease-oriented recovery practice is concerned with the effectiveness of a treatment to 'repair' disease-related deviances or deficits. Patients are victimized by injury or disease, and physiotherapists have been trained to act on disease- or injury-induced changes and are responsible for providing the best available treatment. For example, in cases of ankle sprain, physiotherapists follow a certain procedure in the acute phase, cooling down the bleeding tissues, elevating the leg to reduce oedema, and afterwards gradually introducing specific exercises to restore range of motion and muscle control with the goal of re-establishing former functioning. This type of storyline corresponds well with Frank's (1995) restitution narrative typology and a traditional disease-oriented recovery orthodoxy. Likewise, in lung physiotherapy, procedures are followed to remove mucus from the lungs to improve lung malfunctioning, and both the ill person and the physiotherapist notice an immediate improvement in respiration if the treatment works. These examples illustrate how physiotherapists act on knowledge about the body's biological mechanisms and follow a standardized, 'one-size-fits-all' physiotherapy procedure. Thus, in these examples, a view of recovery focusing on objective and predictable knowledge is applicable.

Contemporary societies worldwide face great concerns and costs related to chronic diseases, illnesses, and disabilities without any known curative or restorative treatment. In such cases, recovery cannot be limited to disease parts and specific functional impairments but should involve the whole person and her or his life project (Cassel, 2004). A personal recovery process differs from protocol-based, 'one-size-fits-all' education defined by professionals teaching ill people how to 'live with their illness', for example, in the form of self-management, lifestyle, or standardized conditioning training programmes. Living with a chronic condition is more complex and intruding than fixed by practising defined techniques, as being ill is fundamentally a social state of affairs. An individualized and differentiated clinical approach is needed, tailored to each person's strengths and opportunities to find a way to come to terms with illness and remake a meaningful life. Such practice calls for information from a scientific knowledge production that is particular, contextual, and situational (Nowotny et al., 2003) and aligned to an interpretive epistemology. Following one of Nicholls' (2018) positions for future education in physiotherapy, we argue for a critical integration of biomedical, psychological, sociocultural, lay, and political knowledge in the curricula of health professions.

Nicholls and Gibson (2010) have argued that an expanded understanding of the body beyond biological deficits is needed. The personal experiential recovery process includes reconnecting with the alienated body. Lupton (2012, Chap. 2) describes the body along two dimensions, as a body-organ object (aligning with disease-oriented recovery) and as a body-self subject (relevant to personal experiential recovery). Accordingly, a body constitutes a duality of being and having

(Crossley, 2006). The mind-body dualism can be overridden through understanding the body as a site of disease, embodied life experiences, and a sense of social self (Lupton, 2012). By discovering the relationship between movements, activities, and daily life, it is possible to make sense of own experiences and reconnect with one's own body and life, as well as to draw new road maps, both for a person's life and for a physiotherapist's understanding. During such an adventurous, often laborious, journey towards a life worth living, a physiotherapist may inhabit the role of co-adventurer and supporter.

In sum, we will argue that disease-oriented and experiential recovery operate in conjunction with each other; the disease-oriented recovery perspective will be privileged for acute or short-term conditions with specific, well-defined problems, where standardized treatment protocols are more likely to work. In contrast, with respect to incurable, long-term conditions that people live with, the personal experiential recovery process will probably take precedence and offer a differentiated treatment approach to meet the complexity of healing a person's suffering or recovery as co-production. Further, supporting a personal experiential recovery process is promoted in the recommended policies of person-centredness, user involvement, self-care, and self-management. However, we worry that the personalization may be veiled by new upcoming technologies aimed to secure human rights through a homogeneous, standardized practice.

## *Predictability and uncertainty in clinical practice*

In the final section, we will explore the interaction of the different understandings of recovery and their positions within evidence-based practice, first in relation to the hierarchical ordering of evidence and then in relation to the logic underpinning EBP.

Originally, the purpose of EBP was to fill a gap between research and clinical practice, thereby reducing clinical malpractice. Today, a kind of 'industry' has been established in order to synthesize randomized controlled trial (RCT) studies to conclude which treatments are on average the most effective (Greenhalgh, 2014). This research has been translated into evidence-based clinical guidelines by expert panels, and based on meta-analysis of effect studies, explicit statements are provided to assist practitioners and patients in making decisions about treatment (Scalzitti, 2001; Feiring & Bonfils, 2019). We argue that results from meta-analysis cannot dictate to professionals what to do in particular cases, but meta-analysis informs clinicians about what the research has to say about effects of interventions.

Research evidence is *hierarchically ordered* according to its design, with the meta-analysis of RCTs at the top; this research aims for unbiased measured effects of standardized treatment by controlling for the influences from persons and context to arrive at generalizable results. The hierarchical order of evidence places knowledge production of particular, contextual, and situational experiences at the bottom of the hierarchy, and sometimes they are excluded entirely. Following our earlier argument that both disease-oriented and personal experiential recovery are likely to operate together, disease-oriented treatment may be more successful in clinical practice if a person finds a treatment meaningful. But according to our argument that standardized treatment is not likely to address the complexity of chronic or long-term conditions, we question whether RCTs can actually tell which treatment is the best. Thus, treatment solutions cannot merely be tied to evidence from RCTs but must be related to a bricolage of various types of knowledge (Shaw & DeForge, 2012).

We argue that disease-oriented recovery practice has a hegemonic position in our society, including in physiotherapy. For example, physiotherapists in clinical practice may ask for appropriate 'tools' developed for research purposes to structure their practice of taking patient histories and for evaluating the outcomes of their practice. As we see it, this is a way to position and legitimize physiotherapy practice within a hegemonic knowledge system in our society. The standardization of practice follows the rational logic illuminating an ordered form of practice that produces predictable results. However, clinical practices are highly social and better understood by interpretative logic. Since clinical practice embraces relationships between people and particularities embedded in clinical meetings, as well as institutional and political contexts (recovery as co-production), practice is social, unstable, and uncertain and may disrupt the stability and predictability of rational logic. Ignoring this may downplay the uniqueness embedded in clinical practice, for example, the healing roles of therapeutic alliances and personal communication, as shown by Hall, Ferreira, Maher, Latimer, and Ferreira (2010).

Paradoxically, placebo studies within a disease-oriented paradigm have shown that disease measures are influenced by a person's thoughts, attitudes, beliefs, expectations, and social relationships (Mestre & Lang, 2017) and thus that the healing power of people's experiences and relationships cannot be ignored. Brun-Cottan, McMillian, and Hastings (2018) argue that some essential components of physiotherapy practice remain a personal tacit 'art'. This artistry should be given a language and incorporated into the body of physiotherapy knowledge. In sum, we argue that treating people in a clinical practice context is an experiential, political, complex, uncertain, and often diffuse endeavour of co-production. It is certainly understandable that people are searching for concretization and predictability. However, in so doing, tensions and ambiguities are likely to occur and need to be understood and managed to create person-centred clinical practice.

## Concluding remarks

In this chapter, we first outlined how two ideal-typical understandings of recovery – recovery as outcome and recovery as experience – have merged into a third type, namely recovery as co-production, promoting both person-centred and evidence-based practice. Disease-oriented recovery builds on a rational, explanatory logic wherein classifications, standardizations, EBP, and 'repairing' disease-related deficits are essential, and recovery outcomes provide measured evidence of effective treatment. On the other hand, a personal recovery process is based on meaning, embracing complexity, diversity, individuality, and humanism, and recovery is seen as a personal healing process relying on an interpretative logic to understand phenomena. Today these two understandings of recovery operate in conjunction, but orthodox physiotherapy approaches have primarily focused on the former, while the latter, heterodox practices seem to be regarded as a kind of personal, tacit knowledge of the 'art' of physiotherapy. We have outlined how health professions, exemplified by physiotherapy, produce different types of knowledge, and we call for a critically reflected integration of the disease-oriented approaches to recovery with the personal, social, and cultural approaches to recovery. We argue that person-centredness and evidence-based practices draw on different understandings of the term 'recovery'. We call for a critical rethink of recovery in clinical practice, educational curricula, and political documents, which we have called co-production of recovery.

## References

Ahlsen, B., Engebretsen, E., Nicholls, D., & Mengshoel, A. M. (2019). The singular patient in patient-centred care: Physiotherapists' accounts of treatment of patients with chronic muscle pain. *Medical Humanities*. doi:10.1136/medhum-2018-011603

Aronowitz, R. A. (1998). *Making sense of illness: Science, society, and disease*. Cambridge: Cambridge University Press.

Boorse, C. (1977). Health as a theoretical concept. *Philosophy of Science*, *44*, 542–573.

Brun-Cottan, N., McMillian, D., & Hastings, J. (2018). Defending the art of physical therapy: Expanding inquiry and crafting culture in support of therapeutic alliance. *Physiotherapy Theory and Practice*, *1*. doi:10.1080/09593985.2018.1492656

Bülow, P. (2008). "You have to ask a little": Troublesome storytelling about contested illness. In L.-C. Hydén & J. Brockmeier (Eds.), *Health, illness and culture: Broken narratives* (pp. 131–153). New York: Routledge.

Bury, M. (1982). Chronic illness as biographical disruption. *Sociology of Health and Illness*, *4*(2), 167–182.

Bury, M. (2005). *Health and illness* (1st ed.). Cambridge: Polity Press.

Cassell, E. J. (2004). *The nature of suffering* (2nd ed.). New York: Oxford University Press.

Charmaz, K. (1991). *Good days, bad days: The self in chronic illness and time*. New Brunswick, NJ: Rutgers University Press.

Crossley, N. (2006). *Reflexive embodiment in contemporary society*. Maidenhead: Open University Press.

Davidson, L., Drake, R. E., Schmutte, T., Dinzeo, T., & Andres-Hyman, R. (2009). Oil and water or oil and vinegar? Evidence-based medicine meets recovery. *Community Mental Health Journal*, *45*(5), 323–332.

Deegan, P. (1997). Recovery as a journey of the heart. In L. Spaniol, C. Gagne, & M. Koehler (Eds.), *Psychological and social aspects of psychiatric disability* (pp. 74–83). Boston: Boston University.

Deegan, P. (2003). Recovering our sense of value after being labeled. In L. Spaniol, C. Gagne, & M. Koehler (Eds.), *Psychological and social aspects of psychiatric disability* (pp. 370–376). Boston: Boston University.

Engel, G. L. (1977). The need for a new medical model: A challenge for biomedicine. *Science*, *196*, 129–136.

Eriksen, T. E., & Risør, M. B. (2014). What is called symptom? *Medicine, Health Care & Philosophy*, *17*(1), 89–102.

Feiring, M. (2013). Politicisation of self-help in Norway. In L. Nicolaou-Smokoviti, H. Sünker, J. Rozanova, & V. Pekka Economou (Eds.), *Citizenship and social development: Citizen participation and community involvement in social welfare and social policy* (pp. 207–220). Frankfurt am Main: Peter Lang Publishing Group.

Feiring, M., & Bonfils, I. S. (2019). The redesigning of neurorehabilitation in Denmark and Norway. In I. Harsløf, I. Poulsen, & K. Larsen (Eds.), *New dynamics of disability and rehabilitation: Interdisciplinary perspectives*. Chapter 5. Singapore: Palgrave Macmillan.

Frank, A. F. (1995). *The wounded storyteller: Body, illness, and ethics*. Chicago: The University Press of Chicago Press.

Garro, L. C., & Mattingly, C. (2000). *Narrative and the cultural construction of illness and healing*. Berkeley, CA: University of California Press.

Gibson, B. E. (2016). *Rehabilitation: A post-critical approach*. Boca Raton, FL: CRC Press, an imprint of the Taylor & Francis Group.

Gibson, B. E., Terry, G., Setchell, J., Bright, F. A. S., Cummins, C., & Kayes, N. M. (2019). The micro-politics of caring: Tinkering with person-centered rehabilitation. *Disability and Rehabilitation*, 1–10. doi:10.1080/09638288.2019.1587793

Gluyas, H. (2015). Patient-centred care: Improving healthcare outcomes. *Nursing Standard*, *30*(4), 50–57.

Grape, H. E., Solbrække, K. N., Kirkevold, M., & Mengshoel, A. M. (2015). Staying healthy from fibromyalgia is ongoing hard work. *Qualitative Health Research*, *25*(5), 679–688.

Grape, H. E., Solbrække, K. N., Kirkevold, M., & Mengshoel, A. M. (2017). Tiredness and fatigue during processes of illness and recovery: A qualitative study of women recovered from fibromyalgia syndrome. *Physiotherapy Theory and Practice*, *33*(1), 31–40.

Greenhalgh, T. (2014). Evidence based medicine: A movement in crisis? *British Medical Journal*, *348*.

Halding, A. G., Wahl, A., & Heggdal, K. (2010). "Belonging": Patients' experiences of social relationships during pulmonary rehabilitation. *Disability and Rehabilitation*, *32*(15), 1272–1280.

Hall, A. M., Ferreira, P. H., Maher, C. G., Latimer, J., & Ferreira, M. L. (2010). The influence of the therapist-patient relationship on treatment outcome in physical rehabilitation: A systematic review. *Physical Therapy*, *90*(8), 1099–1110.

Hammell, K. W. (2006). *Perspectives on disability and rehabilitation: Contesting assumptions: Challenging practice*. Edinburgh: Churchill Livingstone and Elsevier.

Haugen, K. H. (1997). *En utdanning i bevegelse – 100 år med fysioterapiutdanning i Norge* (An education in motion: 100 years of physiotherapy education in Norway). Oslo, NO: Universitetsforlaget.

Herbert, R., Jamtvedt, G., Mead, J., & Hagen, K. B. (2005). *Practical evidence-based physiotherapy*. Edinburgh: Elsevier.

Hofmann, B. (2001). Complexity of the concept of disease as shown through theoretical frameworks. *Theoretical Medicine*, *22*, 211–236.

Jacobson, N. (2004). *In recovery: The making of mental health policy*. Nashville, Tenn, and London, UK: Vanderbilt University Press.

Jasanoff, S. (2004). *States of knowledge: The co-production of science and social order*. London, UK: Routledge.

Johannisson, K. (2004). *Tecknen: Läkaren och konsten att läsa kroppar* (Signs: The physician and the art of interpreting bodies). Stockholm: Norstedt.

Jutel, A. (2011). *Putting a name to it: Diagnosis in contemporary society*. Baltimore: John Hopkins University Press.

Kaltenborn, F. (2003). *Manual mobilization of the joints: The Kaltenborn method of joint examination and treatment: The spine* (4th ed., Vol. 2). Oslo, NO: Nordli.

Kearney, M. H. (1999). *Understanding women's recovery from illness and trauma*. Thousand Oaks, CA: Sage Publications.

Kendall, F. P. (1983). *Muscles: Testing and function* (3rd ed.). Baltimore: Williams & Wilkins.

Kleinman, A. (1988). *The illness narratives*. Cambridge, Massachusetts: Basic Book.

Larson, J. S. (1996). The World Health Organization's definition of health: Social versus spiritual health. *Social Indicators Research, 38*(2), 181–192.

Lau, U., & van Niekerk, A. (2011). Restorying the self: An exploration of young burn survivors' narratives of resilience. *Qualitative Health Research, 21*(9), 1165–1181.

Leplège, A., Barral, C., & McPherson, K. (2015). *Conceptualising disability to inform rehabilitation: Historical and epistemological perspectives*. In K. McPherson, B. E. Gibson, & A. Leplège (Eds.), *Rethinking rehabilitation: Theory and practice*. Chapter 2. Boca Raton, FL: CRC Press.

Lian, O. S. (2007). *Når helse blir en vare: Medikalisering og markedsorientering i helsetjenesten* (When health becomes a commodity: Medicalization and market orientation in health services) (2nd ed.). Kristiansand: Høyskoleforlaget.

Lupton, D. (2012). *Medicine as culture: Illness, disease and the body* (3rd ed.). London, UK: Sage Publications.

Mattingly, C. (1998). *Healing dramas and clinical plots: The narrative structure of experience*. Cambridge: Cambridge University Press.

Mattingly, C. (2010). *The paradox of hope: Journeys through a clinical borderland*. Berkeley: University of California Press.

Mengshoel, A. (2008). Living with a fluctuating illness of ankylosing spondylitis: A qualitative study. *Arthritis Rheumatism* (Arthritis Care and Research), *59*(10), 1439–1444.

Mengshoel, A. M., Bjorbaekmo, W. S., Sallinen, M., & Wahl, A. K. (2019). "It takes time, but recovering makes it worthwhile": A qualitative study of long-term users' experiences of physiotherapy in primary health care. *Physiotherapy Theory and Practice*, 1–11. doi: 10.1080/09593985.2019.1616343

Mestre, T., & Lang, A. (2017). Placebos in clinical trials: Unravelling a complex phenomenon. *The Lancet Neurology, 16*(1), 28–29.

Nettleton, S. (2006). *The sociology of health and illness* (2nd ed.). Malden: Policy Press.

Nicholls, D. A. (2018). *The end of physiotherapy*. Abingdon, UK: Routledge.

Nicholls, D. A., & Gibson, B. E. (2010). The body and physiotherapy. *Physiotherapy Theory and Practice, 26*(8), 497–509.

Njølstad, B. W., Mengshoel, A. M., & Sveen, U. (2019). "It's like being a slave to your own body in a way": A qualitative study of adolescents with chronic fatigue syndrome. *Scandinavian Journal of Occupational Therapy, 26*(7), 505–514.

Nowotny, H., Scott, P., & Gibbons, M. (2001). *Re-thinking science: Knowledge and the public in an age of uncertainty*. Cambridge: Polity Press.

Nowotny, H., Scott, P., & Gibbons, M. (2003). Introduction: "Mode 2" revisited: The new production of knowledge. *A Review of Science, Learning and Policy, 41*(3), 179–194.

Oliver, M. (1990). *The politics of disablement*. Basingstoke, UK: Palgrave Macmillan.

Paterson, B. L. (2003). The koala has claws: Applications of the shifting perspectives model in research of chronic illness. *Qualitative Health Research, 13*(7), 987–994.

Ralph, R. O., & Corrigan, P. W. (2005). *Recovery in mental illness: Broadening our understanding of wellness*. Washington, DC: American Psychological Association.

Roberts, G., & Boardman, J. (2013). Understanding recovery. *Advances in Psychiatric Treatment, 19*(6), 400–409.

Roberts, G., & Wolfson, P. (2006). New directions in rehabilitation: Learning from the recovery movement. In G. Roberts, M. Davenport, F. Holloway, & T. Tattan (Eds.), *Enabling recovery: The principles and practice of rehabilitation psychiatry* (1st ed., pp. 18–37). Trowbridge: Gaskell.

Rose, N. (2006). Governing "advanced" liberal democracies. In A. Sharma & A. Gupta (Eds.), *The anthropology of the state: A reader* (p. 19). Malden, MA: Blackwell.

Rose, S. J. (1988). Description and classification: The cornerstone of pathokinesiological research. *Physical Therapy, 66*(3), 379–386.

Rose, S. J. (1989). Physical therapy diagnosis: Role and function. *Physical Therapy, 69*(7), 535–537.

Sacristan, J. A. (2013). Patient-centred medicine and patient-oriented research: Improving health outcomes for individual patients. *BMC Medical Informatics and Decision Making, 13*, 6.

Sahrman, S. A. (1988). Diagnosis by the physical therapist: A prerequisite for treatment: A special communication. *Physical Therapy, 68*, 1703–1706.

Scalzitti, D. A. (2001). Evidence-based guidelines: Application to clinical practice. *Physical Therapy, 81*(10), 1622–1628.

Shaw, A., & DeForge, R. T. (2012). Physiotherapy as bricolage: Theoretizing expert practice. *Physiotherapy Theory and Practice, 28*(6), 420–427.

Squire, C., Davis, M., Esin, C., Andrews, M., Harrison, B., Hydén, L.-C., & Hydén, M. (2014). *What is narrative research?* London, UK: Bloomsbury Academic.

Stevens, A., Beurskens, A., & Köke, A. (2013). The use of patient-specific measurement instruments in the process of goal-setting: A systematic review of available instruments and their feasibility. *Clinical Rehabilitation, 27*(11), 1005–1019.

Stratford, P. W., Gill, C., Westaway, M., & Binkley, J. M. (1995). Assessing disability and change on individual patients: A report of a patient-specific measure. *Physiotherapy Canada, 47*, 258–263.

Tollefsrud, I., & Mengshoel, A. M. (2019). A fragile normality – illness experiences of working-age individuals with osteoarthritis in knees or hips. *Disability and Rehabilitation*, 1–7. doi:10.1080/09638288.2019.1573930

White, P. (2005). *Biopsychosocial medicine: An integrated approach to understanding illness*. Oxford: Oxford University Press.

Wijma, A. J., Bletterman, A. N., Clark, J. R., Vervoort, S., Beetsma, A., Keizer, D., & Van Wilgen, C. P. (2017). Patient-centeredness in physiotherapy: What does it entail? A systematic review of qualitative studies. *Physiotherapy Theory and Practice, 33*(11), 825–840.

World Health Organization. (1980). *International classification of impairments, disabilities, and handicaps*. Geneva: World Health Organization.

World Health Organization. (2001). *The international classification of functioning, disability and health (ICF)*. Geneva: World Health Organization.

# 6 Physiotherapy for children and the construction of the disabled child

*Kate Waterworth, David A. Nicholls, Lisette Burrows, and Michael Gaffney*

**Introduction**

Discourses of normal child development are commonplace in Eurocentric societies (Smith, 2013). Parents might be asked if their children are walking yet or if they sleep through the night, whether their social interactions are age appropriate or whether their play is at all delayed. Early intervention is available to support children to reach their potential and to address the 'risk' of disability. It is suggested that children can 'catch up'. These practices indicate that a key function of childhood is achieving productive adulthood and that childhood lacks meaning in its own right (Goodley & Roets, 2008). The dominance of this position is problematic for all children, but particularly for those who do not fit normative notions of what a child should be. Disabled children are constructed as such by powerful social, cultural, and discursive practices (Goodley & Runswick-Cole, 2016; Shildrick, 2001). Disabled children are therefore seen as not measuring up: as distinct from normal, as 'other'. This situation has implications for them across their lifespan and dramatically affects the opportunities and constraints available to them.

Discourses are more than mere narratives; rather, they shape and create their subjects (Tremain, 2001). For children who are 'othered', this has significant implications (Campbell, 2009). It is therefore important to explore our notions of childhood and disability, as these have consequences for our rehabilitation practices. This may allow us to bring a more conscious and critical gaze to physiotherapy practices and their unforeseen impacts.

The authors of this chapter bring a range of different perspectives to this question. Kate is a lecturer and researcher currently using Deleuzian approaches to experiment with understandings of disability. Dave is a researcher and writer specialising in critical histories of physiotherapy. Lisette writes and researches in health and physical education from a poststructuralist perspective, and Michael works in early childhood initial teacher education, drawing on sociocultural approaches to understand inclusion and children's rights. Between us, we bring four different lenses to the question of how the disabled child has been constructed in Aotearoa New Zealand in recent years. This chapter derives from early exploratory work from Kate's PhD, along with collaborative conversations with Dave, Lisette, and Michael, Kate's supervisory team. In this piece, we draw on historical surveys and academic literature such as genealogies of childhood, disability, and rehabilitation. We have also used documentary footage and newspaper articles to problematise physiotherapy knowledges acting on disabled children in recent history.

A focus on children's futures (progress, outcomes, etc.), can lead us to take existing customs, knowledges, and practices for granted. Unpacking the history of our ideas can help us to see how and when the knowledges that physiotherapists hold close have arisen and open new avenues for critique (Foucault, 1980). This examination can be facilitated through partnerships with those from beyond the field as well as through philosophical provocations. In this piece, our thinking is aided by the posthumanisms, the new materialisms, and the writings of Foucault, as well as Deleuze and Guattari. These perspectives allow critical and creative analyses and responses to complex issues.

## Tracing the concepts 'child', 'childhood', and 'disability'

Like many other categories taken for granted today, those of disability and the child/childhood emerged in particular social, historical, and cultural contexts (Burman, 2017; Tesar, Rodriguez, & Kupferman, 2016). In this section, we draw out four discourses of childhood that frame physiotherapy practice today: the child coming into attention, the child requiring protection, the child as having potential, and the child as consumer-citizen.

### *The 'child' coming into attention*

Phillipe Ariès's work in the 1960s centred on the emergence of the idea of 'childhood' between the Middle Ages and the end of the 18th century. Ariès (1962, p. 128) suggested that:

> In medieval society the idea of childhood did not exist. This is not to suggest that children were neglected, forsaken or disposed. The idea of childhood is not to be confused with affection for children: it corresponds to an awareness of the particular nature of childhood, that particular nature which distinguishes the child from the adult, even the young adult. In medieval society this awareness was lacking.

Ariès (1962) suggested that children occupied a different phase of time to that of adults (one of growth and development) and that seeing childhood as a distinctive phase of a linear human 'life' was an idea produced by (and that was productive of) a raft of social, cultural, and intellectual changes brought about by the Enlightenment (Corsaro, 2015; James & Prout, 1997). Childhood became delimited from adulthood through interwoven conditions, including the measurement of time (and therefore age), shifts towards a more private nuclear family life, significant changes in infant mortality, and industrialisation (Qvortrup, Corsaro, & Honig, 2009).

72  Kate Waterworth et al.

The bracketing off of childhood from adulthood was underpinned by the first scientific consideration of the 'nature' of children and childhood (James & Prout, 1997; Valentine, 2009). From early 18th century in Europe and across English-speaking countries, children have been variously considered a blank slate (the tabula rasa), innocence personified (the romantic child), and inherently evil and requiring salvation (the evangelical child) (Hendrick, 2009). These understandings persist today, with children being seen in different circumstances as malleable (for example, brain science research around the first three years), as requiring protection (from risky play and social media), and as dangerous (as perpetrators of violence) (Mayall, 2002).

## *The child requiring protection*

Although throughout much of the Western pre- to early industrial periods (15th–18th centuries) children were seen as legitimate agents within the labour market, by the end of the 18th century, it became increasingly untenable for children to be considered this way (Mayall, 2002). The norm shifted from children acting as contributors to the family economy to being seen as requiring protection from exploitation, particularly in newly established factories. Social reformers called for conditions that promoted a 'civilised' and Christian childhood (Corsaro, 2015). In tandem, European state governments sought new means to cultivate appropriate attitudes to authority, with the conduct of mothers and children targeted for special attention. One mechanism to achieve this came with the creation of compulsory schooling (Deacon, 2006).

Formal education meant that children needed to be categorised as either educable or uneducable (Foucault, 1995), with those found to be incompetent, unteachable, disruptive, or otherwise incapable subject to a raft of new educational assessments. Formal education was, and continues to be, a vitally important tool in the construction of the disabled child.

In Australasia, Europe, and elsewhere, children deemed 'imbecile' were housed in asylums and other 'special education' facilities (Stace, 2014) and provided with extensive remedial therapies designed to ward off risks of delinquency, illegitimacy, and alcoholism (Stiker, 2000). Supposedly benevolent social attitudes towards 'retarded' children were also evident in the work of religious and charitable institutions, which began to offer care for 'deserving' orphans and children with conditions such as cerebral palsy in the late 1800s (Tennant, 1996). It is only more recently that this group of children were acknowledged as being entitled to schooling just the same as 'normal' children (Stace, 2014).

## *The child as having potential*

Children and childhood became the object of 'scientific' methods developed by newly formed child studies societies in the late 19th century (Burman, 2017). This novel system of thought placed particular value on objective measurement, categorisation, classification, and standardisation against the norm (Walkerdine,

1993). Science was harnessed to promote particular rationales of care and feeding, focusing in an increasingly granular fashion on mothers' practices, child health, and child mortality (May, 2013).

Accompanying the broader scientific attention on children came medical attention. Early hospitals for children admitted abandoned children in an effort to 'save' them from poverty and enhance their moral and spiritual character (Golden, 1989). New beliefs about the spread of disease, such as germ theory, propelled doctors to take up the work of treating illness and infection in hospitals that better concentrated their power than the earlier bedside medicine (Armstrong, 1995).

The field of developmental psychology also emerged alongside medicine. Darwin's theory of natural selection provided a 'template' against which Victorian societies mapped and measured children, and this attention led to the belief that children's development should follow specific ages and stages (Burman, 2017). In 1925, Arnold Gesell, one of the forebears of developmental psychology, suggested that infancy could be divided into a series of phases in which a child transitions to a more advanced level of cognition (Gesell, 1925). He emphasised that these phases could be used as a tool to identify normal children and those with mental deficiency. In New Zealand, 'backwards' children began to be identified through growth charts and documentation of milestones (May, 2013).

Alongside this focus on child health and development came attention to children's posture and movement – specifically through the application of military drill–style exercises. Armstrong (2002, p. 50) suggests the development of drill without weapons – or physical training, as it was to become known – established techniques of body management that could easily be transferred from military to civilian life. And what better place to start than the growing body of the child?

The demonstration of 'correct' posture and participation in physical exercise became linked to newly dominant values – such as discipline and attitude:

> A virtuous circle linking body, mind and exercise was established in the early decades of the twentieth century. The mind could be trained to manage the movement of the body while movement, in its turn, had positive effects on the mind. Exercises could inculcate habits while the discipline of movement could focus the mind on the task in hand, eliminating stray thoughts – perhaps of a sexual nature – and build up 'character'.
>
> (Armstrong, 2002, p. 55)

Managing the body became a means of managing health through exercise and physical education in schools. Health practitioners began to assess bodies and their potential for movement and search out any potentially detrimental postural defects (Armstrong, 2002). In doing so, they constructed what was to be considered normal, setting up a space for early practitioners of physiotherapy.

The polio epidemics of the mid-20th century encouraged authorities to invest in remedial therapies like physiotherapy and contributed enormously to the establishment of physiotherapy as a trusted ally of the state, especially in the United States and Scandinavia (Nicholls, 2017). The therapy – a system of round-the-clock wet hot packs used to manage the pain and paralysis – was followed by months of physical rehabilitation. It suggested that disabled children had the potential to respond to physical rehabilitation interventions.

This section has shown that it is only in recent history that children (including the disabled child) have been seen to have potential for change – that they are malleable. The following section demonstrates a further shift as human rights discourses began to be applied to understandings of children and disability.

### *The child as consumer-citizen*

Human rights frameworks are often described as outlining essential provisions and freedoms to prevent suffering and promote justice internationally (Brown, 2004). Alternatively, they have been considered a political tool to counter non-democratic (communist) states through defence of the West and its values of freedom and independence (Rasche, 2016). Human rights and their breaches were applied to the individual in the 1970s ('Amnesty International USA', n.d.). More recently, they have been considered an important tool by advocacy groups to demand participation, equity, and justice for 'oppressed' members of society. A rights-based discourse understands disabled children as individual citizens with rights, obligations, and a voice (Qvortrup et al., 2009).

Seeing children as citizens is complicated by a range of competing discourses, including those of capitalism, neoliberalism, and globalisation. Over the last half century, neoliberalism has essentially liberated capitalism from the tempering influence of welfarism through the mechanism of the global 'free market' (Brown, 2004). Today, post-industrial Western capitalism privileges individuals as units of production. Individuals are expected to aspire to be their best self, to work hard, and not to be a burden (Brown, 2015). The intersection of neoliberal globalised capitalism with that of a human rights approach has helped to promote the idea of the child as 'consumer-citizen'. Within this ideology, all children should aspire to be productive, not burdensome; be an independent individual; and be self motivated and competitive, as well as desiring progress and success. In this context, the disabled child not only has potential but is obliged to meet their (economic) potential through active participation in rehabilitation (Sales, 2012).

In this section, we have outlined shifts that have produced varied understandings of the normal child in relation to a number of social, cultural, and historical conditions. We will now go on to look more closely at relationships between physiotherapy and the disabled child.

## Physiotherapy knowledges and the construction of the 'disabled child'

We suggest that physiotherapists rely heavily on two discourses: the disabled child as having 'potential' and the disabled child as not normal. The discourses are problematic, not least because they are relatively uncontested in physiotherapy (Gibson, 2016). In addition, they create a particular social identity for disabled children – that of the 'other' (Shildrick, 2001; Tremain, 2001). Being 'othered' has implications for children's access to the cultural capital that comes with power and control, and this affects children's future status and social positioning, their subjectification in professional practices, and their own sense of being and existence. Being seen as abnormal may be related to disabled children's experiences of discrimination, violence, neglect, and other processes of social exclusion (Campbell, 2009). Remedial interventions may actually *promote* the view that disabled children are not whole or of value as they are. This section closely examines the particular knowledges which are privileged in physiotherapy, which emphasise the construction of 'disability' and in doing so act to 'other' people categorised as such.

Physiotherapy has aligned itself with high-status professions such as medicine to bolster its professional standing (Nicholls, 2017). These disciplines embody the biomedical worldview which prioritises a certain epistemology (in which knowledge is singular, fixed, and discoverable) and a set of values (such as the quest for progress and improvement) (Foucault, 2002). Biomedicine has been credited with much success in terms of population and individual health. If we look closely at dominant physiotherapy knowledges, we can clearly see the influence of biomedicine (Palisano, Orlin, & Schreiber, 2017; Nicholls, 2017).

We referred earlier to how US physiotherapists provided treatment to children affected by the polio epidemic and, in doing so, began to carve out a space for themselves to be recognised as health professionals. In New Zealand, understanding of disabled children as having potential became apparent in the 1930s, driven in part by a shift in the attitudes of health professionals. An orthopaedic surgeon, Dr Alexander Gilles, advocated to the Rotary club for the establishment of the Crippled Children Society (Schorer, 2012). Physiotherapists used hydrotherapy, physical exercise, stretches, and specialised equipment to work with children with physical impairments. A specialised 'garden hospital' facility for children was gifted by the Wilson family, to be controlled by the Auckland Hospital Board in 1937 (Jones, 2012). This was intended for the convalescence of children with polio. Children were resident in the facility for long periods and treated by nursing staff with fresh air and a 'home-like' environment. In the 1950s, the Queen Elizabeth Hospital in Rotorua adapted its facilities to make them suitable for 'cerebral palsied' patients (Visiting Cerebral Palsy Therapists Review Committee, 1984). Children were admitted as inpatients for 'training' to 'meet their potential' (Chilton, 1956).

These developments demonstrate the newfound position that disabled children could be rehabilitated: that they had potential. This perspective was informed by a series of knowledges that emerging physiotherapy practitioners applied in this context. In doing so, these physiotherapists reinforced themselves as healthcare professionals with a distinctive scope, role, and identity. Alongside this, they contributed to the construction of disability that has since permeated social narratives on disability – as warranting intervention to reach potential (as defined by the norm standard). These knowledges included, amongst other things, scientific knowledge around 'normal' development and the body as a machine, the view of people as independent individuals, and the processes derived from scientific methods such as detailed assessment and surveillance and the keeping of records.

Early physiotherapists relied on particular understandings of 'normal development' (Chilton, 1956; Gibson, Teachman, & Hamdani, 2015). Physiotherapists typically understood this as occurring at particular ages and stages, with a linear trajectory towards competent adulthood being 'normal'. Abnormal development demanded further assessment and intervention. Early New Zealand documentary footage demonstrates developmental assessment processes and the resultant institutionalisation of some children (Chilton, 1964). Although these residential institutions have been disestablished, 'knowledges' around normal child development continue to influence service provision criteria (Whanganui District Health Board, n.d.) Ideas on normal development may promote the position that a child can be separated into different domains of function for observation and surveillance and that there are normative standards for gross motor function and cognitive function. These 'functions' are understood to be universal, occurring across cultures, locations, and time periods. Physiotherapists, alongside other professional groups, may continue to lean heavily on these scales in their assessments and understandings of disability (Gibson et al., 2015).

Physiotherapy knowledge has also often assumed the body to be a 'machine' (Nicholls, 2017). The body is something that can be treated and trained in order to 'fix' it or make it work more effectively and efficiently. In New Zealand in the 1960s, some children were offered intensive long-term inpatient intervention in order to promote the development of their cognitive, communicative, and motor function (Chilton, 1964). Service provision has shifted significantly but maintains the position that disabled children can and should be treated with complex rehabilitation procedures such as body weight support treadmill training, the use of ankle-foot orthoses, and functional electrical stimulation in specialist facilities (Palisano et al., 2017). Training is designed and delivered by highly specialised experts, each responsible for a particular function. We now find physiotherapists specialising not just in paediatrics, but in increasingly refined subspecialties like paediatric respiratory, paediatric neurology, and community paediatrics.

Disabled children have often been understood to be individuals in physiotherapy practices. Children are seen not as a valued part of a collective (for example, the family) but as an isolated independent entity. An early documentary demonstrates the arrival of a young boy at the newly inaugurated Child Potential Unit from his rural home (Chilton, 1956). He was delivered into the care of the matron and other nursing and rehabilitation staff (for a stay of several years), and they bade farewell to his family. He was seen as independent from his family, an individual who needed treatment to meet his own potential. It could be said that physiotherapy practice has made attempts to shift this position through the concept of family-centred care and its associated practices (Litchfield & MacDougall, 2002). However, assessment and intervention typically remain focused on the individual child, and goals focus on personal function and participation. Limited attention is paid towards addressing broader social or community issues around equity, racism, or access (Cleaver, Deslauriers, & Hudon, 2018).

The scientific method can also be seen in physiotherapy practice with disabled children. A documentary on the 'Child Potential Unit' shows a child being 'measured' (for head circumference) and 'catalogued' (Chilton, 1956). Although this particular equipment may have been superseded, the processes of observation, measurement, analysis, and recording are still highly valued in today's environment of 'evidence-based practice' (Bjorbækmo & Engelsrud, 2011; Palisano et al., 2017). We can see significant attention to the measurement and recording of details in filing systems and clinical notes regarding body structure and function, with special attention often given to upright, bipedal walking. Walking is prioritised over other forms of ambulation and mobility, such as wheelchair usage or 'bunny hopping'. Functions and structures are given scientific terms like 'gait' and 'ambulation' and removed from everyday life or experience, with assessments often occurring in clinical settings detached from the child's natural surroundings (Palisano et al., 2017). Data is typically analysed with reference to other normative parameters and categorised as normal or abnormal, for example, for gait speed and joint angles. Assessment can reoccur over time periods to enable surveillance over childhood and adolescence at review appointments.

This section has argued that physiotherapists have been heavily influenced by biomedicine and its association with child development. In their use of this set of knowledges and practices, physiotherapists have contributed to the construction of the disabled child as 'other'. Both biomedicine and physiotherapy are associated with humanism, the philosophical worldview associated with the enlightenment-era thinking that values rationality, progress, science, and liberty (or independence) (Braidotti, 2013). Humanism posits that the human is all important and that a particular type of the human is more important than 'lower' beings or things. This hierarchy is implicated in the creation of the norm–other binary and thus is influential (and problematic) in disability discourse (Goodley & Runswick-Cole, 2016).

We have argued that physiotherapy has a complex legacy. Drawing on this particular set of knowledges, values, and practices has contributed to the professional status of physiotherapists, to their position as expert and as professional, to the creation of a space to operate and some 'work to do'. It can be uncomfortable to consider one's occupation in this way, particularly if one strongly feels the desire to make a difference or to help or heal. However, this discomfort may be important if we are able to critique what physiotherapist knowledges and practices do. An orientation to the past may allow us to consider alternative readings of what has previously been taken for granted as 'knowledge', allowing us to explore other possibilities.

## Closing words: alternative constructions of the child, childhood, and normality/disability

Posthuman scholars have attempted to break the binary opposition between the normal child and the other. They hope to influence attitudes around normality and disability, around progress and potential, and therefore social (and rehabilitation) practices (see, for example, Gibson, 2006; Goodley & Runswick-Cole, 2016 or

Shildrick, 2001). Physiotherapists may benefit from engagement with this work. We may be able to imagine and therefore produce alternatives so as to support all children to be accepted, to be valued, to be included, and to thrive.

Posthumanism is considered an active attempt to move ethical and moral concerns beyond human interests. Braidotti (2013, p. 37) comments, 'posthumanism is the historical moment that . . . traces a different discursive framework, looking more affirmatively towards new alternatives'. A posthuman perspective provides a useful space to explore a new framework for understanding relationships between various types of existence. This may be useful when considering the difficulties that humanism has constructed in relationship to disability and childhood. Related to posthumanism, new materialism or neo-materialism has brought together a field of theorists that look to highlight the position of the material, the object, and the real. The work emerging in the field of new materialisms provides an opportunity to rethink disability with explicit attention to matter (Alldred & Fox, 2017).

The breadth of work that has been produced in this space has grown exponentially as academics seek to explore conundrums. Deconstructions inspired by Derrida and Foucault demonstrated the contingent and localised nature of development (Bloch & Popkewitz, 2000), education (Apple, 1995), early childhood education (Cannella, 1997), and even the child itself (Burman, 2017; Tesar, 2014). Others have sought to interrogate the relationship between 'agency and structure, nature and culture, being and becoming' (Prout, 2011). Taylor and Giugni (2012, p. 108) tried to conceptualise relationships in the 'common world' in which children and 'all others in their world, including more-than-human others' are included. Murris (2016, p. 185) argues for a conception of a posthuman child – as '*inhuman becoming iii*'. The work in this area is recent, evolving, and fluid – and is likely to remain contentious given its ontological and ethical positioning.

The field of disability studies has also been influenced by the provocations generated by the work of Foucault, Butler, Barad, and Braidotti. Mitchell and Snyder (2001) have problematised representations of disability in literature and related artefacts. Shildrick (2001) has generated attention with her conceptualisations of leaky bodies and of disability as monstrous and dangerous. Concepts such as the rhizome, interconnectivity, and deterritorialisation drawn from Deleuze and Guattari have also been put to work productively in this area (Alldred & Fox, 2017; Fox, 2002; Gibson, 2006; Gibson, Carnevale, & King, 2012; Goodley & Roets, 2008; Shildrick & Price, 2005; Vehmas & Watson, 2016). These authors have diverse foci that critique dominant notions of disability and make suggestions for creative alternatives, which may be of interest to physiotherapists.

A small group of scholars show particular interest in rethinking the manner in which disability, as it is applied to children, is understood. There have been calls for a distinctive field to emerge – that of disabled children's childhood studies (Curran & Runswick-Cole, 2014). Supporters draw on the work of Deleuze and others to untangle and interrupt typical understandings and ethical positionings of disabled children (Gibson et al., 2012). Goodley and Runswick-Cole (2016, p. 770) advocate for the 'disHuman child . . . a bifurcated complex that allows us to recognise their humanity whilst also celebrating the ways in which disabled children reframe what it means to be human'.

The work of Deleuze and Guattari (and of those they have inspired) appears to have much to offer (Braidotti, 2013; De Landa & Harman, 2017; Morton, 2017; St. Pierre, 2017). Thinking with their concepts can potentially disrupt dominant ideas and associated practices (such as normalisation) in the intersections of childhood studies and critical disability fields, allowing subversive and generative alternatives to be considered and enacted (Cowan, 2017; Fadyl, Teachman, & Hamdani, 2019; Feely, 2016; Gibson et al., 2012; Shildrick & Price, 2005).

The writing of these philosophers and researchers is challenging to read and often uncomfortable to consider – it does not allow the supposed safety nor security of easy answers, quick fixes, or foundational knowledge. However, engaging with philosophy and critical thinking may provoke new, diverse, and interesting constructions and knowledges regarding the child, childhood, and disability. This may provoke physiotherapists to explore questions such as:

- How might physiotherapy/my practices shift if there were no normal, no potential to achieve?
- How might physiotherapy/my practices shift if I understood all beings, including objects and states of being, as ontologically equal and connected?
- How might physiotherapy/my practices shift if I embraced other knowledges, such as that being created in the posthumanisms?

## References

Alldred, P., & Fox, N. J. (2017). Young bodies, power and resistance: A new materialist perspective. *Journal of Youth Studies*, *20*(9), 1161–1175. https://doi.org/10.1080/13676 261.2017.1316362

Amnesty International USA. (n.d.). *History*. Retrieved from www.amnestyusa.org/about-us/history/

Apple, M. W. (1995). *Education and power*. New York: Routledge.

Ariès, P. (1962). *Centuries of childhood: A social history of family life*. New York: Vintage Books.

Armstrong, D. (1995). The rise of surveillance medicine. *Sociology of Health & Illness*, *17*(3), 393–404.

Armstrong, D. (2002). *A new history of identity: A sociology of medical knowledge*. Hampshire: Palgrave Macmillan.

Bjorbækmo, W. S., & Engelsrud, G. H. (2011). Experiences of being tested: A critical discussion of the knowledge involved and produced in the practice of testing in children's rehabilitation. *Medicine, Health Care and Philosophy*, *14*(2), 123–131. https://doi.org/10.1007/s11019-010-9254-3

Bloch, M., & Popkewitz, T. (2000). Constructing the parent, teacher and child: Discourses of development. In L. Diaz Soto (Ed.), *The politics of early childhood education*. New York: Peter Lang Publishing.

Braidotti, R. (2013). *The posthuman*. Cambridge: Polity Press.

Brown, W. (2004). "The most we can hope for . . .": Human rights and the politics of fatalism. *The South Atlantic Quarterly*, *103*(2), 451–463.

Brown, W. (2015). *Undoing the demos: Neoliberalism's stealth revolution*. New York: Zone Books.

Burman, E. (2017). *Deconstructing developmental psychology*. East Sussex: Routledge.

Campbell, F. K. (2009). The project of ableism. In F. K. Campbell (Ed.), *Contours of ableism: The production of disability and abledness* (pp. 3–15). UK: Palgrave Macmillan. https://doi.org/10.1057/9780230245181_1

Cannella, G. S. (1997). *Deconstructing early childhood education: Social justice and revolution: Rethinking childhood* (Vol. 2). New York: Peter Lang Publishing.

Chilton, F. (1956). *The treatment of cerebral palsy in New Zealand*. The National Film Unit, NZ on Screen. Retrieved from www.nzonscreen.com/title/treatment-cerebral-palsy-1955/overview

Chilton, F. (1964). *One in a thousand*. NZ Film Unit, NZ on Screen. Retrieved from www.nzonscreen.com/title/one-in-a-thousand-1964

Cleaver, S., Deslauriers, S., & Hudon, A. (2018). Letter to the editor: Canadian physiotherapists want to talk more about equity. *Canadian Journal of Bioethics*, *1*(3), 90–91.

Corsaro, W. A. (2015). *The sociology of childhood* (4th ed.). Thousand Oaks, CA: Sage Publications.

Cowan, S. (2017). *Choreographing through an expanded corporeality* (Doctoral thesis). ResearchSpace@Auckland. Retrieved from https://researchspace.auckland.ac.nz/handle/2292/36942

Curran, T., & Runswick-Cole, K. (2014). Disabled children's childhood studies: A distinct approach? *Disability & Society*, *29*(10), 1617–1630. https://doi.org/10.1080/09687599.2014.966187

Deacon, R. (2006). From confinement to attachment: Michel Foucault on the rise of the school. *The European Legacy*, *11*(2), 121–138. https://doi.org/10.1080/10848770600587896

De Landa, M., & Harman, G. (2017). *The rise of realism*. Cambridge: Polity Press.

Fadyl, J. K., Teachman, G., & Hamdani, Y. (2019). Problematizing "productive citizenship" within rehabilitation services: Insights from three studies. *Disability and Rehabilitation*, 1–8. https://doi.org/10.1080/09638288.2019.1573935

Feely, M. (2016). Disability studies after the ontological turn: A return to the material world and material bodies without a return to essentialism. *Disability & Society*, *31*(7), 863–883. https://doi.org/10.1080/09687599.2016.1208603

Foucault, M. (1980). *Power/knowledge: Selected interviews and other writings, 1972–1977*. New York: Pantheon Books.

Foucault, M. (1995). *Discipline and punish: The birth of the prison*. New York: Vintage Books.

Foucault, M. (2002). *Archaeology of knowledge*. Abington, UK: Routledge.

Fox, N. J. (2002). Refracting health: Deleuze, Guattari and body-self. *Health*, *6*(3), 347–363.

Gesell, A. (1925). Monthly increments of development in infancy. *The Pedagogical Seminary and Journal of Genetic Psychology*, *32*(2), 203–208. https://doi.org/10.1080/08856559.1925.10534063

Gibson, B. E. (2006). Disability, connectivity and transgressing the autonomous body. *Journal of Medical Humanities*, *27*(3), 187–196. https://doi.org/10.1007/s10912-006-9017-6

Gibson, B. E. (2016). *Rehabilitation: A post-critical approach*. Boca Raton, FL: CRC Press.

Gibson, B. E., Carnevale, F. A., & King, G. (2012). "This is my way": Reimagining disability, in/dependence and interconnectedness of persons and assistive technologies. *Disability and Rehabilitation*, *34*(22), 1894–1899. https://doi.org/10.3109/09638288.2012.670040

Gibson, B. E., Teachman, G., & Hamdani, Y. (2015). Rethinking "normal development" in children's rehabilitation. In *Rethinking Rehabilitation: Theory and Practice* (1st ed., pp. 69–82). Boca Raton, FL: CRC Press.

Golden, J. (1989). *Infant asylums and children's hospitals: Medical dilemmas and developments, 1850–1920*. New York: Garland.

Goodley, D., & Roets, G. (2008). The (be)comings and goings of "developmental disabilities": The cultural politics of "impairment". *Discourse, 29*(2), 239–255. https://doi.org/10.1080/01596300801966971

Goodley, D., & Runswick-Cole, K. (2016). Becoming dishuman: Thinking about the human through dis/ability. *Discourse, 37*(1). https://doi.org/10.1080/01596306.2014.930021

Hendrick, H. (2009). The evolution of childhood in Western Europe c. 1400–c.1750. In J. Qvortrup, W. Cosaro, & M. S Honig (Eds.), *The Palgrave handbook of childhood studies* (pp. 99–113). Hampshire: Palgrave Macmillan.

James, A., & Prout, A. (Eds.). (1997). *Constructing and reconstructing childhood: Contemporary issues in the sociological study of childhood*. London, UK: Falmer Press.

Jones, P. (2012). *The Wilson Home: A celebration of 75 years*. Auckland: The Wilson Home Trust.

Litchfield, R., & MacDougall, C. (2002). Professional issues for physiotherapists in family-centred and community-based settings. *Australian Journal of Physiotherapy, 48*, 105–112. https://doi.org/10.1016/S0004-9514(14)60204-X

May, H. (2013). *The discovery of early childhood. The development of services for the care and education of very young children, mid eighteenth century Europe to mid twentieth century New Zealand*. Wellington: Bridget Williams Books.

Mayall, B. (2002). *Towards a sociology for childhood: Thinking from children's lives*. Philadelphia: Open University Press.

Mitchell, D., & Snyder, S. (2001). *Narrative prosthesis*. Retrieved from www.press.umich.edu/11523/narrative_prosthesis

Morton, T. (2017). *Humankind: Solidarity with nonhuman people*. London, UK: Verso.

Murris, K. (2016). *The posthuman child: Educational transformation through philosophy with picturebooks*. London, UK: Routledge.

Nicholls, D. A. (2017). *The end of physiotherapy*. London, UK: Routledge. Retrieved from http://ebookcentral.proquest.com/lib/aut/detail.action?docID=4930905

Palisano, R., Orlin, M., & Schreiber, J. (2017). *Campbell's physical therapy for children expert consult* (5th ed.). Philadelphia: Elsevier.

Prout, A. (2011). Taking a step away from modernity: Reconsidering the new sociology of childhood. *Global Studies of Childhood, 1*(1), 4–14.

Qvortrup, J., Corsaro, W. A., & Honig, M.-S. (Eds.). (2009). *The Palgrave handbook of childhood studies*. Hampshire: Palgrave Macmillan.

Rasche, C. (2016, August 22). A preface to the genealogy of neoliberalism, part 1 (Carl Raschke). *Religious theory*. Retrieved from http://jcrt.org/religioustheory/2016/08/22/a-preface-to-the-genealogy-of-neoliberalism-part-1-carl-raschke/

Sales, A. P. (2012). History of rehabilitation counseling. In D. Maki (Ed.), *The professional practice of rehabilitation counseling* (pp. 39–60). New York: Springer.

Schorer, M. (2012). *From the New Zealand Crippled Children Society to CCS disability action: A social and political history of a disability organisation in Aotearoa New Zealand moving from charity to social action* (Doctoral thesis). Massey University. Retrieved from https://mro.massey.ac.nz/handle/10179/3844

Shildrick, M. (2001). *Embodying the monster: Encounters with the vulnerable self*. London, UK: Sage Publications.

Shildrick, M., & Price, J. (2005). Deleuzian connections and queer corporealities: Shrinking global disability. *Rhizomes, 11/12*. Retrieved from www.rhizomes.net/issue11/shildrickprice/

Smith, A. B. (2013). *Understanding children and childhood: A New Zealand perspective* (5th ed.). Wellington: Bridget Williams Books Ltd.

Stace, H. (2014). Some aspects of New Zealand's disability history: Part one. *Public Address: Access: Disability and Different Worlds*. Retrieved from https://publicaddress.net/access/some-aspects-of-new-zealands-disability-history/

Stiker, H. J. (2000). *A history of disability* (W. Sayers, Trans.). Ann Arbour, MI: University of Michigan Press. https://doi.org/10.3998/mpub.15952

St. Pierre, E. A. (2017). Deleuze and Guattari's language for new empirical inquiry. *Educational Philosophy and Theory, 49*(11), 1080–1089. https://doi.org/10.1080/00131857.2016.1151761

Taylor, A., & Giugni, M. (2012). Common worlds: Reconceptualising inclusion in early childhood communities. *Contemporary Issues in Early Childhood, 13*(2), 108–119. https://doi.org/10.2304/ciec.2012.13.2.108

Tennant, M. (1996). Disability in New Zealand: A historical survey. *New Zealand Journal of Disability Studies, 2*, 3–33.

Tesar, M. (2014). Reconceptualising the child: Power and resistance within early childhood settings. *Contemporary Issues in Early Childhood, 15*(4), 360–367. https://doi.org/10.2304/ciec.2014.15.4.360

Tesar, M., Rodriguez, S., & Kupferman, D. W. (2016). Philosophy and pedagogy of childhood, adolescence and youth. *Global Studies of Childhood, 6*(2), 169–176. https://doi.org/10.1177/2043610616647623

Tremain, S. (2001). On the government of disability. *Social Theory and Practice, 27*(4), 617–636. JSTOR.

Valentine, G. (2009). Children's bodies: An absent presence. In K. Horschelmann & R. Colls (Eds.), *Contested bodies of childhood and youth* (pp. 22–40). London: Palgrave Macmillan.

Vehmas, S., & Watson, N. (2016). Exploring normativity in disability studies. *Disability & Society, 31*(1), 1–16. https://doi.org/10.1080/09687599.2015.1120657

Visiting Cerebral Palsy Therapists Review Committee. (1984). *Report of the Visiting Cerebral Palsy Therapists Review Committee*. Ministry of Health. Retrieved from www.moh.govt.nz/notebook/nbbooks.nsf/0/320D931C88C0A39D4C2565D70018CBD8/$file/Report_visiting_cerebral_palsy_therapists.pdf

Walkerdine, V. (1993). Beyond developmentalism? *Theory & Psychology, 3*(4), 451–469. https://doi.org/10.1177/0959354393034004

Whanganui District Health Board. (n.d.). *Therapy services*. Whanganui District Health Board. Retrieved from www.wdhb.org.nz/patients-and-visitors/our-departments-and-wards/therapy-services/

# 7 Learning from biology, philosophy, and sourdough bread – challenging the evidence-based practice paradigm for community physiotherapy

*Satu Reivonen, Finlay Sim, and Cathy Bulley*

## Introduction

Physiotherapy interventions are increasingly situated in the community, in people's natural environments. These fluid and dynamic contexts challenge the 'hierarchy of evidence' in the current paradigm of evidence-based practice. Where a highly controlled clinical trial is not feasible, faith in this paradigm may jeopardize the development of 'evidence-based' rationales for the funding of services.

By using the example of a multifactorial intervention – 24-hour postural care – we emphasize the need for a different approach. We explore scenarios where complex care plans function in connection with multiple and intricate systems. To explore these non-linear and symbiotic relationships of systems, and reductionism of viewing 'things' rather than 'processes', we look to applied microbiology. We relate 24-hour postural care to a place where intricate processes unfold over 24 hours – the sourdough microenvironment of an artisan bakery. To guide these connections, we draw on processual ontology of biology and argue that a shift in how we think about biological processes can provide valuable insights into the complexities of physiotherapy interventions. Our aim, through reflecting on concepts from process philosophy, is to emphasize the value of studying the fluid and dynamic interconnections between different systems to improve understanding and delivery of physiotherapy interventions. We highlight the necessity of broadening the nature of evidence required to make a case for funding of a community-based service or intervention.

## Roots and impacts of the evidence-based practice paradigm

Evidence-based practice (EBP) stems from evidence-based medicine (EBM), announced in the early 1990s as the 'new paradigm'. It encouraged clinical decision-making based on formal evaluation of clinical evidence and research rather than on intuition, clinical experience, and pathophysiologic rationale (Guyatt et al., 1992). After extending its arms within health and social care, EBM was re-named EBP, commonly defined as: 'the conscientious and judicious use of current best evidence from clinical care research in the management of individual patients' (Sackett, Rosenberg, Gray, Haynes, & Richardson, 1996). This incorporates patient experience, research evidence, and clinical expertise as partly overlapping components (Haynes, Sackett, Gray, Cook, & Guyatt, 1996). Although each was emphasized as equally important, research evidence has received greatest attention, primarily through development of a hierarchical model to support appraisal and synthesis of research (Guyatt, Rennie, Meade, & Cook, 2008).

In the evidence hierarchy, the pinnacle is research that can most accurately determine a causal relationship between an intervention and its outcome, and syntheses of such studies (Cowen, Virk, Mascarenhas-Keyes, & Cartwright, 2017). The assumption that awards randomized controlled trials (RCTs) their causative high ground is that two randomized groups can be designed to differ only by the variable of interest, and any differences can then be attributed to that variable (Kerry, Eriksen, Lie, Mumford, & Anjum, 2012). These ideas derive from a positivist epistemological view of knowing and are philosophically linked with the biomedical model of health (Shaw, Connelly, & Zecevic, 2010). This reductionist approach 'falls short of capturing the context, complexity, and patient centeredness that characterize expertise in physiotherapy practice' (Shaw et al., 2010, p. 514) and has been widely critiqued (Greenhalgh, Howick, & Markrey, 2014; Goldenberg, 2006).

Despite prevalent critique, such an evidence-based hierarchy often strongly informs influential methodologies for evidence synthesis, such as the Cochrane systematic review process (Higgins et al., 2019). Clinical guideline development also relies on this in relation to which evidence is included and how it is rated within the evidence synthesis. Some guideline development methodologies are more influential than others, such as that of the UK National Institute for Health and Care Excellence (NICE, 2014). Although inclusive of a range of types of evidence as appropriate to different types of questions, when considering intervention effectiveness, RCTs are considered to give the best answer. They state that if RCTs are not available, possible, or appropriate, other forms of trial and experimentation may be needed. This implies that there may be impacts on levels of confidence in the recommendation due to 'suboptimal' study design. Clinical guidelines influence clinical pathways and guidance relating to funding of services (Parkhurst & Abeysinghe, 2016; NICE, 2014), despite the critique that EBP often fails to account for complexity and context (Greenhalgh, Howick, & Markrey, 2014; Shaw et al., 2010).

Hierarchies of evidence continue to have a strong hold in physiotherapy in the structures used to evaluate evidence and make recommendations (Kerry, 2018). This creates an increasing dissonance for physiotherapists pressured to demonstrate 'person-centred healthcare', which stems from thinking that is very different to that of the biomedical model and its positivist roots (WHO, 2016; McCormack & McCance, 2017). Although physiotherapists often learn and practice using more biopsychosocial models for health, such as the International Classification of Functioning, Disability and Health (WHO, 2001), prevailing emphasis on the evidence hierarchy encourages a reductionist approach. The evidence-based movement in healthcare has diligently focused on eliminating bias to discover 'truths'. Yet it has created systematic bias towards certain types of research questions being asked, groups of people included, and types of interventions researched and designed. Multifactorial and highly contextual interventions have received less focus in research, such as many of those designed for people living with long-term conditions. In numerous scenarios where it is not feasible or helpful to do an RCT, other forms of enquiry may be much more informative and should be given appropriate credit in evidence syntheses. If not, this prioritization of certain types of evidence may be contributing to health inequalities.

## A challenge to evidence-based practice – complex and long-term conditions

In many countries, the ageing population is leading to increased prevalence of multiple long-term conditions (LTCs) that are escalating challenges and costs to health systems (Global Burden of Disease Study, 2013 Collaborators, 2015). People with LTCs are often in contact with health professionals for less than one percent of their lives, increasing focus on interventions that facilitate community-based self-management (Department of Health, 2010; Barker, Steventon, Williamson, & Deeny, 2018).

Supporting people living with LTCs can be further complicated where self-management requires coordinated involvement of multiple people and agencies. People who are unable to change their body position without assistance exemplify this. They are at risk of poor habitual and prolonged positioning that can distort body shape and compromise circulation, respiratory function, and digestion (Hill & Goldsmith, 2010). Twenty-four-hour postural care (24hPC) is a preventative and restorative approach incorporating moving and handling, advice and training, adaptive seating, and night-time positioning (Gericke, 2006). 24hPC aims to prevent and correct destructive postures and facilitate good alignment, comfort, function, and participation (Crawford & Stinson, 2015). Careful consideration of the environmental context and views of both service users and carers are imperative (Crawford & Stinson, 2015). Monitoring and adapting provision over time is crucial, highlighting the need for any research design looking at the impacts of 24hPC to be sensitive to context and change.

Reviewers have summarized that good-quality research is lacking around the effectiveness of 24hPC (Robertson, Baines, Emerson, & Hatton, 2016; Blake et al., 2015), which may reflect difficulty achieving the positivist standards inherent in the evidence hierarchy. For example, people who need 24hPC frequently have LTCs with diverse impacts, reflected within a positivist research paradigm as inconveniently heterogeneous samples. Another layer of complexity derives from 24hPC being a multicomponent intervention delivered collaboratively between service user, formal and informal carers, and different organizations. This makes it extremely challenging to define a 'standard intervention' and to justify withholding supportive strategies in a control intervention. Furthermore, outcomes are likely to be fluid due to the dynamic and contextual nature of 24hPC, with different interacting human and non-human agents.

We can look to the Medical Research Council (MRC) guidance for developing and evaluating complex interventions, as 24hPC epitomizes 'several interacting components' (Craig et al., 2006, p. 7). This aims to help researchers address challenges such as standardizing the intervention, considering impact of the local context, and establishing mechanisms of action. Despite revision of this guidance to address criticisms, including its assumption that conventional clinical trials were always optimal and lack of attention to context, there is still priority on the evidence hierarchy. It advocates the use of the best available evidence to build initial theory using systematic review that prioritizes the evidence hierarchy at the outset. The modelling process then takes a positivist approach to testing different elements of the theory, followed by phased pilot testing and evaluation that uses the best available methods for evaluation that clearly prioritizes an experimental approach where possible.

When considering 24hPC, the MRC Framework (Craig et al., 2006) may not address the challenges. The limited literature makes it hard to build initial theory, while the complexity of 24hPC makes modelling elements of theory difficult. Making one specific change, such as adding one piece of equipment, and then seeking to measure change, could give misleading results due to changing care staff who do not use it appropriately. Measurement instruments may not be sensitive enough to detect a meaningful change in the person's life. Equally, one positive change in a person's life might be neutralized by a negative change elsewhere in the overall context of their health and wellbeing. A consequence of this complexity may be that a service or equipment is not funded, and impacts could be substantial in relation to human suffering and likely increased healthcare needs.

Sadly, many people who need 24hPC are in situations where their own financial and social resources are declining over time. The systems of developing evidence and arguing for funding let them down further. If funding decisions prioritize evidence that lends itself to less variable and heterogeneous scenarios, this increases health inequality through an unwillingness to consider different forms of *knowledge*. This thought process led us to consider other debates about ways of knowing – this time through reflections on process philosophy.

## Thinking through processes

Process philosophy has diversified into several different streams of thinking and holds complex theories of metaphysics. Generally speaking, it opposes the predominant favouring of *things* and emphasizes *process* and *becoming* over *being* (Rescher, 2000). Nicholson and Dupré (2018, p. 3) propose that 'the world – at least insofar as living beings are concerned – is made up not of substantial particles or things, . . . but of processes. It is dynamic through and through'. Process ontology opposes the prevalent substantialist philosophy originating from early Greek philosophy, which focuses on a world of things and has dominated research in the West (Seibt, 2012). In contrast, Nicholson and Dupré suggest that *things* can be viewed as abstractions from more or less stable processes (2018). Process thinking in biology stems from a movement starting early in the 20th century – organicism – which suggested that wholes are inherently greater than the sum of their parts. Therefore, to understand how a whole works, instead of having a profound understanding of its parts, significance is in how these parts interact in a specific context (Gilbert & Sarkar, 2000).

Through parallel conversations between the authors over a similar period of time, we saw rich learning that could be applied through process philosophy, challenging the positivist ontology underpinning the evidence-based paradigm. We explore this through examples of working with sourdough bread, an ancient process epitomizing the value of diversity. Unlike other bread, sourdough uses the fermentative activity of wild microbes to leaven bread rather than commercial baker's yeast. The basis of a sourdough is the *levain* or the *starter*, a mixture of flour and water that ferments over time with lactic acid bacteria (LAB) and wild yeast. It consists of a rich microbial mingling, with a symbiotic relationship between yeast and LAB that persists through bakers continuously propagating or 'feeding' their starters. These associations are so robust that they create a stable microenvironment, which prohibits other invasive strains of bacteria and yeast from competing (De Vuyst et al., 2014). This stability is dependent on constant flow of activity within the starter and its environment.

The microbial community and its evolution are based on the raw materials: what type of grain has been used, how the grain was milled, what part of the world it has been grown in, soil health, and the house microenvironment where the starter is kept. Key roles are also played by parameters of the sourdough propagation itself, temperature and fermentation time, how often it is 'fed', the percentage distribution of each raw ingredient, and starter acidity (De Vuyst, Kerrebroeck, & Leroy, 2017). Moreover, some suggest that the microbes of the baker enter an interchanging of microbes with the sourdough starter (Patterson, 2018).

A *levain* is continuously developing, as for the starter to maintain its fermentative capacity, more water and flour must be added to it regularly. Bacteria and yeast then undergo their growth and reproduction cycles, feasting on the starches from the flour as their food. As a baker, you become responsible for the maintenance of the starter, learning how intricately the fermentation will vary and how to play with the conditions for different flavour, texture, and smell. In this respect, developing a sourdough starter takes time, trial and error, intuition, and understanding of several processes outside of the bakery.

## Nonlinear and symbiotic relationships of systems

In the argument for a process stance in biology, Nicholson and Dupré (2018) discuss ecological interdependence, whereby the persistence of entities and their behaviours and capacities is dependent on a complex web of relations. In substance thinking, *things* are defined by their boundaries and a level of independence or autonomy (Nicholson & Dupré, 2018). Since the development of new technologies in biology, complex systems and symbiotic relationships between and within diverse microscopic and macroscopic forms of life have been discovered. These discoveries have transformed classical ideas of individuality within biology, shifting focus to interactions (Gilbert, Sapp, & Tauber, 2012). Thinking more about processes challenges the idea of being able to explain or predict a *whole* by examining its *parts* in isolation. This is exemplified by *emergent properties* that develop from a complex and contextualized system without having the potential to be predicted from the properties of the system's *parts* (O'Connor & Wong, 2015). Philosophers Deleuze and Guattari (1987) illustrate this complexity by describing a rhizome – a network of multiple lateral off-shooting connections, always in the middle, always becoming something else. The rhizome defies binary logic and challenges hierarchical structures. A rhizome is always connected to anything other, and these connections can be with diverse 'modes of coding' (e.g. political, biological, social) in the words of Deleuze and Guattari (1987).

While a sourdough may initially seem like a simple interaction between flour and water, the ingrained intricacy, experienced in practice, evokes curiosity amongst sourdough bakers. To illustrate the power and sensitivity of context, one of the authors (FS) shares an experience from a sourdough bakery where a basic test led to unexpected realizations:

> One particular afternoon, we were keen to explore aspects of dough elasticity and extensibility (rheology). My co-worker decided to test the effects of the resting time of water and flour on the rheological properties of dough during mixing. He set out by letting a mixture of flour and water rest overnight for ca. 12 hours rather than the usual 30–60 minutes. We expected to find relaxed dough with an improved mixing potential. Instead, the following day we found that the dough had expanded to twice its size and blown the container's top off. Confused at first, we then realized that the dough had spontaneously become a starter – a process which usually takes a week to occur. The experience gave us insight into how a bakery can become inoculated with the microbes in the sourdough itself, contributing to the activity and resilience of the microbial environment of the bakery – the 'house microbiota'.

Due to this sensitive nature of microbes, enabling great diversity and adaptability in varying environments, bakers and scientists have begun to look beyond the baking process – including fields of agroecology. Understanding the processes taking place before, during, and after the baking is what allows for skill and adaptability in the unpredictable microbial world.

In 24hPC, there are multiple connected and overlapping processes. We can consider ecological interdependence, for instance, through positioning. The term 'positioning' suggests a one-way process, while, more carefully examined, there is a collaborative process with sensitive intermingling between the carer(s), service user, equipment, and the wider environment. The 'physical' interaction is a coming together of several unmeasurable aspects, such as past experiences, thoughts, feelings, touch, and surroundings. The consideration of *physical attributes* of posture could be seen as a merging of processes, blurring the boundaries between different systems such as the biological, psychological, and social. The environment where postural care is happening includes broader political and social systems. Milligan and Wiles (2010) describe these through the concept of 'landscapes of care', involving social arrangements of care; work arrangements; changing policies at local, national, and international levels; and ideological beliefs around care. The overlapping processes involved are so diverse that an exploration of complexity is necessary to understand, develop, and adjust postural care.

Quantitative research designs guide researchers to look at single components of 24hPC. Refracting a component of postural care and using pre-specified outcomes to see whether it is *effective* is problematic. Whether a *part* of the intervention has a positive impact on someone's life is a complex question of previous events and experiences, how, with whom, where, and when it is used, and what else takes place over 24 hours. Viewing these components of 24hPC as processes encourages an engagement in context. The principle and thinking behind 24hPC is that for the intervention to meet its aims, we must look beyond the body and beyond a part of a person's day. Due to the dynamic and highly contextual nature of the intervention, it must be distorted to enable selection of one component that is treated as static and measured using a single outcome measure.

## Reductionism and fallacy of misplaced concreteness

During the Enlightenment, there was a movement towards 'substantialist' philosophy, exemplified by Galileo: 'Count what is countable, measure what is measurable, what is not measurable, make measurable' (Galileo Galilei, 1664–1642; in Kaydos, 1999). This substance ontology has largely influenced, along with much of the way we think and communicate, the evidence-based paradigm. To describe the overarching manifestation of substance ontology, Seibt (2018) refers to the 'myth of substance' – a set of presuppositions emphasizing static entities. This overreliance on substance in science has implied that to explain complex phenomena, it is necessary to reduce these to simpler structures (Mazzocchi, 2011). Process ontology of biology holds that mechanistic descriptions of living organisms are inadequate, as they rely on substance ontological assumptions of fixed entities (Nicholson & Dupré, 2018).

It is common in healthcare research to separate out the discrete units that form variables: those being held as static as possible and those being changed. These 'things' are either measured through specific scales or administered in 'doses' of intervention. The problem, according to process thinking, is when or if this abstraction is mistaken for 'truth'. Alfred Whitehead calls this 'The Fallacy of Misplaced Concreteness', through which we 'neglect the degree of abstraction involved when an actual entity is considered merely so far as it exemplifies certain categories of thought' (1978, p. 7). Thompson (1997) describes this in relation to inquiry always involving the picking out of certain features, epitomizing value-based judgements of what is important. This becomes problematic when the abstraction is mistakenly thought to carry the full meaning of the situation, underrating the complexity and the value-based decisions made in the process.

In the world of sourdough baking, complexity is a topic of relevance, and research continues to highlight the value of diversity within microbes (Urien, Legrand, Montalent, Casaregola, & Sicard, 2019). Sourdough is one of the oldest known biotechnologies, used to leaven bread since the beginning of civilization, becoming neglected after Louis Pasteur isolated baker's yeast in the late 19th century (Cappelle, Guylaine, Gänzle, & Gobbetti, 2013). Baker's yeast allowed for a substantial reduction in the amount of time for which bread was fermented and reduction in the depth of knowledge required in comparison to complex sourdough matrices. As a knock-on effect, the type of flour used for these formulas with baker's yeast could be standardized for greater consistency. The standardization of bread is tied to years of innovation in agriculture and industry. And, whilst these innovations have been large-scale logistical achievements, they have ignored aspects of nutrition, taste, sustainability, and equity and led to a bottleneck of crop diversity (Steavenson, 2019). Nowadays, with the public's renewed interest in how food is made, sourdough baking is also recognized as a movement involving revival of alternative cereal varieties with potential to maintain nutrients and flavour (Steavenson, 2019). Related research, progressive milling technology, and ecological farming practices favour flour with higher nutritional profiles, rich and diverse soils, plants resilient against abrupt environmental changes, healthier guts, and more ethical practices. Bread is recognized as a combination of biological processes which are culturally, historically, and politically imbedded. This was recognized in the annual GrAiNZ Gathering in 2019, which brought together farmers, researchers, and bakers. Process thinking comes across within sourdough as an example of the way a healthy world works through a set of relationships in a cyclical, non-linear, symbiotic way (Whitley, 2014).

24hPC is temporal and dynamic. In other words, postural care is an *open system*, which Biesta (2010a) describes as a system that depends on its interaction with its environment for its function. Biesta (2010a) refers to the efficacy deficit of EBP within the field of education, where interventions do not generate effects in a mechanistic way but rather through open processes, making the relationship between the intervention and its effect non-linear. Through categorization, the drawing of boundaries begins to lose sight of interactions between *parts* that are essential in explaining the capacities and behaviours of those parts. The risk of fallacy of misplaced concreteness comes into play where the *lack of evidence* is taken as *lack of effectiveness* and the underlying abstractions are not adequately engaged in. The sourdough movement, through the examination of complexity of the microbial world, sees that the microbial diversity is very much connected to the processes in other systems. This recognition is guiding interdisciplinary research and is an approach to be learnt from within physiotherapy. Instead of trying to eliminate complexity from processes, the sourdough movement is about immersion in, and reclaiming of, diversity.

Healthcare and related research has been following a similar journey to that of modern baking towards a culture of standardization. To facilitate this, the person has been removed from their context and boundaries have been drawn around different parts, which are assigned numerical value. Based on these principles, clinical recommendations are made, services are designed, and funding is allocated. This does not intuitively allow for an understanding of the processes and connections that are the precondition for what we view as distinct *parts* in the first place. Physiotherapy, and healthcare more broadly, are now trying to find ways to reintegrate the person within care and research systems that are based on ideals of standardization and consistency. To study open systems as closed ones, the number of *available options for action* for the elements within a system is limited, referred to as complexity reduction (Biesta, 2010b). This thinking challenges research into an intervention such as 24hPC, which is never uniform, as it is suited to people with diverse conditions, abilities, and care plans.

## Researching processes

The critique of EBP is not new, and movement beyond use of the traditional evidence hierarchy is taking place in many fields (Satterfield et al., 2009). Different ways of doing research (and practice), including aspects of process thinking, have also been suggested within physiotherapy and rehabilitation (Gibson, Nicholls, Setchell, & Synne Groven, 2018; Nicholls et al., 2016; Gibson, 2018). We have aimed to highlight the value of process thinking more broadly in physiotherapy. Instead of modifying the current model of EBP, we suggest there is a need to go further to examine the underlying philosophy of EBP. This is necessary to address complexities and inequalities within physiotherapy interventions and service development. A processual way of looking at the world welcomes an exploration beyond the categorization and boundaries that characterize much of physiotherapy practice today. As the processes of interest are reciprocally dependent and interconnected, exploring one process without taking account of the greater picture might give limited insights that do not account adequately for complexity.

There are many developing types of research processes that may already reflect aspects of process philosophy to an extent. Implementation science aims to address research not only at the 'patient' level but also looking at the providers, wider organizations, and healthcare policy (Bauer, Damschroder, Hagerdorn, Smith, & Kilbourne, 2015). This incorporates ideas around reciprocal dependencies and dynamic processes through emphasis on the people affected by the research and the journey. Strategies are encouraged to ensure that findings are meaningful and contextualized and to accelerate the route to decision-makers and practice. Another example is 'Experience-based co-design', a quality improvement method which focuses on co-production of creative solutions to key issues identified by people who experience services. Creative solutions for that context are forged by these people together with others who can make the changes happen (Donetto, Pierri, Tsianakas, & Robert, 2015). In relation to synthesis and evaluation of research, there could be greater credibility given to methods like Realist Review and Evaluation which focus on exploring how mechanisms interact with contexts to produce outcomes (Rycroft-Malone et al., 2012).

Individual studies could incorporate greater exploration of the context and consciously map interdependent processes with an awareness of the simplifications made. There should be analysis of how the relevance of insights might be influenced by changing circumstances. This may call for more practice-based and creative, less structured methods. Law (2004) discusses 'dealing with mess' in the context of social science and argues that instead of standardization and regularities, we need to move towards heterogeneity and variation in research methods. He suggests going beyond evaluating the rules used within research and critically examining the need for rules in the first place. Similarly, to make physiotherapy more inclusive and diverse, we need to greatly broaden our ideas of method and ways of *knowing*.

Perhaps when synthesizing a field of study, more emphasis should be given to different perspectives, with further exploration of how research findings have changed over time as the context has changed. Design of synthesis studies should build a picture of interconnected contextual insights, with judgements about validity of the research reflecting a much more inclusive view of different ways of knowing about the world. Pallesen (2017) discusses re-examining concepts such as validity through process philosophy. As process thinking emphasizes the singularity of experience and multiplicity, she suggests that validity becomes more about taking a further step to engage in variation rather than trying to control it. She further suggests that if we consider processes as fundamental, then relating to the vagueness and multiplicity brought by these processes is necessary when approaching them in research.

An interesting example of how process philosophy is paving its way through changing the world of research is in education, where Deleuze and Guattari's rhizomatic thinking has been explored in some depth (Mazzei & McCoy, 2010; Masny, 2016). Through what has been termed rhizoanalysis, the traditional qualitative research processes are disrupted and an opportunity to acknowledge more variable types of data is suggested (St. Pierre, 1997). Clarke and Parsons (2013) discuss rhizomatic research as an open system allowing for interrelations that may not have been traditionally considered. They describe a movement away from binaries and a focus on the researcher becoming embedded within the research. Much like the world of sourdough, rhizomatic research celebrates chaos and creativity, embracing diversity.

## Conclusion

Process philosophy has much to offer in the area of healthcare research and in building up momentum to diversifying ways of knowing. There are clearly many fascinating directions for exploration when reading about process philosophy and considering how so much of physiotherapy and its pursuit of EBP derives, without intention, from substance thinking. Evolving our mind-sets and our use of evidence is crucial in our rapidly changing world; physiotherapy cannot stand still – it is also a merging of many active and interconnected systems.

The dominance of EBP in physiotherapy has led to a tendency to take what we read in meta-analyses and systematic reviews as facts. Education in physiotherapy focuses on skills to critically review evidence, but less emphasis is placed on critically reviewing the foundations underlying what we consider *evidence* in the first place. To transform and acknowledge complexity in the world, it is useful, if not necessary, to look to the philosophy underpinning our models of research and practice.

While there is a growing wave of different and creative research practices, the privileging of quantifications and numerical outcomes still dominates and steers development of services. There is a need to broaden the definitions of *knowledge*, and process philosophy may be a valuable tool for inspiring and enabling a more appropriate way of researching the dynamic and complex world of physiotherapy.

## References

Barker, I., Steventon, A., Williamson, R., & Deeny, S. R. (2018). Self-management capability in patients with long-term conditions is associated with reduced healthcare utilisation across a whole health economy: Cross-sectional analysis of electronic health records. *BMJ Quality and Safety, 27*(12). doi:10.1136/bmjqs-2017-007635

Bauer, M. S., Damschroder, L., Hagerdorn, H., Smith, J., & Kilbourne, A. M. (2015). An introduction to implementation science for the non-specialist. *BMC Psychology, 3*(1), 31. doi:10.1186/s40359-015-0089-9

Biesta, G. J. J. (2010a). Why "what works" still won't work. *Studies in Philosophy and Education, 29*, 491–503. doi:10.1007/s11217-010-9191-x

Biesta, G. J. J. (2010b). Five theses on complexity reduction and its politics. In D. C. Osberg & G. J. J. Biesta (Eds.), *Complexity theory and the politics of education* (pp. 5–14). Sense Publishers. doi:10.1163/9789460912405

Blake, S. F., Logan, S., Humphreys, G., Matthews, J., Rogers, M., Thompson-Coon, J., . . . Morris, C. (2015). Sleep positioning systems for children with cerebral palsy (review). *Cochrane Database of Systematic Reviews 2015*, (11) doi:11.10.1002/14651858. CD009257.pub2

Cappelle, S., Guylaine, L., Gänzle, M., & Gobbetti, M., (2013). History and social aspects of sourdough. In M. Gobetti & M. Gänzle (Eds.), *Handbook on sourdough biotechnology* (pp. 1–10). New York: Springer.

Clarke, B., & Parsons, J. (2013). Becoming rhizome researchers. *Reconceptualising Educational Research Methodology, 4*(1), 35–43. doi:10.7577/rerm.685

Cowen, N., Virk, B., Mascarenhas-Keyes, S., & Cartwright, N. (2017). Randomised controlled trials: How can we know "what works"? *A Journal of Politics and Society, 29*(3), 265–292. doi:10.1080/08913811.2017.1395223

Craig, P., Dieppe, P., Macintyre, S., Michie, S., Nazareth, I., & Petticrew, M., for the Medical Research Council. (2006). Developing and evaluating complex interventions: New guidance. *MRC*. Retrieved from www.mrc.ac.uk/complexinterventionsguidance

Crawford, S., & Stinson, M. (2015). Management of 24hr-body positioning. In I. Söderback (Ed.), *International handbook of occupational therapy interventions* (pp. 189–198). Springer. doi:10.1007/978-3-319-08141-0

Deleuze, G., & Guattari, F. (1987). *A thousand plateaus: Capitalism and schizophrenia*. Minneapolis, MN: University of Minnesota Press.

Department of Health. (2010). *Improving the health and well-being of people with long term conditions*. London, UK: Department of Health, 2010. Retrieved from www.yearofcare.co.uk/sites/default/files/pdfs/dh_improving%20the%20h&wb%20of%20people%20with%20LTCs.pdf

De Vuyst, L., Kerrebroeck, S. V., Harth, H., Huys, G., Daniel, H.-M., & Weckx, S. (2014). Microbial ecology of sourdough fermentations: Diverse or uniform? *Food Microbiology, 37,* 11–29. doi:10.1016/j.fm.2013.06.002

De Vuyst, L., Kerrebroeck, S. V., & Leroy, F. (2017). Microbial ecology and process technology of sourdough fermentation. *Advances in Applied Microbiology, 100,* 49–160. doi:10.1016/bs.aambs.2017.02.003

Donetto, S., Pierri, P., Tsianakas, V., & Robert, G. (2015). Experience-based co-design and healthcare improvement: Realizing participatory design in the public sector. *The Design Journal, 18*(2), 227–248. doi:10.2752/175630615X14212498964312

Gericke, T. (2006). Postural management for children with cerebral palsy: Consensus statement. *Developmental Medicine and Child Neurology, 48*(4), 244. doi:10.1017/S0012162206000685

Gibson, B. E. (2018). Post-critical physiotherapy ethics: A commitment to openness. In B. E. Gibson, D. A. Nicholls, J. Setchell, & K. Synne Groven (Eds.), *Manipulating practices: A critical physiotherapy reader* (pp. 35–52). Cappelen Damm Akademisk. Retrieved from https://press.nordicopenaccess.no/index.php/noasp/catalog/book/29

Gibson, B. E., Nicholls, D. A., Setchell, J., & Synne Groven, K. (Eds.). (2018). *Manipulating practices: A critical physiotherapy reader.* Cappelen Damm Akademisk. Retrieved from https://press.nordicopenaccess.no/index.php/noasp/catalog/book/29

Gilbert, S. F., Sapp, J., & Tauber, A. I. (2012). A symbiotic view of life: We have never been individuals. *The Quarterly Review of Biology, 87*(4), 325–341. doi:10.1086/668166

Gilbert, S. F., & Sarkar, S. (2000). Embracing complexity: Organicism for the 21st century. *Developmental Dynamics, 219,* 1–9. doi:10.1002/1097-0177(2000)9999:9999<::AID-DVDY1036>3.0.CO;2-A

Global Burden of Disease Study 2013 Collaborators. (2015). Global, regional, and national incidence, prevalence, and years lived with disability for 301 acute and chronic diseases and injuries in 188 countries, 1990–2013: A systematic analysis for the Global Burden of Disease Study 2013. *Lancet, 386*(9995), 743–800. doi:10.1016/S0140-6736(15)60692-4

Goldenberg, M. J. (2006). On evidence and evidence-based medicine: Lessons from the philosophy of science. *Social Science and Medicine, 62*(11), 2621–2632. doi:10.1016/j.socscimed.2005.11.031

Greenhalgh, T., Howick, J., & Markrey, N. (2014). Evidence based medicine: A movement in crisis? *BMJ, 348*(g3725). doi:10.1136/bmj.g3725

Guyatt, G. H., Cairns, J., Churchill, D., Cook, D., Haynes, B., Hirsh, J., . . . Tugwell, P. (1992). Evidence-based medicine: A new approach to teaching the practice of medicine. *JAMA, 268*(17), 2420–2425. doi:10.1001/jama.1992.03490170092032

Guyatt, G. H., Rennie, D., Meade, M. O., & Cook, D. (Eds.). (2008). *Users' guides to the medical literature: Essentials of evidence based clinical practice* (2nd ed.). McGraw Hill Medical, JAMA evidence, and American Medical Association. Retrieved from www.ebcp.com.br/simple/upfiles/livros/005EEBM.pdf

Haynes, R. B., Sackett, D. L., Gray, J. M., Cook, D. J., & Guyatt, G. H. (1996). Transferring evidence from research into practice: 1: The role of clinical care research evidence in clinical decisions. *BMJ Evidence Based Medicine, 1*(7), 196–198. doi:10.1136/ebm.1996.1.196

Higgins, J. P. T., Thomas, J., Chandler, J., Cumpston, M., Li, T., Page, M. J., & Welch, V. A. (Eds.). (2019, July). *Cochrane handbook for systematic reviews of interventions.* Version 6.0. Cochrane. Retrieved from www.training.cochrane.org/handbook

Hill, S., & Goldsmith, J. (2010). Biomechanics and prevention of body shape distortion. *Tizard Learn Disability Review, 15*(2), 5–32. doi:10.5042/tldr.2010.0166

Kaydos, W. (1999). *Operational performance management: Increasing total productivity.* Boca Raton, FL: CRC Press LLC.

Kerry, R. (2018). Reconceptualising causation in evidence-based physiotherapy. In B. E. Gibson, D. A., Nicholls, J. Setchell, & K. Synne Groven (Eds.), *Manipulating practices: A critical physiotherapy reader* (pp. 77–100). Cappelen Damm Akademisk. Retrieved from https://press.nordicopenaccess.no/index.php/noasp/catalog/book/29

Kerry, R., Eriksen, T. E., Lie, S. A., Mumford, S. D., & Anjum, R. L. (2012). Causation and evidence-based practice: An ontological review. *Journal of Evaluation in Clinical Practice, 18*(5), 1006–1012. doi:10.1111/j.1365-2753.2012.01908.x.

Law, J. (2004). *After method: Mess in social science research.* Routledge and Taylor & Francis. Retrieved from www.leofoletto.info/wp-content/uploads/2016/08/john_law_after_method_mess_in_social_science_research_international_library_of_sociology__2004.pdf

Masny, D. (2016). Problematizing qualitative research: Reading a data assemblage with rhizoanalysis. *Qualitative Inquiry, 22*(8), 666–675. doi:10.1177/1532708616636744

Mazzei, L. A., & McCoy, K. (2010). Thinking with Deleuze in qualitative research. *International Journal of Qualitative Studies in Education, 23*(5), 503–509. doi:10.1080/09518398.2010.500634

Mazzocchi, F. (2011). The limits of reductionism in biology: What alternatives? *E-Logos: Electronic Journal of Philosophy.* Retrieved from https://nb.vse.cz/kfil/elogos/science/mazzocchi11.pdf

McCormack, B., & McCance, T. (2017). *Person-centred practice in nursing and healthcare: Theory and practice.* West Sussex: Wiley-Blackwell.

Milligan, C., & Wiles, J. (2010). Landscapes of care. *Progress in Human Geography, 34*(6), 736–754. doi:10.1177/0309132510364556

National Institute for Health and Care Excellence. (2014). Developing NICE guidelines: The manual. *NICE.* Retrieved from www.nice.org.uk/process/pmg20/chapter/introduction-and-overview

Nicholls, D. A., Atkinson, K., Bjorbækmo, W. S., Gibson, B. E., Latchem, J., Olesen, J., . . . Setchell, J. (2016). Connectivity: An emerging concept for physiotherapy practice. *Physiotherapy Theory and Practice, 32*(3), 159–170. doi:10.3109/09593985.2015.1137665

Nicholson, D. J., & Dupré, J. (Eds.). (2018). *Everything flows: Towards a processual philosophy of biology.* Oxford University Press. Retrieved from www.researchgate.net/publication/322836323_Everything_Flows_Towards_a_Processual_Philosophy_of_Biology

O'Connor, T., & Wong, H. Y. (2015, Summer). Emergent properties. In E. N. Zalta (Ed.), *The Stanford encyclopedia of philosophy.* Metaphysics Research Lab and Stanford University. Retrieved from https://plato.stanford.edu/archives/sum2015/entries/properties-emergent/

Pallesen, E. (2017). Documenting the invisible: On the "how" of process research: (Re)considering method from process philosophy. *Methodological Innovations, 10*(3), 1–10. doi:10.1177/2059799117745781

Parkhurst, J., & Abeysinghe, S. (2016). What constitutes "good" evidence for public health and social policy-making? From hierarchies to appropriateness. *Social Epistemology, 30*(5–6), 665–679. doi:10.1080/02691728.2016.1172365

Patterson, L. (2018, November 12). The salt: What's on your plate: Sourdough hands: How bakers and bread are a microbial match. *NPR.* Retrieved from www.npr.org/sections/thesalt/2018/11/12/665655220/sourdough-hands-how-bakers-and-bread-are-a-microbial-match?t=1577794577536

Rescher, N. (2000). *Process philosophy: A survey of basic issues.* University of Pittsburgh Press. doi:10.2307/j.ctt6wrc3b

Robertson, J., Baines, S., Emerson, E., & Hatton, C. (2016). Postural care for people with intellectual disabilities and severely impaired motor function: A scoping review. *Journal of Applied Research in Intellectual Disabilities, 31*(S1), 11–28. doi:10.1111/jar.12325

Rycroft-Malone, J., McCormack, B., Hutchinson, A. M., DeCorby, K., Bucknall, T. K., Kent, B., . . . Wilson, V. (2012). Realist synthesis: Illustrating the method for implementation research. *Implementation Science, 7*(33), 1–10. doi:10.1186/1748-5908-7-33

Sackett, D. L., Rosenberg, W. M., Gray, J. A., Haynes, R. B., & Richardson, W. S. (1996). Evidence based medicine: What it is and what it isn't. *BMJ, 312*(7023), 71–72. doi:10.1136/bmj.312.7023.71

Satterfield, J. M., Spring, B., Brownson, R. S., Mullen, E. J., Newhouse, R. P., Walker, B. B., & Whitlock, E. P. (2009). Towards a transdisciplinary model of evidence-based practice. *The Milbank Quarterly: A Multidisciplinary Journal of Population Health and Health Policy, 87*(2), 368–390. doi:10.1111/j.1468-0009.2009.00561.x.

Seibt, J. (2012, Summer). Stanford encyclopedia of philosophy: Process philosophy. In E. N. Zalta (Ed.), *The Stanford encyclopedia of philosophy*. The Metaphysics Research Lab and Stanford University. Retrieved from https://plato.stanford.edu/entries/process-philosophy

Seibt, J. (2018). The myth of substance and the fallacy of misplaced concreteness. In D. J. Nicholson & J. Dupré (Eds.), *Everything flows: Towards a processual philosophy of biology* (pp. 113–136). Oxford University Press. Retrieved from www.researchgate.net/publication/322836323_Everything_Flows_Towards_a_Processual_Philosophy_of_Biology

Shaw, J. A., Connelly, D. M., & Zecevic, A. A. (2010). Pragmatism in practice: Mixed methods research for physiotherapy. *Physiotherapy Theory and Practice, 26*(8), 510–518. doi:10.3109/09593981003660222

Steavenson, W. (2019, October 10). Flour power: Meet the bread heads baking a better load. *The Guardian*. Retrieved from www.theguardian.com/food/2019/oct/10/flour-power-meet-the-bread-heads-baking-a-better-loaf

St. Pierre, E. A. (1997). Methodology in the fold and the irruption of transgressive data. *Qualitative Studies in Education, 10*(2), 175–189. doi:10.1080/095183997237278

Thompson, H. E. (1997). The fallacy of misplaced concreteness: Its importance for critical and creative inquiry. *Interchange, 28*(2–3), 219–230. doi:10.1023/A:1007313324927

Urien, C., Legrand, J., Montalent, P., Casaregola, S., & Sicard, D. (2019). Fungal species diversity in French organic bread sourdoughs made of organic wheat flour. *Frontiers in Microbiology, 10*(201), 1–17. doi:10.3389/fmicb.2019.00201

Whitehead, A. (1978). *Process and reality*. New York: The Free Press.

Whitley, A. (2014, May 6). Sourdough: More than a bread, it's a philosophy. *Natural Health News*. Retrieved from www.naturalhealthnews.uk/article/sourdough-more-than-a-bread-its-a-philosophy

World Health Organization. (2001). *International classification of functioning, disability and health (ICF)*. World Health Organisation. Retrieved from www.who.int/classifications/icf/en/

World Health Organization. (2016). *Framework on integrated, people-centred health services*. World Health Organization. Retrieved from http://apps.who.int/gb/ebwha/pdf_files/WHA69/A69_39-en.pdf?ua=1&ua=1

# 8 Mâmawi-atoskêwin, "working together in partnership" – challenging Eurocentric physical therapy practice guided by Indigenous Métis worldview and knowledge

*Liris Smith, Sylvia Abonyi, Liz Durocher, TJ Roy, and Sarah Oosman*

> Note: We use Cree and Michif language throughout the chapter text. A glossary of terms and definitions is provided at the end of the chapter.

## Mâmawi ("altogether")

We acknowledge the traditional Indigenous territories that include treaty lands, unceded lands, and Métis homelands on which we (the authors) live, work, teach, and learn. We pay our respects to the First Nation, Métis, and Inuit ancestors of the land we currently call Canada and to all Indigenous ancestors of lands globally. We (the authors) engage in our work together on Treaty 6 and Treaty 10 territory and the Homeland of the Métis and affirm our commitment to respectful relationships with one another and the land that nurtures us all.

As we maintain that all things are relational, we begin our chapter in this book by describing who we are in relation to one another and to the research collaboration that informs the thoughts we share here on new epistemologies for physical therapy. We are five individuals, two of whom are Métis (LD, TJR) and three of whom are non-Métis (LS, SO, SA), with diverse cultural, historical, geographical, social, and academic backgrounds.

Liz (LD) is a third-generation Métis woman with French ancestry on her dad's side of the family. Her parents were from the community of Île-à-la-Crosse, and she is the 11th of 13 children. Before she was 5 years old, she was learning the Michif language and participating in many Métis cultural activities and practices that were taught to her by her parents, grandparents, aunties, uncles, and Elders. She is a social worker and community developer with a particular passion for working with young adults in her community.

TJ (TJR) is a Plains Cree and Métis man, having a bloodline with two rich cultures. His mom was a Cree First Nation woman from Canoe Lake and a Treaty

Indian; his dad was Métis with French and Irish heritage and a strong connection to the land. TJ grew up speaking Cree and Michif and engaging in rich Cree and Métis teachings, practices, and activities. TJ is a community developer who, in recent years, has worked closely with older adults and Elders in the community to address their diverse needs and build on strengths that exist within his community.

Together, Liz and TJ work to support wellness of Métis youth, young adults, and older adults in their northern Saskatchewan (Canada) Métis community and continue to emphasize the critical importance of teaching young Métis about their language and culture as they work through challenges in their lives. They believe strongly that young people need to learn from older adults, who are the knowledge keepers in the community, in order to keep Métis language and cultural practices strong and alive. In their partnership with us (LS, SO, SA), they integrate Métis culture, knowledge, and worldview in relation to the health and wellness of their community and ensure we privilege Métis perspectives.

Liris (LS) is a mother of two adults and a physical therapist who has worked for almost three decades in rural/remote/northern practice and leadership. She is a first-generation Canadian on her mother's side and third generation on her father's side. She is now a graduate student, working with older Métis adults to understand how they experience physical activity through their life journey. She believes that as physical therapists it is incumbent on us, when working within Indigenous communities, to use reflective practice within an ethical space of engagement and thereby find transformative ways to support health and wellness.

Sylvia (SA) is a first-generation Canadian, wife, mother of two boys, and a medical anthropologist at the University of Saskatchewan. She has worked closely with First Nation and Métis peoples and communities in Canada for most of her career, having received tremendous teaching and mentorship through these collaborations. The long-term relationships that have been developed have shaped her personal and professional contributions to redressing colonization impacts on the health and wellbeing of the first peoples of the land in which we live and work.

Sarah (SO) is a first-generation settler Canadian, mother of two children, a physical therapist, an associate professor (University of Saskatchewan, Canada), and an ally to Indigenous people and priorities. She has had the honour of working with Métis community members from northern Saskatchewan (Canada) for over 10 years and is on a continual learning journey in finding new and innovative ways to ground research and practice in ways that privilege Indigenous knowledge. She values the relationships with the first peoples and this land as she contributes to the practice of reconciliation necessary to enhance health equity in our country and around the globe.

As a group of five (niyânowak), we strive to do our work together in a safe, ethical space that honours our individual strengths and knowledge systems while respecting mutual morals, values, and boundaries (Ermine, 2007). We argue that we need to re-think/re-examine how physical therapists practise, research, and teach. This re-examination is particularly important in light of health inequities that disproportionately impact Indigenous peoples. Engaging within an ethical space, integrating the practice of cultural humility, and cultivating culturally safe environments are foundational to our collaborative research that supports and privileges the emergence of Métis worldview. This chapter describes our practices as niyânowak, which we feel are necessary for, and transferable to, clinical physical therapy practice when working with Indigenous peoples. Throughout the chapter, we examine the practice of physical therapy embedded in strong biomedical roots and suggest a layered concept of embodiment that may help us to evolve and grow the physical therapy profession in the context of Indigenous health. We highlight our process of engaging in an ethical space as a framework for integrating a new epistemology for physical therapy that recognizes different ways of knowing. Finally, we conclude by mobilizing knowledge shared in this chapter that was gained from our collaborative work to inform the practice and profession of physical therapy.

## Mâmawi-atoskêwin, "working together in partnership", in an ethical space

Our current partnership has developed over the past six years as we have collaborated on an intergenerational healthy aging in-place research project among the Métis peoples of Sakitawak Territory in northern Saskatchewan, Canada. Two of the authors (SO & SA) have been the academic co-leads on this project and travel to and from the northern Métis community of Île-à-la-Crosse up to 10 times per year. The community is located approximately 470 km northwest of Saskatchewan's largest urban centre, Saskatoon. It takes just over five hours to drive north from Saskatoon to Île-à-la-Crosse. The landscape changes from prairie and farmland to boreal forest speckled with lakes that are interconnected with rivers, a geographical representation of the transition to the north. More than this, LD and TJR mark the crossing into this boreal forest as coming home. For SO, LS, and SA these five hours and the terrain changes represent a space to mindfully transition our Euro-Western orientations to Métis values that include spending time in the community, visiting with Métis Elders and adults, and truly hearing the stories that inform our understanding of their aging experiences and aspirations. The community is on Treaty 10 Territory and the Sakitawak Métis homeland, situated at the meeting point of three rivers. In the Michif (Métis) language, Sakitawak means "where the rivers meet". The lakes and rivers define the Métis people of Sakitawak, as, historically, the water provided opportunities for travel and access to food and resources. Métis people from Île-à-la-Crosse have always built their own boats, canoes, and toboggans (particularly before road access), and this is a practice maintained to this day across generations. These activities represent the ethic of hard work and being self sufficient that are important to being Métis. Historically, the Sakitawak Métis have experienced a very different Canada to those of us who identify as settlers to this land. In addition, the Métis experience of colonization is different from First Nations and Inuit peoples, a distinction that is rarely recognized in a conflation of identity as collectively Aboriginal (Truth and Reconciliation Commission, 2015a). It is paramount that those of us who spend the large majority of time embedded in a Eurocentric worldview and practice setting (SO, SA, and LS) recognize the need to place such worldviews to the side in order to make space for the emergence of Métis worldview and perspectives such as those shared with us during our time in community. We are often greeted in Île-à-la-Crosse by our Métis co-authors, LD and TJR, who are deeply integrated into Sakitawak Métis culture, language, practice, and daily life. The tangible language translation that LD and TJR provide, for example, is on the surface just that, translating Michif and Cree to English and vice versa. However, these translations, which convey important concepts not readily captured in the English language, are also symbols of deeper-rooted bridges that are being built between us and the Métis community to support us in finding common ground (or ethical space).

Throughout this chapter, we will refer to the concept of ethical space that is defined by Indigenous lawyer Willy Ermine (2007). Ermine describes ethical space as the space that exists between two societies with distinctive worldviews, a space that contributes to the development of a framework to support relevant discussion to create new knowledge (2007). The ethical space creates opportunity for us to confront any hidden interests, attitudes, and assumptions that can influence communication and behaviours (Ermine, 2007). Meeting with LD and TJR is important to ensuring we work in a good way, grounded in uplifting Métis knowledge and experience, locating who we are and what we do together in a safe, ethical space.

Transitioning into an ethical space provides an example of what we, the academic members of the team, are continually working towards in our collaboration. These processes are not linear, simple, or easy to do in practice. Navigating between two worlds/worldviews is something that is required of Indigenous peoples daily and not a common experience among non-Indigenous peoples who function optimally in a dominant Eurocentric society. Practicing in a mindful, present way that is in a mutually beneficial ethical space means that we have to take a step back from our role as experts and recognize that there is essential knowledge, expertise, and lived experience in the Métis community that we do not have. In this chapter, we clarify the need for practicing in an ethical space and provide exemplars from our collaborative work of how we apply the ethical space concept. It is our responsibility, as non-Indigenous researchers and practitioners, to create a space for this essential Métis knowledge to emerge and inform our practice.

## Acknowledging the truths of colonization

Practising in an ethical space has provided our team a practical and rich approach to ensuring that we privilege Métis worldview over the more dominant Eurocentric perspective pervasive in society. As we have been doing this, it has become clearer that this approach is transferable to clinical practice. In order to clarify why practicing within an ethical space is necessary, we believe it is pertinent to share a brief background on the historical and political context of colonization and its impact on Indigenous peoples and their health and wellness.

In Canada, racism and discrimination stemming from colonization are entrenched throughout diverse social, cultural, and political systems, including the health system. The history of colonization in Canada, and its continued negative impact on the lives and health of Indigenous people, is too large to cover in the context of this chapter (Truth and Reconciliation Commission, 2015b). Therefore, we provide a list of suggested readings at the end of this chapter for those who may be interested in learning more. In brief, Indigenous peoples populated the territory currently known as Canada long before the arrival of European explorers and settlers (Employment and Social Development Canada (Beatty), 2018). The people who lived in this territory were diverse and autonomous, and each community and/or cultural group had its own name and identity for themselves and the peoples living around them. Each unique community maintained its own distinct language, culture, spirituality, beliefs, political system, and health system (Blackstock, 2009; Employment and Social Development Canada (Beatty), 2018; Indian and Northern Affairs Canada, 2002; Truth and Reconciliation Commission, 2015b). Although there is much diversity between Indigenous peoples and communities, there is a shared and common belief (Indigenous epistemology) that all things are interconnected and related, communal rights are prioritized, and the knowledge that is handed down from generation to generation is highly valued and passed forward in a sacred trust (Blackstock, 2009). Indigenous knowledge, philosophies, and systems of care successfully sustained Indigenous communities, families, and individuals until the arrival of the European settlers (Blackstock, 2009; Kovach, 2015). Colonization led to many efforts to eradicate Indigenous peoples through the intentional introduction of diseases, dislocation of Indigenous peoples from their lands and territories, and imposed restrictions on freedom of movement (Blackstock, 2009; Truth and Reconciliation Commission, 2015b). The Métis people were uniquely impacted by colonization through policies like 'scrip' designed to terminate Métis title and identity (University of Saskatchewan Archives, Our Legacy Kinanaskomitin, 2008) (University of Saskatchewan, 2008). Further, as land was opened to homesteading and settlers were given land to farm, Métis people were forced to retreat to live in shacks on 'road allowances' (30-foot-wide strips of government-owned land located on either side of a road) (Truth and Reconciliation Commission, 2015a). Indigenous peoples in Canada have endured (and continue to endure) a long history of trauma and loss as a result of colonization, racism, and discrimination, all of which have fragmented their family and kinship structures (Waldram, 1997; Roberts, 2013; Wesley-Esquimaux & Smolewski, 2004) and intergenerational knowledge transfer and negatively impacted their health and wellness over time. These historical truths included silencing Indigenous perspectives, voice, and worldview. Further, colonization has created health inequities such that Indigenous peoples experience greater health challenges that appear earlier in life and track into older adulthood (Wilson, Rosenberg, & Abonyi, 2011; Cooke & Long, 2016). Presently, Indigenous peoples and non-Indigenous allies are focused on revitalizing Indigenous knowledge systems and practices, cultures, and languages. Our health system and the physical therapy profession are implicated in this important process for improving Indigenous health and wellness.

There are epistemological, cultural, and linguistic strengths and strong spirit among the Sakitawak Métis that have been interrupted through colonization. However, there is a keen desire to 'come back to [our] Métis ways', to re-connect families and communities and young Métis people to their culture, language, and strengths of Métis perspectives of wellness. The teachings that are embedded in the Michif language and cultural practices are being revitalized, as they are all present in the community (maintained by knowledge keepers) and will inform healing and wellness of the Métis. As we (SO, SA, LS) learn to enter an ethical space as learners and listeners, and step away from roles of expert researchers/practitioners and doers, a space opens for Métis perspectives and worldview. This is the middle ground, the ethical space of engagement that our team functions within, which we believe is transferable to physical therapy practice.

## E-ti-miyoyat, "on a journey towards wellness" – enhancing physical therapy practice

An increasing interest in refining, re-defining, and evolving the physical therapy profession has been taking place over the past several years (Gibson, Nicholls, Setchell, & Groven, 2018; Dean, 2009a, 2009b) as health challenges become multifaceted and more complex. Physical therapy has much to offer individuals and populations in the realm of health promotion. However, there are a number of modifiable limitations that prevent physical therapy care and services from being accessible to all. Indigenous populations experience disproportionately greater health challenges compared to the general Canadian population, while at the same time, physical therapy services are not as accessible to Indigenous peoples. Changes at individual physical therapy practice and health system levels must take place, such as finding a path towards practising in an ethical space, in a culturally safe environment, and with cultural humility. Further to this is the need to re-examine the deeper epistemological underpinnings that inform physical therapy practice in order to evolve the profession in ways that are meaningful to the populations in most need of relevant physical therapy care.

In the following section, we demonstrate why physical therapists need to consider individual practice– and health systems–level change. Our research team not only focuses on capturing stories, experiences, and aspirations of aging among Métis Elders and adults, but we have also been inspired to create experiential learning practicum opportunities for physical therapy students within a community setting (Oosman et al., 2019). Physical therapy students spend four to six weeks in the Métis community of Île-à-la-Crosse in northern Saskatchewan (Canada), outside of a health facility and fully embedded in the community in an ethnographic-style placement. The details of the practicum are outlined elsewhere (Oosman et al., 2019). Physical therapy students are required to write field notes on their experiences. One pair of students had the opportunity to spend a small portion of their practicum in a local physical therapy department. These students observed several 'no shows' (individuals who have been booked but do not attend their appointment) while in clinic and initially described feeling frustrated that the community members 'did not bother to show up'. The assumptions underlying their initial response were evident in the tone and language of their field notes. As the students spent time in the community getting to know many Métis Elders and older adults throughout the duration of their community-based practicum, their reflections started to shift. They observed the strong kinship support that existed within the community; as one community member experienced hardship or required support, many others would step in and help out, often at the sacrifice of their own self-care (such as missing a physical therapy appointment). It did not take long for the physical therapy students to realize that the way care is delivered in the community is actually not in keeping with how Métis community members structure their everyday lives. They started asking questions like, "Why do we continue to deliver care in this way if we know it is not working?" When they explored this question in greater detail with the physical therapy practitioners in the neighbouring community, it became clear that the answer was complex. One of the reasons they grappled with was that the health system structures did not allow for a modified approach to service provision (as one reason of many). Furthermore, they also observed that the structure and function of the clinic/health facility was not the same as how people lived and accessed other community services on a daily basis. This led to an in-depth reflective discussion on the feeling of safety Indigenous peoples have/do not have as they enter into Eurocentric-dominant institutions (health facilities) that may bring back traumatic experiences from their past. As we debriefed their experiences and reflections, topics of practicing cultural humility and informing culturally safe health environments were explored as important factors in evolving the physical therapy profession and health system.

## Cultural humility and cultural safety support the creation of an ethical space in practice

In our work, we take time to listen to stories shared by Métis Elders, stories that reignite Métis knowledge and practices. We have learned that we do not merely interview an Elder one time and expect to capture their story of wellness and aging, but rather we are invited back repeatedly to listen to numerous stories over periods of time. We are often told, "I will tell you more next time", which is an invitation and also mentorship to us that there is more to the story, the story is not finished, and there is an expectation that we will continue to engage. It is not up to us, the academic researchers, to decide whether enough information has been gathered in order to move forward (such as is the practice when taking a subjective history in clinic), but rather the decision is made by community members. As we spend time in the (Métis) community, we have learned to create space for just being present in the community without an agenda or a task-list of data that needs to be collected. An Indigenous approach is one that can bring both Indigenous and non-Indigenous scholars to move beyond the binary approach to place of mutual dialogue and action (Kovach, 2009; Canadian Institutes of Health Research, 2010; Ermine, Sinclair, & Jeffery, 2004). We are continually taught and guided by community members that we cannot rush this important work and the messages/teachings they are sharing with us. Instead, we now sit back and "be" in order to listen, observe, and hear Métis voices share their perspectives of meaningful and culturally relevant solutions. Using Michif and Cree words, they share their vision and support a different way of thinking, which relocates and centralizes expertise between practitioner and community members. We now spend more time at the kitchen table, sharing tea; attending cultural gatherings; and observing movement, health, and well-being in the broader sense of community.

This engagement is different than traditional physical therapy interactions and provides examples of how our team practices cultural humility. Stepping out of the Eurocentric practices that we have been trained within and being open to approaching practice in ways that are guided by a Métis perspective, practice that is more aligned with what Métis community members expect, is how we exemplify cultural humility. Cultural humility requires time for consistent self-critique and self-reflection in order to examine the role a practitioner/researcher may play in perpetuating or mitigating racism and discrimination (Oosman et al., 2019; Beagan, 2015). It requires a lifelong commitment to self-critique in order to redress power imbalances that often exist in relationships between practitioners and clients (Oosman et al., 2019; Tervalon & Murray-Garcia, 1998). Cultural humility supports the deconstruction, or "decolonization", of underlying assumptions and aspects of practice that practitioners assume to be true but are actually perpetuating racism, discrimination, and the creation of unsafe cultures of care. Bringing the physical therapy student experience back into light, as they described the tension in clinic when individuals chose not to show up for a clinical appointment, a culturally humble approach would be to pause, to avoid jumping to the conclusion that the individual did not value the physical therapist's time (or treatment), but rather create space to better understand the situation from a different perspective. Engage with the individual in ways that strengthen the relationship, that do not impose judgement but create opportunities for conversation to gather their narrative and experience in order to learn about Métis lived experience, including culture, language and practice, and what Métis wellness looks like for them (in the moment). The reality of what today looks like is fluid and may look quite different tomorrow. If judgements are made, these will continue to create barriers to accessing physical therapy (PT) care/services for Métis community members.

We have discovered that as we create a safe space for conversation and dialogue, and with sharing back-and-forth over time, that Métis knowledge emerges and ancestral knowledge is revitalized. As Métis knowledge emerges, excitement to share this knowledge and move it forward becomes a priority within the community. Métis Elders and youth share stories that give us teachings and messages in different ways that must be shared; it is through gatherings and recurrent conversations that Métis practices re-emerge and are shared with the younger generation. There is a wealth of knowledge in the community, so it is not always relevant to tell community members how to be well, but rather it is supporting them to bring their strengths and knowledge to inform holistic wellness. This practice of repeated conversations, spending time with people, and the importance of gathering and sharing has informed our research practices and methodologies, all of which are relevant to informing how physical therapists practice in Indigenous communities. Developing long-term, long-lasting relationships with community members builds a trusting healing environment.

Interestingly, as practitioners develop cultural humility skills, there is a strong link to creating culturally safe health environments and spaces. Many physical therapy services require clients to enter health environments/facilities that do not always feel comfortable or culturally safe. Healthcare facilities typically represent Eurocentric, government-led institutions that are reminiscent of the past and have potential to ignite trauma associated with historical colonized acts. This, in turn, limits access to care for many Indigenous people. Furthermore, in current Eurocentric models of care, time is limited in appointments and does not create a climate of trust to be established, which, in turn, greatly impedes therapeutic relationship building and comfortable (safe) health contexts. Indigenous knowledge systems and practice see time and experiences as not being separated or compartmentalized as they are in Eurocentric cultures (Duran & Duran, 2000; Little Bear, 2000). A Eurocentric care model of service delivery, with a structured, time-limited approach, with set appointments and limited tolerance for lateness for appointments, may be challenging to Indigenous peoples seeking care. These policies and practices maintain the power imbalances that are inherent in our healthcare system, creating inequitable and limited access to physical therapy services for Indigenous peoples. Practicing cultural humility within these care settings is an important first step in learning how practitioners and health managers can modify how health services are delivered in ways that are culturally responsive and relevant to Indigenous ways of doing and knowing. Honouring and developing relationships and connections through the practice of cultural humility is an essential step in providing relevant and respectful healthcare services for Indigenous peoples. This may take more time and energy, which does not often fit within our current system of public and/or private healthcare provision.

In our current healthy aging work, we have been guided through a learning process informed by Métis worldview where observing, listening, and doing occur simultaneously (Wilson, 2008; Smith, 1999; Roberts, 2013). We have heard stories from Elders and older adults that share experiences and aspirations for aging well while being taught how to bead moose hide. We have been taught words in Cree and Michif while learning how to make bannock or to filet fish. We have also heard about experiences of growing up and aging well from the Métis youth while sewing medicine bags and working with our hands and on the land. It became clear that the richness of information shared among Elders, researchers, and community members was enhanced when learning was created and guided in an active way by Métis community members. These contexts for learning/engagement ensured opportunities for reciprocity, to share knowledge and to receive knowledge, that supported mutual learning (Kovach, 2009; Canadian Institutes of Health Research, 2010; Kovach, 2015). The use of Cree and Michif languages is an important way in which Métis knowledge, practice, and culture is passed down to the next generation. As language is spoken and knowledge is shared, they become internalized and embedded among Métis youth and young adults, thus securing Métis ways of knowing and doing, the Métis social code of conduct (Little Bear, 2000). Seeking to learn and understand language is an essential skill within physical therapy practice when working in Indigenous communities. This can be done through learning

106  *Liris Smith* et al.

basic words and turning to community members to seek the meaning of terms, phrases, and customs. Reciprocal sharing of knowledge, rather than simply imparting our biomedical knowledge onto an individual, and being open to diverse treatment practices can support good relationships and honouring of cultural practices, including traditional medicines and therapies. We can create an ethical space in practice if physical therapists use action-oriented skills to engage in activities and conversations that are meaningful to the Métis people seeking treatment, by doing activities together and by spending more time listening and practicing reciprocity.

To this point, we have introduced the idea of improving physical therapy practice with Indigenous peoples through engagement in an ethical space, offering some of our experiences of what that looks like in a practical way. The encounters with knowledge that take place there suggest we need to think more deeply about what that knowledge means and how it is constructed. This is the epistemological challenge that the PT profession faces. Epistemology is about how we come to know what we believe to be real and is embedded in iterative interactions between the knower and the known. This process of knowing and finding out is guided by characteristics, principles, and assumptions that merit reflection. We turn now to a consideration of epistemology in physical therapy and suggest a means to advance our knowledge and view of reality in an ethical space that also includes Indigenous epistemologies.

## Miyo-mâmti-nitsigan, "thinking clearly in a good way towards wellness" – evolving physical therapy practice towards embodiment

Re-examining the deeper epistemological underpinnings that inform PT practice and approaches requires a brief summary of the history and the strong biomedical values informing the physical therapy profession. Physiotherapy in Canada is almost 100 years old, is based on a European model of isolated and specialized training, and remains relatively unchanged since its inception (Cameron, 2011; Nicholls, 2018). Physiotherapists acknowledge that their training is fundamentally biomedical and biomechanical in nature (Sanders, 2014). Biomedicine gained prominence in the 19th century when biological, objective experimentation (in laboratories) was applied to treatment and healing practices within public health (Quirke & Gaudilliere, 2008). Standardization of medical practice emerged as the dominant biomedical approach to healthcare which also dissociated the human body from the reality of peoples' lives and lived experiences (Lock & Nguyen, 2018). The binaries of "normal"/"not normal", and "well"/"not well" silenced diversity, including the social, cultural, and political factors that influence health. These binaries have been recently critiqued as problematic in a variety of diverse situations by several authors in the first critical physical therapy reader, *Manipulating Practices: A Critical Physiotherapy Reader* (Gibson et al., 2018). While biomedicine honours new knowledge developed through innovation and discovery, it places little value on knowledge brought forward from the past. Numerous biomedical technologies developed with the assumption they would be universally effective in promoting health, preventing disease, and diagnosing and treating diseases and disabilities (Lock & Nguyen, 2018). Biomedical philosophy and knowledge underpin physical therapy practice at the individual level and also inform the design and policies that are enacted within our health system. A limitation of a biomedical and biomechanical approaches is that they focus on health and wellness of a physical body but do not account for sociopolitical or cultural factors that are expressed through that body. In more recent years, PT has also embraced the biopsychosocial (BPS) model, which has broadened the perspective of the profession to include elements beyond the biomechanical framework (Nicholls, 2018). The BPS model suggests that there is an interconnection between an individual's biology, psychology, and socioenvironmental factors that all, in turn, influence an individual's health (Bath, 2015; Borrell-Carrio, Suchman & Epstein, 2004). The BPS model is also informed by Eurocentric knowledge paradigms and epistemology, similar to the underpinnings of the biomedical model that work within a structured classification system based on norms and binaries that silence unique and diverse cultures and worldviews (Nicholls, 2018). Further, as with the biomedical model, the BPS model does not necessarily account for the context of colonization, racism, and discrimination that are often invisible and that influence perceptions of health and wellness. It is helpful, here, to think of these factors as becoming embodied, which provides the means to conceptualize and integrate understandings of the lived sociocultural experiences that shape individuals' perception and experience of their bodies, their self, and their self-expression (Nettleton, 2005).

The concept of embodiment extends the physical body beyond its biological, anatomical, and physiological limits to encompass the idea that the body is also socially constructed and shaped by social, cultural, political, and economic forces (Nettleton, 2005; Hughes & Lock, 1987; Nicholls & Gibson, 2010). Applying an anthropological lens, Dr. Margaret Lock describes the body as being made up of three bodies: (1) the individual body (made up of the body, mind, psyche, soul, self, and their relations to one another), (2) the social body (the role of the body as a symbol in nature, society, and culture), and (3) the political body (referring to the regulation, monitoring, and control of individual and collective bodies). Others have applied the concept of these three bodies to health and wellness (Fox, 1999; Williams, 2006; Williams, 2003) and more recently within the profession of physical therapy (Nicholls & Gibson, 2010; Hay, Connelly, & Kinsella, 2016). These three threads are interconnected and embodied in individual and collective experiences, behaviours, and perceptions of health and wellness. For Métis and Indigenous people, the political body includes the impact of colonization. The social body is expressed through language and practices that reflect both a quotidian lived reality linked to social determinants of health and the revitalization of Métis culture and its transmission between generations. In addition to the individual body, which is the usual purview of physical therapy practice, a new epistemology would also acknowledge and account for these other bodies. Physical therapists are movement specialists, focusing on the outward physical movement of the human body, and although the biological requirement of movement for the human body is universal, the cultural and political context of how activity or movement is perceived, defined, and measured is not universal. An epistemology of the three bodies is one way to expand or enhance a biomedical and biomechanical approach to understanding movement and providing care.

Health and wellness for Métis people, for example, requires an intergenerational approach that honours relationships with one another and the land, and the Michif language holds many essential teachings that have been passed down from previous generations. These concepts, also highlighted by other Indigenous scholars in Canada (Blackstock, 2011; Wilson, 2008; Ermine et al., 2004), embody wellness in the community, where wellness is not just physical wellness but is also informed by relationships and kinships (whakotowin), relationship to the land, practices and protocols, and sharing and helping one another, whether it be through sharing of story, cultural teachings, living on the land, and/or procuring food. It is also important to note that when Métis people seek healthcare in health facilities that are designed and structured in a primarily Eurowestern worldview, Métis perspectives are often marginalized, and the experience is framed within a sociopolitical context of colonization (both of which impede delivery of optimal care). Biomedicine and the application of a predominantly biomechanical approach to treatment does not privilege, acknowledge, or recognize the diverse constructs of Métis health and wellness that are at play in an interrelated way through all three bodies.

As niyânowak, we reflect on our collaborative healthy aging research, where we are working in an ethical space that is laying the foundation for bringing different worldviews together. We have come to appreciate the layered complexity that is embodied in the Métis individuals and peoples with whom we work. The epistemology of three bodies is helpful for us in a health research role, and we believe can also be helpful as the physical therapy profession reshapes itself to better meet the health treatment and promotion needs of Indigenous peoples.

## Miyo-kisinahamowat – mobilizing knowledge to improve physical therapy practice

Our team has practice recommendations that physical therapists (and researchers and other healthcare providers) may find helpful when engaging with Indigenous communities and providing healthcare services in Indigenous communities:

- Be visible and present in the community; be physically present;
- Build trusting relationship(s) with a local individual in the community. When people see someone from the community whom they trust engaging in the work, then others will be more comfortable engaging in collaborative work as well;
- Be open to community cultural practices and participate in these with community members; this builds insight into how people live and function day to day;
- Learn some of the words and key phrases from Cree and Michif languages that are relevant to health and wellbeing; listen to people in the community using their traditional language and be curious; culture goes hand in hand with language, so the more you understand, the deeper your comprehension of cultural concepts;

- Work collaboratively with a local community member to provide language translation support and enhance communication within the community;
- Consider "opening" yourself up and share your own lived experiences and stories to support relationship and rapport building;
- Consider how people in community access services and care in ways that are meaningful for them and try to apply these learnings to your own practice and service delivery; consider wellness booths at a community event to expand beyond in-clinic appointments;
- Gather (Kehokatowin) with community members and connect with community members in this way; good things happen when people gather and share stories and knowledge;
- Bring multiple generations together to enhance wellness across diverse generations;
- Expand activities and treatment to the land; the water and the trees are healing, and being on the land can support health, wellness, and healing;
- Engage in cultural activities as you share and receive knowledge; and
- Be comfortable with uncertainty.

In this chapter, we have highlighted how our current health service provision in Canada is clearly not meeting the needs of Indigenous people, and the physical therapy profession must consider an evolution in its practice. In order to support health equity and universal access to healthcare for all citizens in Canada, physical therapists must critically re-examine the dominant Euro-centric paradigms embedded in physical therapy practice. Changing physical therapy practice in partnership with Indigenous communities and individuals is at the heart of evolving practice. The physical therapy profession has a responsibility to dismantle underlying assumptions and aspects of practice that many assume to be true but are actually perpetuating racism, discrimination, and the creation of unsafe cultures of care. This is possible by creating an openness to change within physical therapy, to "expose the taken-for-granted truths" (Gibson et al., 2018, p. 21), to challenge how we approach assessment, prescription, treatment, and intervention design in the context of Indigenous worldview. Not only is this practice evolution ethically important as the physical therapy profession strives to be accessible to all, the evolution is necessary in the colonized context in Canada. All citizens and professions in Canada are being challenged at a societal level by the Truth and Reconciliation Commission of Canada's Calls to Action to do better.

## Glossary of Michif and Cree terms

**E-ti-miyoyat.**   Moving forward, getting well; to make an effort to be well; a general statement of wellness; starting to change into wellness; on the journey towards wellness; being well/achieving wellness over time

**Kehokatowin.**   Gathering to share and communicate; gathering here and there to be well

**Mâmawi.**   All together

**Mâmawi-atoskêwin.** Working together in partnership
**Miyo-kisinahamowat.** Passing on teachings of wellness; sharing positive teachings
**Miyo mahcihowin.** Physical, mental, emotional, and spiritual wellness
**Miyo mâmti-nitsigan.** Thinking clearly in a good/positive way; thinking wellness
**Niyânowak.** A group of five; our group of five
**Pimatsiwin.** Living a good life; living in a good way; being grounded
**Sakitawak.** Where the rivers meet
**Whakhotowin.** Family; community; kinship

## References

Bath, B. (2015). Biopsychosocial predictors of short-term success among people with low back pain referred to a physiotherapy spinal triage service. *Journal of Pain Research, 8*, 189–202.

Beagan, B. L. (2015). Approaches to culture and diversity: A critical synthesis of occupational therapy literature. *Canadian Journal of Occupational Therapy, 82*, 272–282.

Borrell-Carrio, F., Suchman, A. L., & Epstein, R. M. (2004). The biopsychosocial model 25 years later: Principles, practice and scientific Inquiry. *Annals of Family Medicine, 2*(6), 576–582.

Blackstock, C. (2009). The occasional evil of angels: Learning from the experiences of Aboriginal peoples and social work. *First Peoples Child and Family Review, 4*, 28–37.

Blackstock, C. (2011). The emergence of the breath of life theory. *Journal of Social Work Values and Ethics, 8*.

Cameron, A. (2011). Impermeable boundaries? Developments in professional and interprofessional practise. *Journal of Interprofessional Care, 25*, 53–58.

Canadian Institutes of Health Research. (2010). *Tri-council policy statement: Ethical conduct for research involving humans* (G. O. Canada, Ed., Chapter 9). Ottawa, CA: Canadian Institutes of Health Research.

Cooke, M., & Long, D. (2016). A way forward in efforts to support the health and well-being of Canada's Aboriginal peoples. In D. Long & O. P. Dickason (Eds.), *Visions of the heart: Issues involving Aboriginal peoples in Canada* (4th ed.). Don Mills, ON: Oxford University Press.

Dean, E. (2009a). Physical therapy in the 21st century (Part 1): Toward practice informed by epidemiology and the crisis of lifestyle conditions. *Physiotherapy Theory & Practice, 25*, 330–353.

Dean, E. (2009b). Physical therapy in the 21st century (Part II): Evidence-based practice within the context of evidence-informed practice. *Physiotherapy Theory & Practice, 25*, 354–368.

Duran, B., & Duran, E. (2000). *Applied postcolonial clinical and research strategies.* Vancouver, BC: University of British Columbia Press.

Employment and Social Development Canada (Beatty, B.). (2018). *Social isolation of seniors: A focus on Indigenous seniors in Canada.* Canada.

Ermine, W. (2007). The ethical space of engagement. *Indigenous Law Journal, 6*, 193–203.

Ermine, W., Sinclair, R., & Jeffery, B. (2004). *The ethics of research involving Indigenous peoples: Report of the Indigenous Peoples' Health Research Centre to the Interagency Advisory Panel on Research Ethics (PRE).* Regina, SK: Indigenous Peoples' Health Research Centre.

Fox, N. (1999). *Beyond health: Postmodernism and embodiment.* London, UK: Free Association Books.

Gibson, B., Nicholls, D., Setchell, J., & Groven, K. S. (2018). Working against the grain: Criticality for an otherwise physiotherapy. In B. Gibson, D. Nicholls, J. Setchell, & K. S. Groven (Eds.), *Manipulating practises: A critical physiotherapy reader.* Oslo, NO: Nordic Open Access Scholarly Publishing.

Hay, M., Connelly, D., & Kinsella, E. (2016). Embodiment and aging in contemporary physiotherapy. *Physiotherapy Theory & Practice, 32,* 241–250.

Hughes, N., & Lock, M. (1987). The mindful body. *Medical Anthropology Quarterly, New Series, 1.*

Indian and Northern Affairs Canada, I. (2002). *Words first, an evolving terminology relating to Aboriginal peoples in Canada.* Ottawa, CA: Government of Canada.

Kovach, M. (2009). *Indigenous methodologies: Characteristics, conversations, and contexts.* Toronto, ON: University of Toronto Press.

Kovach, M. (2015). Emerging from the margins: Indigenous methodologies. In S. Strega & L. Brown (Eds.), *Research as resistance: Revisiting critical, indigenous, and anti-oppressive approaches.* Toronto, ON: Canadian Scholars' Press.

Little Bear, L. (2000). *Jagged worlds colliding.* Vancouver, CA: University of British Columbia Press.

Lock, M., & Nguyen, V.-K. (2018). *An anthropology of biomedicine.* Oxford, UK: Wiley-Blackwell.

Nettleton, S. (2005). The sociology of the body. In C. WC (Ed.), *The Blackwell companion to medical sociology.* London, UK: Blackwell.

Nicholls, D. (2018). *The end of physiotherapy.* Abingdon, UK: Routledge.

Nicholls, D., & Gibson, B. (2010). The body and physiotherapy. *Physiotherapy Theory & Practice, 26,* 497–509.

Oosman, S., Durocher, L., Roy, T., Nazarali, J., Potter, J., Schroeder, L., Sehn, M., . . . Abonyi, S. (2019). Essential elements for advancing cultural humility through a community-based physical therapy practicum in a Métis community. *Physiotherapy Canada, 71,* 146–157.

Quirke, V., & Gaudilliere, J. P. (2008). The era of biomedicine: Science, medicine, and public health in Britain and France after the Second World War. *Medical History, 52,* 441–452.

Roberts, R. (2013). *Connection to the land as a health determinant.* Saskatchewan, CA: Canadian Nuclear Safety Commission Participant Funding Program.

Sanders, T., Bie Nio, O., Sowden, G., & Foster, N. (2014). Implementing change in physiotherapy: Professions, contexts and interventions. *Journal of Health, Organization and Management, Bradford, 28,* 96–114.

Smith, L. (1999). *Decolonizing methodologies: Research and Indigenous peoples.* Dunedin, Nea Zealand: Zed.

Tervalon, M., & Murray-Garcia, J. (1998). Cultural humility versus cultural competence: A critical distinction in defining physician training outcomes in multicultural education. *Journal of Health Care Poor Underserved, 9,* 117–125.

Truth and Reconciliation Commission. (2015a). *Canada's residential schools: The Métis experience.* Montreal and Kingston: McGill-Queens University Press.

Truth and Reconciliation Commission. (2015b). *Truth and Reconciliation Commission of Canada: Calls to action.* Winnipeg: Man.

University of Saskatchewan Archives. (2008). *Our legacy Kinanaskomitin.* Saskatoon, Saskatchewan: University of Saskatchewan.

Waldram, J. B. (1997). *The way of the pipe*. Peterborough, ON: Broadview Press.

Wesley-Esquimaux, C. C., & Smolewski, M. (2004). *Historic trauma and Aboriginal healing*. Ottawa, ON: Aboriginal Healing Foundation.

Williams, S. (2003). *Medicine and the body*. London, UK: Sage Publications.

Williams, S. (2006). Medical sociology and the biological body: Where are we now and where do we go from here? *Health, 10*, 5–30.

Wilson, K., Rosenberg, M. W., & Abonyi, S. (2011). Aboriginal peoples, health and healing approaches: The effects of age and place on health. *Social Science & Medicine, 72*, 355–364.

Wilson, S. (2008). *Research is ceremony: Indigenous research methodologies*. Black Point, NS: Fernwood.

# 9 Feeling good about yourself? An exploration of FitBit "new moms community" as an emergent space for online biosociality

*Alma Viviana Silva Guerrero and Wendy Lowe*

## Introduction

The rise of technologically mediated exercise provides a challenge for physiotherapists because professional boundaries can become blurred with the personal and patients can negotiate their own way through rehabilitation and perhaps may trust traditional healthcare providers less (Setchell, Nicholls, Wilson, & Gibson, 2018). Traditional assumptions (held by physiotherapists) that they are the best providers of post-baby recovery assessment and treatment are challenged by technologically savvy mothers who prefer to engage with online communities via devices like the now ubiquitous FitBit wearable device and its supporting apps. This chapter engages with critical scholarship on the subject of FitBit communities by exploring the sociological and philosophical literature exploring how physiotherapists engage critically with the technological material and reflecting on participants' technological, cultural, material, and social aspects of fitness practice. We will explore notions of competition and self-policing to re-conceptualise how physiotherapists can engage with the world of technologically mediated exercise. By doing so, we hope to challenge taken-for-granted assumptions, and therefore power, around expert versus novice knowledge (Eakin, 2016).

One of the main motivations for writing this chapter was the recent motherhood experience of one of the authors (AVS). Having trained as a physiotherapist but also finding some of the biomedical language used by health professionals dehumanising and depersonalising, I felt ambivalent about physiotherapy when applying what I knew I should do as a new mother. However, when I turned to FitBit to increase my fitness post-delivery, I felt challenged by the competitive online environment and worried that participants could do more harm than good. I struggled to reconcile these different perspectives. This struggle is explored in the following text, with the acknowledgement that the biomedical scaffolding is useful in some respects, yet it is not the whole story. In our experience, this is a common struggle for healthcare professionals – how to write and live different discourses once exposed to wider horizons of knowledge. Whilst FitBit provides an opportunity for user empowerment, the users' perceptions of themselves as empowered consumers may be at odds with the sense that their subjectivity is being co-opted by these types of technology.

In addition, the second author (WL) also struggled with integrating knowledge from different disciplines. I went from physiotherapist, to researcher, to educator, and completed my PhD on health professional training drawing on critical pedagogy and sociology. In practice, I went from a biomedical domination to the opposite end of the spectrum, decrying all neo-liberalism and instead identifying with a post-structuralist deconstruction of healthcare. However, now I am working in a medical school, I have been challenged again by having to bring sociology into my teaching whilst grappling with the context that does not always appreciate this perspective (Lowe, 2018). Relating different paradigms to each other is hard and is much easier when outside the location one is critiquing. But I recognise that this is a crucial movement, a process which deserves commitment if we are to change healthcare for the benefit of patients and marginalised people.

This work is unique because it brings together the critical scholarly work on online communities, fitness, motherhood, and our health professional perspectives. To our knowledge, there has been no critical scholarship in the physiotherapy field to date that examines the interaction between health professional perspectives and mothers' use of a FitBit app. This is in spite of digital eHealth being seen as a panacea for organisational issues across many sectors of present and future healthcare (Blixt, Solbrække, & Bjorbækmo, 2019).

## What is the FitBit 'New Moms' community?

FitBit's 'New Moms' community has a dual character. First, it is a fitness app connected through a wearable device, essentially a digital watch with motion-tracking capabilities, and second, it is an online discussion forum. This means that users can access a peer community with the benefits of sharing experiences and finding support from others (Lupton & Maslen, 2019), whilst also monitoring their heart rate, steps taken, and other physiological events in a practice of self-digitised self-tracking. However, the nature of this dual characteristic of both self-monitoring and social support actively engenders a competitive environment through the achievements of targets such as the 'Workweek Hustle' or the 'Weekend Warrior'. The competitiveness in these campaigns contrasts with a less overtly competitive approach traditionally taken by physiotherapists.

Here we come to our first exploration of assumptions underpinning practice from a critical scholarship perspective. The words in use for FitBit tend to be framed in terms of pushing, aggression, fight, hero, bravery, courage, and strength. These words imply that fitness is something to be fought for, in a duel, with one ultimate winner. The assumption for FitBit is that one cannot become fit without being in a battle, against the self or others, which could include family or members of the online community. For example, the following text message highlights the nature of the battle:

> I wanted to keep walking today. I was close to 10,000 steps! But it was getting hot and bubs needed to nurse. I'm sure the FitBit doesn't account for these needs. So, what wins: good motherhood or fit motherhood? I know this is a

ridiculous binary, but I'm still left feeling guilty. The power of the discursive pressing upon my every day!

(Clark & Thorpe, 2019, p. 6)

Clark and Thorpe (2019) are well aware of the way in which they describe their dilemma in terms of a binary. These structuring binaries make situations into an either/or choice, with one choice usually taking precedence over the other, and by these choices, making structures or habits of practice.

Another binary is that healthcare tends to be spoken about as caring; caring for and caring about, as Julianne Cheek argues, 'Here, care is often reduced to what must be done to people in order to care for them' (Cheek, 1999, p. 61). There are expectations about how carers will behave as well as cultural and social expectations of what is normal and what is right. Further, there are what are described as 'soft' cultural supplements that bridge the gap between binaries such as those between biological representations of illness and subjective aspects of the lived experience, such as walking or exercise (Kristeva, Moro, Odemark, & Engebretsen, 2018).

Both of these sets of assumptions show the 'effect *of* cultural systems of values *on* health outcomes' (Kristeva et al., 2018; emphasis original). These sets of assumptions reinforce the divide between objective and subjective data in both the FitBit and health professional realms. The compartmentalization of knowledge and information is perhaps motivated by a need to reduce internal conflict; yet the paradox is that it may actually increase the battle between different perspectives. Both sets of assumptions limit internal coherence, are subject to confirmation bias (about being a warrior vs being a carer), and are implicitly seen through a lens of relevance to participants' lives.

For example, FitBit targets are often conceptualized as 'competitions' that promote exercise. From a physiotherapy perspective, these exercises are in opposition to, or in competition with, caring for women who are vulnerable in a post-operative post-delivery period. The biomedical evidence shows that a slower walking speed and strategies to evenly distribute loads over the sides of the body may be beneficial for their pelvic floor muscles. In addition, walking has been added to a short list of vital functions including heartbeat, respiration, blood pressure, and temperature. But these ideas can be in opposition to the need to belong to a community focused on achieving steps and winning competitions. These different discourses on exercise and walking compete with each other for dominance in the mind of the beholder.

## *Motherhood and mothering*

Further assumptions that require unpacking are those surrounding motherhood. Whilst this is a vast field of scholarly activity, we have chosen to focus on the different imperatives that act upon mothers and are themselves acted upon by mothers. Simone de Beauvoir asks us to consider 'What is a woman?'(De Beauvoir, 1997, p. 15). Likewise, we are compelled to consider 'What is a mother?' since there are biological, cultural, and social imperatives that act on women to produce the materiality of the (mother's) body. Moreover, these imperatives intersect with other social categories, such as social class, to produce ideals to which women feel they must conform (Lupton, 2012, p. 102). For example, whilst women from middle classes may speak about health from the point of view of participating in exercise, eating the right food, and being fit and active, many of those from the working class talk more about survival and getting through the day without feeling ill (Lupton, 2012). Therefore, the types of activities engaged in by women show an intersection between gender and class, as well as other sociodemographic characteristics. These imperative ideas intersect with the assumptions explored previously about competitive fitness and caring, in addition to gender identity and professional roles.

Our interest in this research focused on the dynamic between health professional advice and motherhood. Stewart (2020) suggested that mothers are set up to fail by the prevailing intensive mothering ideology which appears to escalate unrealistic and idealistic standards: these are impossible to meet, and so they lead to feelings of guilt and inadequacy. Her research demonstrates that the dynamic between a professional (social worker) and a mother serves to reinforce the ideology of intensive mothering and that this ideology is both the norm and the mechanism through which women do as they are expected.

Part of the intensive mothering ideology is the notion that mothers must focus solely on children (Stewart, 2020). Intensive mothering fits within neo-liberal ideas of individual responsibility and risk management and is based on middle-class values of self-governance and self-improvement (Stewart, 2020). At the same time as this emphasis on individual autonomy, there is a cut in social welfare budgets and state responsibility for collective social problems, such as poverty or inequalities in health (Romagnoli & Wall, 2012).

There is also an increased policy focus on risk and risk management through the preventive identification of, and intervention with, high-risk groups (Romagnoli & Wall, 2012). Children are seen as most at risk and therefore in greater need of increasing protection from these risks. Further, there are increasing portrayals of parents as risk factors in children's lives, which only serves to multiply the mechanisms through which prescriptive, regulative risk targeting, education, and surveillance interventions act.

Therefore, health professionals may find themselves co-opted by neo-liberal policies to not only identify so-called high-risk groups but also to intervene in ways that perpetuate a middle-class intensive ideology when applied to new mothers. One of the ways in which this co-option can be manifested is through the disappearance of the subject – the mother – with the health professional focus being on a cluster of risk factors. Health professionals would do well to understand how their training has inculcated them to follow prevailing norms and how they are potentially a reinforcing factor for ideologies that may unwittingly intensify the sense of the mothers' being at risk. One of the ways in which health professionals can work against this tide is by understanding the experience of mothers from their own perspective, which is inextricably embedded in the context of their lives (Romagnoli & Wall, 2012). This is particularly necessary for disadvantaged people, embedded in poverty, whose experiences do not necessarily fit the health professionals' messages, where diet and exercise are oversold clinically as remedies for chronic illness (Mendenhall, 2019). But this is a tricky dilemma for health professionals, knowing, on the one hand, that these biomedical solutions can work to address features of an illness, and thereby improve quality of life and, on the other hand, not wanting to be complicit with a neo-liberal regime that relies on individual self-management or improvement and risk reduction. Perhaps the key to moving forward is understanding the reductionism inherent in both perspectives?

Therefore, this research questioned how new mothers used the FitBit community to increase their motivation to return to pre-baby fitness levels, what some of the consequences of this were, and how physiotherapists can critically engage with and learn from FitBit communities to address the perspectives of new mothers. We drew on praxiography (Bueger, 2013; Bueger & Gadinger, 2018; Clever & Ruberg, 2014; Kingod, 2018; Littig, 2013) in order to specifically include the materiality of the body in how new mothers managed the dilemmas they were faced with.

Thirteen participants agreed to take part and allowed access to their online postings over a period of four months from June to September 2019. From those whose country could be identified, participants were from the United States (69%), Canada (8%), and Australia (8%). Ages ranged from 23 to 42 years, whilst the number of children for each mother ranged from one to three. Table 9.1 shows the participant characteristics in full. We identified three main categories of comments – 'competition', 'wanting to feel good about yourself', and 'enjoying their senses and/or physical accomplishments'.

*Table 9.1* Participant characteristics.

| Participant number | Age | Location | # kids | Average number of steps per day | Member of other FitBit communities | Member since pregnancy or before | Number of friends in the community |
|---|---|---|---|---|---|---|---|
| 1 | 35 | USA | 1 | 12,819 | N | N | 157 |
| 2 | 42 | Australia | 2 | 8,362 | N | N | 26 |
| 3 | 29 | Canada | 1 | 8,565 | Y | N | 80 |
| 4 | | | | 5,687 | N | N | 9 |
| 5 | | USA | | 6,947 | N | N | 13 |
| 6 | 38 | USA | 2 | 7,358 | Y | N | 30 |
| 7 | 25 | USA | 3 | 4,914 | Y | Y | 27 |
| 8 | | USA | 1 | 9,839 | Y | Y | 22 |
| 9 | 26 | USA | 2 | 7,483 | Y | y | 27 |
| 10 | | | | 6,102 | N | N | 19 |
| 11 | 29 | USA | 1 | 8,258 | Y | N | 12 |
| 12 | 23 | USA | 1 | 8,382 | Y | N | 24 |
| 13 | 27 | USA | 3 | 6,236 | Y | Y | 32 |

## Competition

Competition manifested in participants through such activities as multitasking; reaching goals, such as number of steps, target heart rate, or calories burned; and competitions won or participated in: 'tonight, I simultaneously worked on my laptop [while walking on the treadmill] by placing a board across the armrests. I know – a lot going on, lol' (Participant 1). Other participants spoke directly of the competitiveness they felt, often against themselves, or a condition they termed 'postpartum': 'after being LAST last week. I pushed for the first place this week. F*** your postpartum' (Participant 8). Competition was also manifested in frustration with equipment or the perception that they were cheating in some way by using the device in a particular way: 'frustrated that it registered my heart rate that high so that it shows I burned far more calories than I actually did' (Participant 1). These feelings of pushing, frustration, and guilt at the idea they might be cheating, lends weight to the idea that the main person they were in competition with was themselves, in order to try being better.

This perspective of striving to be better could be seen as fuelled in part by the notion of celebrity mom profiles setting standards. Douglas and Michael (2005) suggest that celebrity mom profiles have reinforced and romanticised intensive mothering, the expectations around which regulate women's behaviours (Douglas & Michaels, 2005). Celebrity moms are perceived as emphasising corporeality through their promotion of maternal body management in 'slender-pregnant' profiles to encourage body work pre- and postpartum, enhancing the desire to 'have it all' (Hallstein, 2015). McRobbie has argued that,

> As feminism (in a variety of its forms) has re-entered political culture and civil society, there is, as though to hold this threat of new feminism at bay, an amplification of the control of women, mostly by corporeal means so as to ensure the maintenance of existing power relations.
>
> (2015, p. 1)

Women could be engaging with this celebrity culture more once they are mothers, regardless of the prior state of their body, in an effort to aspire to the type of transcendence on show by celebrities, in order to rise above the contradictions inherent in being a mother – contradictions such as having to do basic tasks like cooking, cleaning, and childcare whilst also appearing glamorous and appealing, without any apparent effort or attempting to hide the reality of their lives (they hire domestic service and chefs in order to achieve their glamorous status; they are not really like themselves).

Transcendence (Mahendran, 2019), in this case, may mean rising above the perceived limitations of the body through the pursuit of exercise and fitness. In addition, transcendence may also mean rising above the material limitations of one's life context, towards the concept of the ideal perfect mother. For example, one mother stated: 'Had my baby on Saturday morning. Trying to heal. So, I can lose weight . . . but my feet/ankles are swollen. My body hurts an sore. . . . any ideas on how to heal quicker or that helps? This is my 2nd baby' (Participant 10; six days post-delivery). This participant wanted to rise above the pain, swelling, and the embodied reality of a post-delivery baby body. Transcendence can be seen as wanting a life beyond the limits of ordinary experience, or just avoiding or disconnecting from what is actually happening. While wanting to avoid pain is normal, the point is that the context of this woman's life is being ignored or displaced in terms of a technological device is engaged with instead of one's own senses and perceptions.

Focusing on a digital application, whilst ignoring or transcending the social material context of one's life, could be seen as a neo-liberal strategy, with its emphasis on self-governance and self-improvement. This could be how women are actively co-opted into the neo-liberal ideal as a way to escape their circumstances. Part of the transition to motherhood involves negotiating a new identity based on how new mothers think they are seen and how they see themselves through a 'lens' of perfection. This complex transition between identities may be negotiated as mothers come to see themselves in different ways. However, since the prevailing attitude of intensive mothering is increasing, it seems likely that identities will fall within this ideology. Health professionals may unwittingly collude with this ideology.

## *Wanting to feel good about yourself*

In this section, we identify instances where the participants were clearly knowledgeable about what they needed, in contrast to the first theme, which seemed more driven by FitBit. Implicit in this knowledge about self was that in order to feel good *about* themselves, participants needed to feel good *in* themselves. Hence participants described how physical activity, such as exercise, was seen as providing a way of moving 'through' feelings of 'being stuck':

> It's hard for me to get up and out sometimes but it feels so good after getting some fresh air on a nice walk. One day at a time! Yes, it sure does just need to keep pushing so I'm a better mum for it in the long run.
>
> (Participant 2)

The physical activity was a way of 'feeling myself', what we interpret to mean feeling the embodied sense of *being* good because they *felt* good in themselves. For example, Participant 3 said: 'First Zumba class since pregnancy. Missed it so much! I appreciate my body and being able to move so much more now'. Their physical sense of themselves appears to have been tied to their biomedically framed mental health. For example, Participant 6 said: 'not been doing great lately been a bit depressed but trying to get back to eating better and working out'. Statements such as: 'despite me struggling with depression/postpartum not today satan [sic], not today, not tomorrow, not ever!! My baby needs me!!!' (Participant 8) were a way of pushing through the lurking depression that threatened their sense of self.

Being a part of an online community focused on physical activity seemed to be a way of addressing the social isolation the participants experienced as a direct result of new motherhood. Gaining support from others in a similar situation was an enabling factor in their sense of well-being. The digital technologies provided a platform for belonging that the new mothers may otherwise not have experienced (Ogden, 2002). Other members of the participants' families were rarely mentioned or photographed, so the mothers seemed to be doing this activity in isolation. The steps the mothers took appeared to be an enabling way to address what was potentially a debilitating sense of isolation.

*Enjoying their senses and/or physical accomplishments (photographs)*

In this section, we explore how participants emphasised the materiality of their bodies and lives by posting photographs of themselves exercising or of food they had prepared (two participants). In addition, photographs were included of their babies (five participants) or of recent achievements such as number of steps and weight loss (two participants), completing a marathon (three participants), aerobic workouts with heart rates mapped on a graph (eight participants), daily goals accomplished, weekly goals accomplished (two participants), pregnancy photos (four participants), sleep graphs (four participants), positive affirmations, inspirational quotes (three participants), YouTube workouts (one participant), and photos of natural spaces/outdoors (three participants) (See Figures 9.1, 9.2 and 9.3).

The majority of photos posted are related to their senses. For example, the smell and taste of their food or the sight, sound, and touch of nature. However, these photos also express the feeling of more than two or three senses. For example, the photos with their babies are exemplification of the touch – expressing the sense of contact and togetherness – they are not just touching their babies, but they are looking, hearing, smelling, and even tasting them. These photos are immersed in the emotional and sensory experiences of motherhood. They are (re)discovering their bodies and the new sensations that motherhood is bringing them.

However, it was also noticeable that the pictures posted were of desirable lifestyles, such as outings with children in nature or fun-filled destinations. Again, there seems to be a focus on an ideal lifestyle which they, as perfect mothers, can manifest for their children. There seemed to be less questioning in this forum of the intensive mothering ideology, and there was a noticeable tone of consumerist culture. There seemed to be fewer instances of struggling or of poverty on display, perhaps for obvious reasons.

### Both sides of the same neoliberal coin?

In this chapter, we have explored how mothers engage with an online community and wearable devices, perhaps seduced by the idea of improving their fitness post-delivery of their baby. We noted that there were three main themes: competition with themselves to achieve specific fitness levels, feeling good about themselves, and the presentation of a sensory record of their lifestyles through photographs.

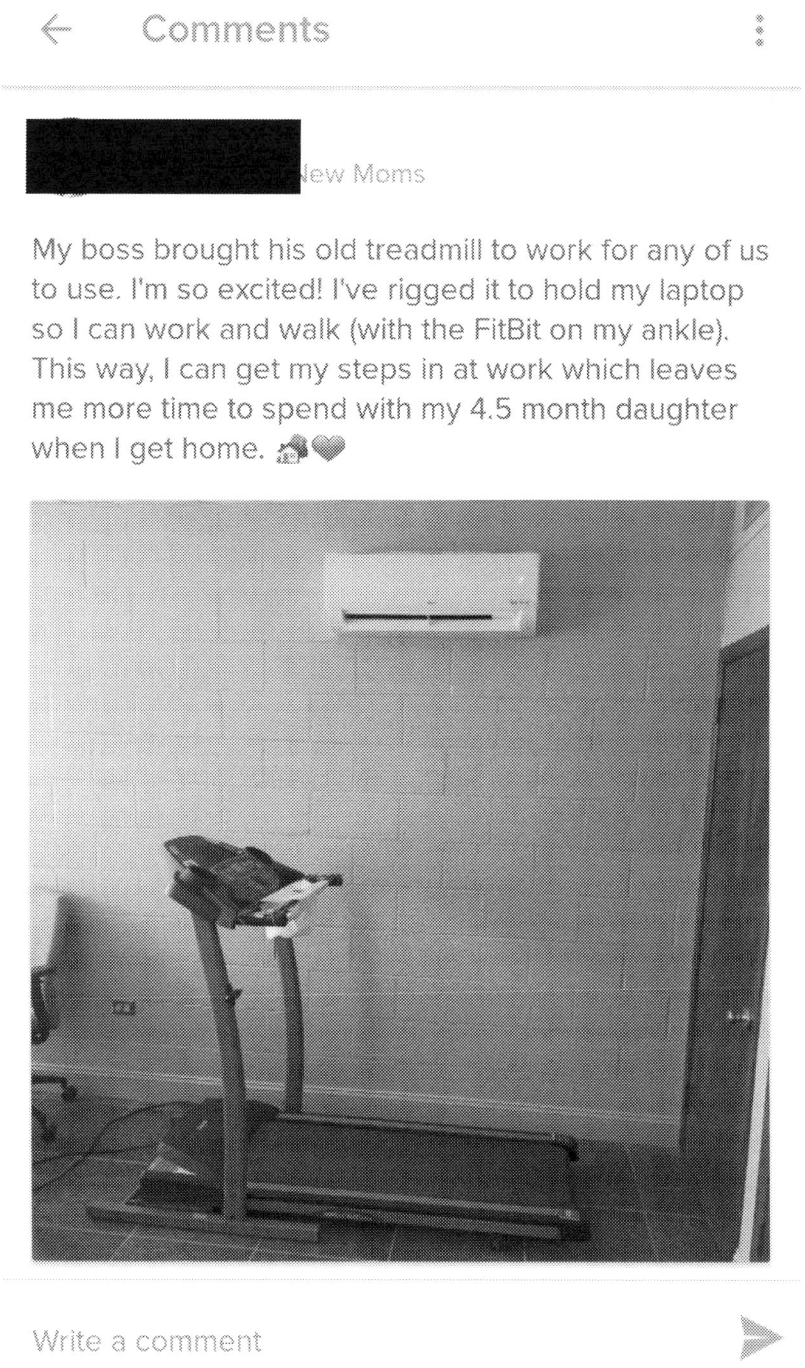

New Moms

My boss brought his old treadmill to work for any of us to use. I'm so excited! I've rigged it to hold my laptop so I can work and walk (with the FitBit on my ankle). This way, I can get my steps in at work which leaves me more time to spend with my 4.5 month daughter when I get home. 🏠❤️

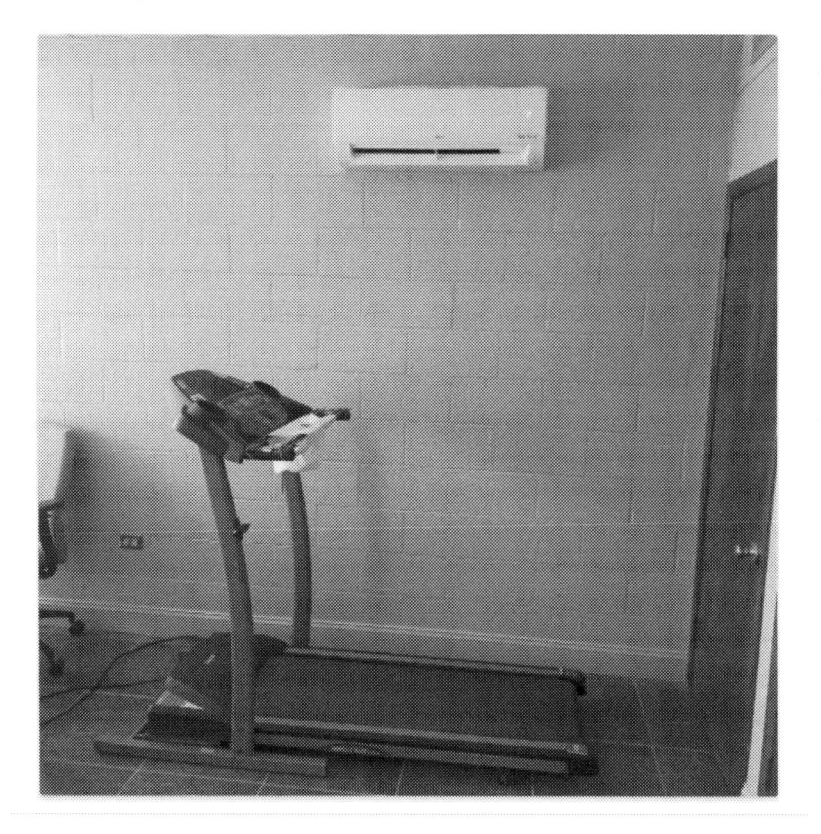

*Figure 9.1* Participant 1.

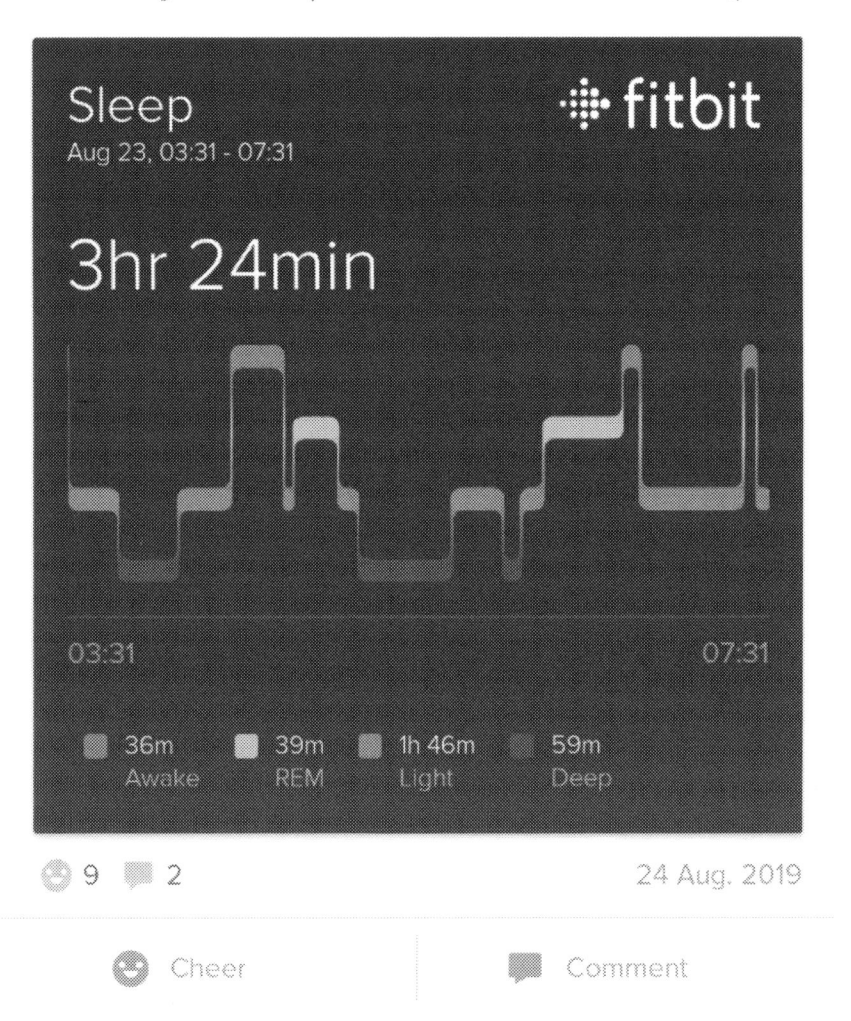

*Figure 9.2* Participant 5.

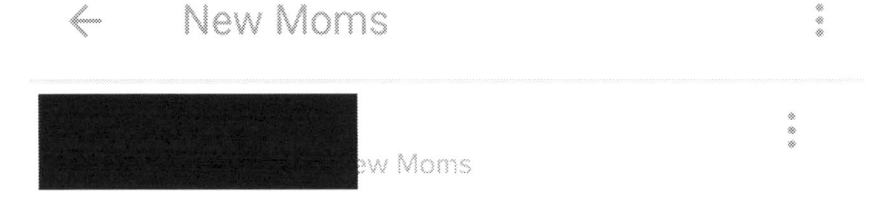

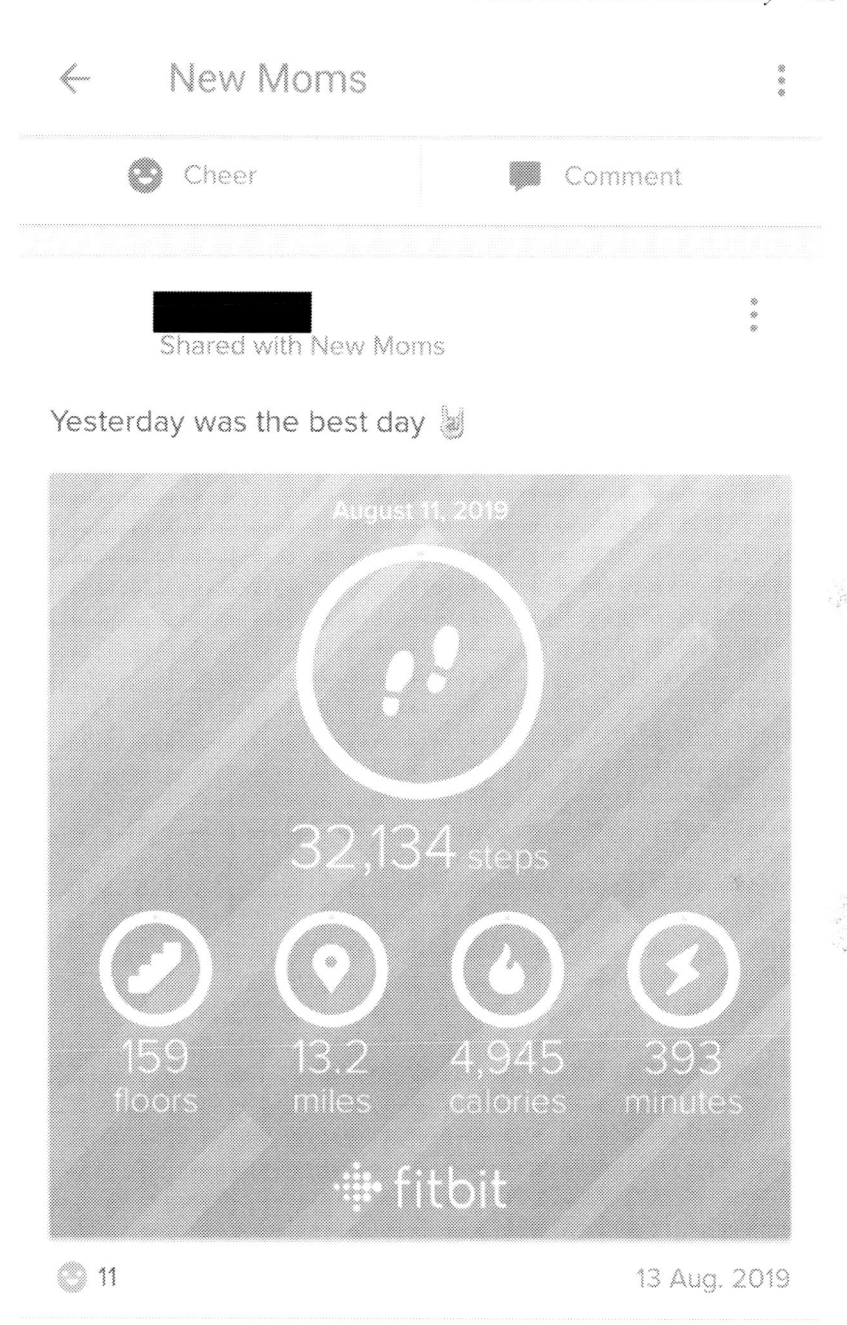

*Figure 9.3* Participant 12.

Throughout the text, we have woven critical analyses of the assumptions about what a good mother is and how fitness can be seen as a battle to be fought, with competing bodies of knowledge between mothers and health professionals. We suggest that health professionals may be complicit with the intensive mothering ideology and that, in fact, biomedical risk management is as reductionist and as much a part of neo-liberal ideology as that of good mothering(Petersen & Lupton, 1996). Having explored these assumptions, we now consider how to proceed with a critical scholarship that identifies contradictions, idealisations, and the ways women can be complicit with neo-liberal regimes whilst also working with biomedical knowledge that may be of benefit.

Working between and within different paradigms whilst trying to find a way forward within a context that prefers one ideology over another is an extremely challenging task. One way through this perplexing situation is to stay with the troubling nature whilst connecting with the humanity of the people involved and not to try to erase any difficulties but instead take them on board and struggle with them. This means trying to explain matters without necessarily being a psychologist or a social worker or a sociologist but being able to validate and normalise the struggle between different ideologies. It is the singularity of dominant ideologies that can be exclusionary and prevent further analysis, speech, connection, and deeper thinking.

It was interesting to note that health professionals did not feature much in the texts by participants. Health professionals' advice was perceived as being outside the community, whilst allies were generally seen as inside that community. There may be some distrust of health professionals as being part of an 'expert' community and potentially more reinforcing of intensive mothering ideals than these participants want compared with advice seen on social media platforms.

The key point seems to be that there are at least two potentially conflicting positions – the ideal and the reality of lived experience. The ideal position is the one that is explicitly aimed for as a way of reducing internal conflicting thoughts, desires, and expectations; yet this may also actually increase frustration as efforts fall short of achieving the ideal. The participants demonstrated this in their frustration and competition between the reality of their day-to-day lives and what they felt drawn to achieve. Likewise, health professionals may have a strong body of biomedical knowledge and yet feel frustrated with enacting this in the world of patients' lived experience. The contrasting bodies of knowledge and experience provide an uncertain experience, and the responses to this can include compartmentalization of knowledge; splitting off from lived experience (Le Breton, 2017); ignoring or discounting thoughts, beliefs, and feelings; or polarizing between one and the other. The act of holding knowledge where both can be true and yet both come from different disciplinary places, so they are not the same, means that neither can ever be the whole story. There must always be a relationship of tension between the two.

For example, knowing that intensive mothering is a socially constructed ideology does not detract from the lived experience of mothers trying to reach this ideal and transcend their material reality. Both are reductionist in terms of usually feeling like you have to choose one way over the other or, conversely, feeling like you have no choice at all. The relationship between the two seems characterized by self-policing (O'Grady, 2005) as a way of managing the difference. At times, health professionals may need to engage with an ideology that, for a particular person, in particular circumstances, may be a resource for them. If that is the case, then in terms of critical scholarship, what we are being asked to do requires more discernment of both the biological and material reality of peoples' lives. How do we resolve this tension and reconcile ourselves to this reality? One way is through an engagement with the person through their self-presentation.

Butler talks about an ethical response to impingement on self and other:

> Perhaps most importantly, we must recognize that ethics requires us to risk ourselves at moments of unknowingness, when what forms us diverges us from what lies before us, when our willingness to become undone in relation to others constitutes our chance of becoming human.
>
> (2009, p. 136)

As health professionals, we need to learn more about this ethics: 'an ethics relative to how one responds and emerges' in the moment (Mahendran, 2019, p. 33). Perhaps in this way, we could refuse the inculcation of a norm and show a different way beyond ideology with patients and mothers. Health professionals could explore what happens when we fall off the cliff edge of certainty, guidelines, and policy when crossing the invisible border between routine and the unexpected.

Physiotherapists may need to relinquish their role of expert to become more of a guide that enables mothers to question their mantle of responsibility within an intensive mothering ideology. Do people know how to trust their own bodies – how do they know when they have done too much exercise? How do they know when they can push through tiredness or when they need to honour that? How do they know when the pain should be heeded or ignored? Suspending judgement as experts in knowing what is 'good' for others, and what those practices are doing to them, without knowing the nuances of power that those women entangled within seems to be a way forward. It is a radical shift in the nature of professionalism that will challenge the knowing what is 'good' for a patient in a way that has been central to our professional identity in the past. There are many pressures on mothers, so they can resist in a variety of ways. They can also be complicit in other ways. Sometimes it seems counterintuitive in that they are risking their own health. However, the pressure imposed by societal stereotypes to 'care', for themselves and others, need to be considered.

What is needed is a way of working towards a relationship between the two, to see how sustained engagements with power can be achieved for the benefit of patients, whilst not being complicit with biomedical truths. As Foucault wrote, 'the ethico-political choice we have to make every day is to determine which is the main danger' (Tamboukou & Ball, 2003, p. 9). Being mindful of an ethical response within a neo-liberal ideology seems to be a way through transcendent approaches in order to take into account the lived experience of both mothers and health professionals.

We noted silence in relation to any birth trauma or lingering ill effects from encounters with the health system in people's postings. The silence could be for a number of reasons, for example, wanting to maintain a public profile without disclosing perhaps more intimate vulnerable details. We mention this silence because trauma or iatrogenic illness may be an area within health and fitness that is not easily outsourced to a peer community at present. Walking may provide a safe embodied experience for women who have undergone trauma who otherwise would not have the kind of affirmation and resourcing necessary to enable them to function. There was no data in our study that answered questions such as: With whom do these women share their experiences, and will online forums take over where confidential conversations with trusted healthcare practitioners once provided an outlet? It is important for physiotherapists to look at ways to engage women in conversations about trauma related to pregnancy, miscarriages and later pregnancy loss, delivery, and post-natal experiences. What is certain is that the lived experience of health professionals and mothers will be different, yet these differences need not be exclusionary. Critical reflection means learning where others are coming from and not necessarily reinforcing dominant ideologies (Delany & Watkin, 2009).

## Acknowledgements

The authors thank Adele Pavlidis, PhD, Griffith University, for her help in reviewing and editing of some sections.

## References

Blixt, L., Solbrække, K. N., & Bjorbækmo, W. S. (2019). Physiotherapists' experiences of adopting an eTool in clinical practice: A post-phenomenological investigation. *Physiotherapy Theory and Practice*, 1–13.

Bueger, C. (2013). Pathways to practice: Praxiography and international politics. *European Political Science Review*, 6(3), 383–406. doi:10.1017/s1755773913000167

Bueger, C., & Gadinger, F. (2018). Doing praxiography: Research strategies, methods and techniques. In *International practice theory* (pp. 131–161). Dortrecht, Germany: Springer.

Butler, J. P. (2009). *Giving an account of oneself*. New York, NY: Fordham University Press.

Cheek, J. (1999). *Postmodern and poststructural approaches to nursing research*. London, UK: Sage Publications.

Clark, M. I., & Thorpe, H. (2019). Towards diffractive ways of knowing women's moving bodies: A Baradian experiment with the FitBit: Motherhood entanglement. *Sociology of Sport Journal*, 1(aop), 1–15.

Clever, I., & Ruberg, W. (2014). Beyond cultural history? The material turn, praxiography, and body history. *Humanities*, 3(4), 546–566.

De Beauvoir, S. (1997). *The second sex*. New York, NY: Vintage Books.

Delany, C., & Watkin, D. (2009). A study of critical reflection in health professional education: "Learning where others are coming from". *Advances in Health Sciences Education*, 14(3), 411–429.

Douglas, S., & Michaels, M. (2005). *The mommy myth: The idealization of motherhood and how it has undermined all women.* New York, NY: Simon and Schuster.

Eakin, J. M. (2016). Educating critical qualitative health researchers in the land of the randomized controlled trial. *Qualitative Inquiry, 22*(2), 107–118.

Hallstein, L. O. B. (2015). *Bikini-ready moms: Celebrity profiles, motherhood, and the body.* New York, NY: SUNY Press.

Kingod, N. (2018). The tinkering m-patient: Co-constructing knowledge on how to live with type 1 diabetes through Facebook searching and sharing and offline tinkering with self-care. *Health,* 1363459318800140.

Kristeva, J., Moro, M. R., Odemark, J., & Engebretsen, E. (2018). Cultural crossings of care: An appeal to the medical humanities. *Med Humanit, 44*(1), 55–58. doi:10.1136/medhum-2017-011263

Le Breton, D. (2017). *Sensing the world: An anthropology of the senses.* London, UK: Bloomsbury Publishing.

Littig, B. (2013). On high heels: A praxiography of doing Argentine tango. *European Journal of Women's Studies, 20*(4), 455–467. doi:10.1177/1350506813496397

Lowe, W. (2018). Reflecting with compassion on student feedback: Social sciences in medicine. *Journal of Perspectives in Applied Academic Practice, 6*(3).

Lupton, D. (2012). *Medicine as culture: Illness, disease and the body.* London, UK: Sage Publications.

Lupton, D., & Maslen, S. (2019). How women use digital technologies for health: Qualitative interview and focus group study. *Journal of Medical Internet Research, 21*(1), e11481. doi:10.2196/11481

Mahendran, A. (2019). *Moments of rupture: The importance of affect in medical education and surgical training: Perspectives from professional learning and philosophy.* Abingdon, Oxon: Routledge.

McRobbie, A. (2015). Notes on the perfect: Competitive femininity in neoliberal times. *Australian Feminist Studies, 30*(83), 3–20.

Mendenhall, E. (2019). *Rethinking diabetes: Entanglements with trauma, poverty, and HIV.* Ithaca, NY: Cornell University Press.

Ogden, J. (2002). *Health and the construction of the individual.* Hove, UK: Psychology Press.

O'Grady, H. (2005). *Woman's relationship with herself: Gender, Foucault and therapy.* Abingdon, Oxon: Routledge.

Petersen, A., & Lupton, D. (1996). *The new public health: Health and self in the age of risk.* London, UK: Sage Publications.

Romagnoli, A., & Wall, G. (2012). "I know I'm a good mom": Young, low-income mothers' experiences with risk perception, intensive parenting ideology and parenting education programmes. *Health, Risk & Society, 14*(3), 273–289.

Setchell, J., Nicholls, D. A., Wilson, N., & Gibson, B. E. (2018). Infusing rehabilitation with critical research and scholarship: A call to action. *Physiotherapy Canada, 70*(4), 301–305. doi.org/10.3138/ptc.70.4.gee

Stewart, S. (2020). A mother's love knows no bounds: Exploring "good mother" expectations for mothers involved with children's services due to partner violence. *Qualitative Social Work.* doi:10.1177/1473325020902249

Tamboukou, M., & Ball, S. J. (2003). Genealogy and ethnography: Fruitful encounters or dangerous liaisons. *Dangerous Encounters: Genealogy and Ethnography, 17,* 1–36.

# 10 Disability as expertise

Mobilizing a critique of school-based physical therapy for integrating disability studies into physical therapy professionalization

*Devorah Shubowitz*

**Introduction**

In the United States prior to 1975, disabled children had few options for attending school. Children who did not conform to able-bodied norms were sent to live in institutions, where, segregated from society, they were left to languishment and abuse. Since the enactment of The Education for All Handicapped Children Act in 1975, which mandated a "free and appropriate education" for disabled children throughout the United States, ninety percent fewer disabled children are institutionalized and segregated from their families and communities (Colker, 2013, p. 6). Currently, the educational policy of "inclusion" in the United States means ideally educating disabled children together with their non-disabled peers in the same classrooms and curriculums. In this chapter, I reflect on the application of inclusion policy to physical therapy as a related service for children in special education. I focus on the language used in the federal education law of educating children in the "least restrictive environment" and the physical therapy (PT) practices that emerge from this legal language. I argue that this language maintains the possibility of institutionalization, in that the best disabled children can aspire to is to be least restricted. Restriction, therefore, is always possible, if not desirable. I argue that this framework is founded upon the requirement for disabled children to attain able-bodied norms. I discuss why the standards of able-bodied norms are untenable in the practice of school-based physical therapy and that understanding disability as expertise and integrating disability studies into PT professionalization would move physical therapy in more just directions.

In my three years as a physical therapist in Brooklyn, New York, public schools, I have seen inclusion educational policy result in empathy, kindness, love, and friendship between able-bodied and disabled children in integrated co-teaching kindergarten classes. But there are differences that lock disabled children into the reprimand cycle, end inclusion beyond kindergarten for children who do not sufficiently keep up, and harm disabled children who do well academically but are made miserable trying to socialize with uneducated non-disabled peers who react to overt differences with fear, distancing, or mockery. As I will discuss, for the current system of inclusion to work, disabled children must regulate themselves and muster great effort to learn in curriculum designed for their able-bodied peers. Inclusion does not require that disabled populations determine how curriculum, teaching, and policy are designed in the first place. What knowledge, expertise, and values would disabled children and adults bring to physical and academic education that able-bodied educators lack access to because we are devaluing disability to push through normative agendas?

While my training as a physical therapist at the New York City Department of Education (NYC DOE) inspired me to explore the connections between education policy, physical therapy, and the expertise of disabled embodiment, I have been thinking about the ethics of physical therapy practice in relation to disability since I entered PT in 1991. From the beginning of my career, it seemed problematic to me that although I studied the neurobiology and biomechanics of walking, jumping, running, and transitioning to gain expertise, I could apply what I studied to teach these movements to people with bodies that did not follow the neurobiological and biomechanical sequences I studied. I wondered how I, who did not have to cognitively or with awareness learn to perform such movements with my own body, could model for others who did have to exert great effort. My ethical unrest became acute when working with children born with bodies that would not conform to able-bodied forms, postures, and gross motor skills, when the main tool I had for movement was persistence toward the same typically developing movement goals.

As a new therapist, I instinctively drew from my dance training, where movement was meant to feel good, express creativity, and was meaningful in itself. I drew from my training in Erik Hawkins dance technique and Tai Chi Chaun that codified a connection between sensation and movement, along with movement improvisation, exploring what I was learning with disabled populations. When working with children, I followed and developed the movements they initiated and desired, encouraged fun and playful interactions, and validated their movement choices and problem-solving. For example, if a child climbed up onto a trampoline using their hands and feet, I did not insist they climb without their hands but enjoyed how children with disabilities moved. In my personal practice, unilateral stance in this instance emerged within the context of play with unspoken hand-held support or an unspoken facilitated reach integrated into the play.

Despite developing an improvised practice, I struggled with physical therapy's language of working to improve poor function, fix impairments, or adapt and compensate for limitations to describe the robust intricate movements and lives of the people I worked with. In 2002, I decided to leave full-time physical therapy and entered a master's in religious studies, completing a PhD in social-cultural anthropology while working part-time in early intervention to support myself and subsequently my son. While my research was not in physical therapy or disability, classes and readings introduced me to disability studies, where I reflected upon physical therapy practice.

For example, Gail Heidi Landsman's book, *Reconstructing Motherhood and Disability in the Age of "Perfect" Babies* provided me perspectives to understand how physical therapy upholds able-bodied dominance as a mechanism that promises through hard work, disabled children can become "normal." When that does not happen, the child is considered to have "plateaued," which parents interpret as being given up on (2009, pp. 118–119). I recognized the events Landsman explained of how mothers of disabled children search for toys that will help their children gain normative skills like pincer grasping, rather than getting a toy their children may enjoy (185). But these same mothers were most concerned that their children's disabled hands, bodies, and speech would preclude meaningful, loving, respectful relationships rather than not being able to perform this or that function (195). These readings provided me with language and insights I did not receive in PT school but directly related to my work as a PT.

In Landsman's discussion on the interconnectedness of impairment and disability, she provides a basis for understanding the mechanisms by which the practice of physical therapy creates disability in viewing and comparing disabled children through the lens of normative function. Landsman applied Kevin Paterson and Bill Hughes's (1999, pp. 602–603) concept of impaired bodies "dys-appearing" or becoming visible as disabled when in the company of normative children or when these mothers received information about their children from doctors (Landsman, 2009, pp. 199–203). She explained that when the mothers she interviewed were home caring for their children, they viewed them as uniquely themselves. It is when these same mothers went to the playground or supermarket and were around able-bodied children performing activities their own children could not do, or when doctors told them all the ways their children's bodies were faulty, that their children become disabled to them. In experiences of comparison, their children's bodies dys-appear, or appear to them as dysfunctional and defective. As physical therapists, we are trained to compare children's gross motor functioning to a normative age standard to work toward achieving gross motor milestones and, in this way, also create disability.

Disability scholars have for decades critiqued rehabilitation for trying to fix impairments that cannot be fixed and are experienced as self and driving normalizing intervention programs that adults with disabilities experience as oppressive (Finkelstein, 1980; Oliver, 1990; Oliver & Barnes, 2012). However, recently, disability scholars are reconsidering rehabilitation as an area that can be reformed. Tom Shakespeare and other scholars have reconsidered the rehabilitation fields to require research precisely because these practices deeply affect disabled people and to ensure "rights-based rehabilitation" policies that can only be formulated based on how disabled people experience rehabilitation (Shakespeare, Cooper, Bezmez, & Poland, 2018, p. 61). Shakespeare describes how some who participate in rehabilitation experience the process as helpful, while others do not (66–68). Shakespeare's approach is qualitative and ethnographic, deriving primary data from individual experience and circumstances to draw commonalities by which to direct reform. Shakespeare understands disability as a normative human experience that most able-bodied people will go through with bodily age-related or other circumstantial changes (2013, p. 221).

David Mitchell and Sharon Snyder are disability scholars who approach the problem of rehabilitation from historical, political, philosophical, literary, and cultural perspectives. These scholars do not think that reform will emerge from a rehabilitation worldview that favours those who can approximate able-bodied function (2015, pp. 6–8). They assert that disabled people have expertise that is directly informed by physical, emotional, and intellectual differences. This expertise can be accessed through studying and attending to histories, literatures, art, and learning approaches of the diversely disabled that provide a more complete and accurate understanding of all humanity. For these scholars, disabled knowledge is not a response to normative healthcare practices but devised in the failure of rehabilitation and inclusion practices. Their focus is on recognizing the unique cultures of crip individuals and communities, developing curricular cripistemology that requires disability perspectives and values to be included in all school curriculums, hiring crip/queer instructors, and using universal design teaching methods for all students to benefit (2015, pp. 82–92).

I argue that both of these approaches and others are necessary to understand how diverse populations experience physical therapy and how to reconceive the profession. While Mitchell and Snyder speak about academic education, prioritizing disability expertise is equally relevant to play, problem-solve, move, and function. For example, I have witnessed a pre-school child teach herself how to button her sweater with one hand, adamantly refusing instruction to use her other hand as a stabilizer. This child figured out a strategy and did not care that it took time. Disabled movement strategies for dressing, transitioning, and mobility are not necessarily encumbered by biomedical concerns of symmetry, expedience, or hyper-vigilant safety measures. Able bodies can learn about creativity, desire, and innovation from understanding how disabled individuals move. For example, a blind dancer has taught me about listening for the other dancers' steps and feeling air displacement generated by other dancers' movements to know where I am in space in relation to others. These are experiences I would not have known to attend to without her disabled expertise. Both "rights-based rehabilitation" and cripistemology are necessary for restructuring, redesigning, and reauthorizing what are currently the rehabilitation professions.

Currently, there are PT scholars who integrate disability studies and expertise into physical therapy professionalization. For example, Barbara Gibson (2016) argues for expanding the concept of movement beyond the physical body, and Karen Yoshida et al. (2015) details how to create ethical PT programs by collaborating with individuals and communities with disabilities. Both of these PT scholars are at the University of Toronto. However, in the United States, PT departments and programs continue in the biomedical model. For example, in 2019, I attended a lecture in a New York physical therapy department where I listened to a disabled guest lecturer pleading for the students to listen to their patients because they are the experts of their bodies, detailing how she prefers to transfer, which was not how her physical therapist instructed her to transfer. The students subsequently moved to a lesson on transfers without this expertise. The students also simulated a disabled person's experience by spending time blindfolded or in a wheelchair, unaware that simulations do not provide accurate information about what it is like to be disabled (French, 2007).

Disabled expertise is also continually undermined by the language PTs use. The premise of paediatric physical therapy is that there are children with impaired bodies defined as weak, tight, imbalanced, misaligned, uncoordinated, asymmetrical, and disorganized, such that they do not perform daily functional activities as do their typically developing peers. Disability scholars have long cited the harm negative characterizations of disabled bodies cause in social, cultural, political, economic, and emotional terms, and while we are in a period when therapy fields have recalibrated language, to use words such as "typical and atypical" instead of "normal and abnormal" and focus on abilities, function, and participation, these efforts prove hollow without a disability scholarship approach. Vehmas and Watson (2014) assert that language and discourse as its central concern cannot address ethical care, which is always material, a critique directed to discursive approaches in critical disability studies that applies equally well to the linguistic tinkering that substitutes "atypical" for "abnormal" as social progress. To change the material consequences of the language of defect requires, in part, acknowledging that being able-bodied is not the highest form of human development, gross motor or otherwise. Seeking to understand disability expertise is necessary to change the material consequences of defect language.

As a point of entry into rethinking physical therapy's reliance on aspirations of becoming able-bodied, I will analyse the guidelines for practice that the NYC DOE implemented for school-based physical and occupational therapists. Beginning about ten years ago, the NYC DOE changed the practice of PT, requiring therapists to solely work on improving participation and not on remediation of impairments. In the NYC DOE, children with disabilities are not deemed eligible for physical therapy and other related services to remediate impairments; rather, PT is only indicated to address the gross motor functions required for children to participate alongside their classmates in school. At first glance, this appears to be a progressive disability policy that argues for a participation rather than impairments definition of disability. However, because this seemingly progressive effort is not grounded in disability studies and advocacy, critiques of health-related rehabilitation, alterative models of embodiment, and valued codifiable movement differences, I will demonstrate that this change to school-based PT practice has conflicting ramifications for therapists schooled in the medical model, as well as for children who require more than school-based participation to develop their movement potential.

The social model of disability, which states that society, not individual impairments, disables people through structural barriers and social stigma, has been grossly applied to the NYC DOE's adoption of a participation model to determine whether children with disabilities are eligible for physical therapy services required to benefit from their education. This gross application includes using the School Functional Assessment (SFA) to translate into PT goals to address six areas of motor activities children are asked to perform at school. These six areas are: transportation to and from the school building, hallway transitions between classrooms, in-classroom transitions and seating, lunchroom activities, recess participation, and gym class participation. Requiring school-based physical therapy to address only six areas of school activity, as opposed to motor function in all areas of the child's life or remediate impairments, limits services because as long as children keep up with their peers in these contexts, PT is not indicated. Deeming children ineligible for PT may allow for movement innovations and acceptance of movement differences simply by leaving disabled children to go about their school days in the bodies they have without intervention.

But, for many disabled children, the six areas of school activity either prove impossible or demand low expectations. For example, PTs may have goals for disabled children to keep up in gym class where the children cannot even tolerate the music or are too fearful of the able-bodied students' basketball and soccer free play to even try to participate. This PT goal of gym participation would be impossible for the child without revamping the gym class for everyone. Further, a school is supposed to be a training ground for life beyond school walls. When gross motor participation at school narrowly means walking in line to get from one class to another, climbing stairs, and getting by in gym class, how does this support children with very different movement requirements and aspirations outside of their particular school building and classroom layout? A more detailed analysis of the physical therapy school-based participation model will further explicate these problems and contradictions. I begin this discussion with the legal foundations of how disabled children receive PT in school.

## Idea

Advocacy and public reckoning of the abusive institutional system led to the Education for All Handicapped Children Act of 1975 that required all states to provide a "free and appropriate public education" to all disabled children. Congress has since modified the law through reauthorizations in 1986, 1990, 1997, 2002, and 2004, changing the name of the Act in 1990 to Individuals with Disabilities Education Act (IDEA) and attempting to rectify problems that educators, students, parents, and communities experienced having lived through iterations of the law. Along with the changes and additions to federal education law, some basic provisions of the original 1975 Act remain in IDEA, including: "educating children with disabilities in least restrictive environments with supplementary aids and services, as needed" (2002, pp. 1–2). This, along with all of IDEA's provisions, provides general language for each of the 50 states and their local governments to interpret. The general mandates of IDEA that are locally interpreted include related service provisions (Section 300.34 Related services).

IDEA lists physical therapy as one of the professional fields within related services that could make it possible and therefore required for a child to benefit from their education. However, IDEA does not provide a detailed framework for why a child would be eligible for physical therapy, what goals to address, where, when, how long physical therapy is to be provided, what methods physical therapists and related service providers should employ, or how related service providers should function as members of an educational team. It is up to state education departments and local educational agencies to debate and establish their own guidelines.

I will next discuss the particular guidelines of the NYC DOE for school-based PT, including its distinction from clinical PT, the least restrictive environment application, and testing to illustrate how able-bodied norms and a connection to institutionalization underlie this particular participation model.

### *Clinical vs. school-based physical therapy*

Beginning around 2008, Suzanne Sanchez, then occupational therapy (OT) Director and Carlo Vialu, then PT Director spearheaded the publication of *The PT/OT DOE Practice Guide* (2011) to standardize PT/OT school practice. The guide asserts that PTs may not practice as clinicians remediating impairments but assist a child with a disability to access their educational curriculum and participate alongside their peers at school (3). But because this distinction is not grounded in discussion or critique of the medical model, it dissolves under scrutiny. For example, treatments are not regulated by these guidelines. A PT may, therefore, remediate an impairment such as muscular and soft tissue restrictions as compared with norms for a child to maintain balance when walking around toys scattered around the classroom floor during free play, in which case the degrees of hip and foot range of motion and strength measurements (impairment model) are goals. Although an impairment goal cannot be included in the school Individualized Education Program (IEP) goals, PTs may still work to remediate them if they are determined to be the cause of a limitation in participation. The guide does explain that there may be different reasons for a lack of participation that may or may not be based on an impairment (8). There may be environmental or personal factors such as lack of interest or motivation (8). It is then determined whether PT would be the professional area to address the problem that causes a lack of participation (9–10).

A PT will be the professional identified as necessary if the root cause of the participation problem is an impairment such as weakness, impaired balance, and incoordination. However, although PTs remediate impairments in service of improving participation, because they cannot write impairment goals for an IEP, this has the effect of easily deeming them irrelevant for school participation if students display other causational factors such as lack of interest, attention, and cognitive limitations. When instructed to leave impairments alone when it is not clear they are the primary reason for the limitation in participation, therapists have the opportunity to observe how children come up with innovating movement as a result of their impairments. For example, I have observed a child with a club foot gracefully and speedily step over her non-clubfoot when running in the playground. I have observed a child with fluctuating muscle tone roll himself seamlessly in and out of desired spaces.

Determining whether an impairment be remediated or accepted and left alone in school should be based on factors that demonstrate a broader understanding of the connections between impairment, participation, and disability that emerge from the lives of disabled people and disability scholarship, which is not the case. It appears that PT schools follow the biomedical model that impairments cause disability, locating the limitation within the individual to be fixed. In contrast, by deemphasizing impairments as significant for participation, the DOE grossly follows the social model where disability is created by society's limits to accessibility. While the impairment model of disability has been oppressive, the social model of disability has also been critiqued as ignoring impairments altogether. For example, Tom Shakespeare explained:

> Any researcher who does qualitative research with disabled people immediately discovers that in everyday life it is very hard to distinguish clearly between the impact of impairment and the impact of social barriers (Watson, 2002; Sherry, 2002). In practice, it is the interaction of individual bodies and social environments, which produces disability. For example, steps only become an obstacle if someone has a mobility impairment: each element is necessary but not sufficient for the individual to be disabled. If a person with multiple sclerosis is depressed, how easy is it to make a causal separation between the effect of the impairment itself; her reaction to being oppressed and excluded on the basis of having an impairment; other unrelated reasons for her to be depressed? In practice, social, and individual aspects are almost inextricable in the complexity of the lived experience of disability.
> 
> (Shakespeare, 2013, p. 218)

Understanding the complexity of embodiment in society is vital for those in the rehab professions. But currently in the United States, we are instructed to identify the primary root cause of impairment and disability rather than the connections between human systems.

For example, in my time working with children with disabilities, I have noted that young disabled children do not consider their bodies impaired no matter their diagnoses and will protect and care for their bodies as they are. A child's perception of her body will change in relation to her social treatment and will then influence how she moves. I have witnessed a middle schooler processing her body as different for the first time in my presence, having worked together for many months. This occurred when the child became upset because able-bodied peers laughed when a ball hit her when she was playing basketball at an adjoining hoop to these able-bodied peers. When I entered the gym to greet this child for PT, she was curled up in the corner in tears. After telling me what happened, she then transferred to her wheelchair and left the gym. I remained to ask those who laughed to make amends. A boy followed her and apologized while the others went on playing.

Upon the boy's return to the gym, this child listed diagnoses she heard about herself to me, including learning and physical disabilities, stating, "I have [X], [Y], and [Z]." I read her listing as her relaying to me how her impairments affect how she is treated by others, how she feels as a result, and how she views herself. I listened and expressed my appreciation of her many talents and intelligence. But I would be a more ethical PT if I were trained to understand how disabled advocates and scholars view the connections between impairment and disability, how to discuss these connections with children when they experientially discover them, and how to support disabled children to love their impaired bodies in our current society.

## *Least restrictive environment*

The IDEA's language of "least restrictive environment" (LRE) underlies the rationale for distinguishing between "clinical" and "school-based" PT. Education law both coins and defines "least restrictive environment," explaining that LRE means: to the extent possible, children with disabilities should be educated in the same classrooms as their non-disabled peers. However, there is a glaring dissimilarity between the word "restrictive" and this definition. To restrict means to put a limit on, to control, to confine. This term, coined in the 1975 education law, harkens to institutionalization, where disabled people were cruelly bound to beds and chairs. Extending this language to mean separate classrooms and special educational programs assumes that anytime a child with a disability is separated from her able-bodied peers, she is restricted and controlled in ways that deny her the freedom an able-bodied education would bring.

The principle of "least restrictive environment" is extended in the *NYC DOE OT/PT Practice Guide* to mean that PTs should ideally work in educational contexts, including classrooms, gymnasiums, recess locations, lunchrooms, hallways, and stairwells, as the child goes through their day with their peers. PTs must also minimize therapy frequencies and durations so that children are not separated from interacting with their classmates (2011, p. 14). In contradiction to these recommendations, a recent study demonstrated that having a therapist shadow a student in real time in the context of a school activity and having therapy in least restrictive groups correlated negatively with SFA outcomes, while higher student participation during (more restrictive) individual therapy correlated with higher SFA outcomes (Westcott McCoy et al., 2018). This shows that it may be ideal in terms of meeting school functional independence to work one on one for a short interval away from peers, but this ideal would be considered "restrictive."

In this same vein, LRE applications also become illogical under conditions where children prefer to work with a PT individually, considering the alternative. For example, schools may have few spacious indoor recess locations and require children to remain in crowded classrooms such that children prefer moving and playing in a therapy room or empty hallway separate from their peers at recess. There may also be instances where gym and assisted physical education (APE) classes are crowded and loud or, in some charter schools I have worked in, consist solely of child-led basketball, where basketballs are grabbed without a moment's notice, thrown hard and fast in random directions, and fly quickly through the air in ways that make some disabled children run for cover.

Children who feel unsafe or uncomfortable in gym and APE classes bolt toward the PT holding a yoga mat at the door with relief, knowing they can seek refuge in an empty classroom to exercise. I have also noted through my work in autism educational programs that autistic kids learn well and enjoy being together with other autistic kids, so they do not experience learning separate from their able-bodied peers as "restrictive." This discrepancy of applying the term "least restrictive environment" to related services and education curriculums demonstrates that the IDEA language of institutionalization does not reflect actual circumstances children with disabilities must contend with and indicates nothing about the conditions any child needs to thrive in.

*Testing*

The focus on participation in school for disabled children occurs within a context of disability rights movements working to shift societies from defect categorizations of disease and impairment to more whole-person characterizations of abilities, function, and participation. In 2001, the United Nations World Health Organization and its Assembly agreed on common language for classification of individuals with disabilities in terms of function, participation, and ability with the International Classification of Functioning, Disability, and Health (ICF). This shift requires different tests and measures that observe children in their daily living environments that are not comparisons to normative bodies rather than in controlled testing environments that do compare results with normative bodies.

However, in the past 10 years, tests that standardize performance in terms of time in comparison to normative bodies have been developed, which backsteps from viewing disabled bodies more holistically. These include Timed Up and Down Stairs (TUDS), Timed Up and Go (TUG), Timed Floor to Stand-Normal (TFTS-N), Thirty-Second Walk Test (30sWT), and the Shuttle Run (SR). These tests measure timeliness for walking, stair climbing, transitioning to stand and sitting, and running in comparison to able-bodied children of the same age.

By definition, standardized tests determine where a child ranks among their same-age able-bodied peers. Standardization also by definition means that the test must be administered in the same way, using the same verbal cues, modelling, and materials in comparable settings for all. Disabled children, therefore, score much lower than highly athletic able-bodied children. Recent studies have shown that when administering standardized tests, physical therapists do not use the required testing procedures but incorporate imaginary play, cueing, and specific demonstrations so that the children who do not find these tests easy can succeed in demonstrating what they can physically do (Fay et al., 2018). Fay et al. also explained that the primary reasons therapists have for modifying the test related to how the child responded to test administration in terms of non-cooperation, language ability, attention, and cognitive ability. Therapists find disabled children respond better with engaging cues and contextualizing games. Fay argued that PTs must not change the instructions and conditions in standardized testing because this makes the test ranking meaningless (2018).

Yet we can read the major finding to ask whether standardized movements and function are possible, desirable, useful, interesting, and motivating for children who find them difficult, too difficult, and impossible. We can change orientation to how the child is experiencing the test rather than how the test is evaluating her. For decades, I have heard therapists say that a child is resisting because the test is hard and that the child should persist. When children resist normative testing but respond when testing is contextualized with meaningful play, it is useful to understand the basis for this resistance beyond determining that all of these many children are too lazy to exert more effort.

David Mitchell and Sharon Snyder explain standardization in political terms, asserting that inclusion structured to standardize disabled children's incapacities is part of the neoliberal agenda of hyper-consumption that privatizes public institutions to for-profit interests that deem under-consumptive bodies unworthy of investment and voice (2015, p. 79). By standardizing children in comparison to what is normal (ascending and descending stairs in a set number of seconds) children with disabilities are canonized as failures, and resources are siphoned to those who succeed. These scholars assert that the failure students with disabilities exhibit is not scientific evidence of defect but "an agentive form of resistance, a purposeful failure to accomplish the unreal (and, perhaps unrealizable) objectives of normalization" (80). Children with disabilities are agentive when they clearly express that they are not interested in performing a normative bodily act or standardized tests. PTs would benefit from understanding how disabled children experience physical testing when being compared to normative standards so as not to create disability by comparing children who must exert enormous effort to children who perform standardized movements such as jumping over six-inch hurdles using a two-foot take-off and landing or standing on one leg for 10 seconds effortlessly.

## Conclusion

In *The Biopolitics of Disability: Neoliberalism, Ablenationalism, and Peripheral Embodiment*, David T. Mitchell and Sharon L. Snyder explain, "Meaningful inclusion is only worthy of the designation 'inclusion' if disability becomes more recognized as providing alternative values for living that do not simply reify reigning normalcy" (2015, p. 5). For these scholars, inclusion in school does not mean that children with disabilities train with supports to become as able-bodied as they can possibly be but that lived differences and expertise of disabled embodiments need to be included in every aspect of general education curriculum. What rehabilitation applications would result from a robust engagement with disability scholarship? I have demonstrated in this article that despite distinguishing between "clinical" and "participation" models for school-based PT practice, normative ideals continue to drive physical therapy in the United States because the profession is rooted in biomedicine, with little or no professional engagement with disability studies and expertise. School-based models of "least restrictive environment" and standardized testing requirements continue in the same language as institutionalization that demands disabled children do what their able-bodied peers do to be worthy of inclusion. An interdisciplinary professionalization of physical therapy that integrates disability scholarship in the United States would be a step toward a more just PT practice on the path toward achieving equitable participation and authentic inclusion for all.

# References

Colker, R. (2013). *Disabled education: A critical analysis of the Individuals with Disabilities Education Act*. New York: NYU Press.
Fay, D., Brock, E., Peneton, S., Simon, R., Splan, M., Sullivan, L., & Weiler, A. (2018). Physical therapists' use and alteration of standardized assessments of motor function in children. *Pediatric Physical Therapy*, *30*(4), 318–325.
Finkelstein, V. (1980). *Attitudes and disabled people*. New York: World Rehabilitation Fund.
French, S. (2007). Simulation exercises in disability awareness training: A critique, disability. *Handicap & Society*, *7*(3), 257–266.
Gibson, B. (2016). *Rehabilitation: A post-critical approach*. New York: Taylor and Francis.
IDEA. Retrieved from https://sites.ed.gov/idea/regs/b/a/300.34
Landsman, G. H. (2009). *Reconstructing motherhood and disability in the age of "perfect" babies*. New York and London: Routledge.
McEwen, I. R. (2002). A great IDEA. *Physical and Occupational Therapy in Pediatrics*, *22*(2), 1–6.
Mitchell, D. T., & Snyder, S. L. (2015). *The biopolitics of disability: Neoliberalism, ablenationalism, and peripheral embodiment*. Ann Arbour, MI: The University of Michigan Press.
Oliver, M. (1990). *The politics of disablement*. Basingstoke, UK: Palgrave Macmillan.
Oliver, M., & Barnes, C. (2012). *The new politics of disablement*. Basingstoke, UK: Palgrave Macmillan.
Paterson, K., & Hughes, B. (1999). Disability studies and phenomenology: The carnal politics of everyday life. *Disability & Society*, *14*(5), 597–610.
School-based physical therapy and occupational therapy practice guide. (2011, Fall). NYC Department of Education.
Shakespeare, T. (2013). The social model of disability. In *The disability studies reader* (4th ed., L. J. Davis, Ed.). New York and London: Routledge.
Shakespeare, T., Cooper, H., Bezmez, D., & Poland, F. (2018). Rehabilitation as a disability equality issue: A conceptual shift for disability studies. *Social Inclusion*, *6*(1), 61–72.
Sherry, M. (2002). *If I only had a brain* (Unpublished PhD dissertation). University of Queensland.
Vehmas, S., & Watson, N. (2014). Moral wrongs, disadvantages, and disability: A critique of critical disability studies. *Disability & Society*, *29*(4), 638–650.
Watson, N. (2002). Well, I know this is going to sound very strange to you, but I don't see myself as a disabled person: Identity and disability. *Disability and Society*, *17*(5), 509–528.
Westcott McCoy, S., et al. (2018). School-based physical therapy services and student functional performance at school. *Developmental Medicine & Child Neurology*, *60*, 1140–1148.
Yoshida, K. K., Self, H. M., Renwick, R. M., Forma, L. L., King, A. J., & Fell, L. A. (2015). A value-based practice model of rehabilitation: Consumers' recommendations in action. *Disability and Rehabilitation*, *37*(20), 1825–1833.

# 11 A person-centred and collaborative model for understanding chronic pain. Perspectives from a pain patient, a practitioner, and a philosopher

*Christine Price, Matthew Low, and Rani Lill Anjum*

**Evidence-based healthcare, in practice and theory**

*A patient's perspective on being treated according to the best available evidence*

It is hard to believe that a simple manual handling injury could change my life in such a dramatic and traumatic way, but it did. It was the summer of 2008, and I had spent two weeks clearing out a loft in an old Victorian house. It was a beautiful sunny Saturday morning and so my husband and I decided to venture out to a local beauty spot. As I sat in the car, I could feel a niggling pain in my leg, but not enough to bother me unduly. However, the pain that started as a niggle gradually increased, until by the time I arrived home for lunch I just knew I was in trouble. I headed for the pain killers and waited, hoping the pain would go away. Instead of the normal dissipation of pain with pain killers, the pain continued to grow. By early evening, the pain had escalated to the point that I could no longer walk. The pain was now in both my back and my leg and was excruciating. I don't remember ever experiencing pain this bad, not even when giving birth.

Somehow, I managed to get through the night, and the next day a GP was called. I was given strong pain killers and left in the hope that the pain would resolve. Twenty-four hours later, I was still unable to walk and still in excruciating pain. I was in urinary retention, and so an ambulance was called to take me to hospital, where I stayed for five days. I was told that a disc in my lower back had prolapsed. The disc was compressing the S1 nerve root, causing sciatica, and I was suffering from severe neuropathic pain.

I was discharged from the hospital with a variety of pain medications, including liquid morphine. Although I could now walk a few metres, my pain, distress, and disability levels remained high. I remained in often-excruciating pain. I was unable to sit or stand long enough to shower. I couldn't fully dress myself, and I found it difficult to function. It took weeks before I could walk much further than a few metres and longer before I could sit for more than a few minutes. The pain was invasive and affected every aspect of my life. I actively sought healthcare support. I knew I couldn't get through this on my own; I couldn't control the pain. I continued to try to work and continued to try to live my life the best I could, but I was struggling. I needed strong pain medications to help get me through the day, but the side effects were making me ill. Looking back, I can't imagine how I coped.

In terms of quantity, I was receiving quite a lot of healthcare. In terms of effectiveness, I'm not so sure. I was treated 'conservatively' before having spinal decompression surgery 17 months after the injury. I had a number of epidural injections, a nerve root block, and large quantities of medications. I was put onto a spinal cord stimulator pathway, which I eventually declined.

My pain clinic input was minimal. My appointments were merely a precursor to injections or for spinal cord stimulator assessment. I was not given any pain education input or offered other treatments such as acupuncture. I received a reasonable amount of physiotherapy. Two episodes before surgery and then four afterwards. I would describe my first four episodes of physiotherapy care – two before surgery and two within a year of surgery – as 'routine'. Although they were delivered by four different therapists, they were similar in nature, and I'm sure similar to the physiotherapy care given to many, maybe most, other patients with a similar diagnosis. None of these four episodes of care proved effective enough for me.

My first episode of physiotherapy care closely followed my hospital discharge. The outpatient reception area was only a short walk from the car park, but it was a walk I struggled to do. Sitting on the seats in the reception area was more than I could manage, and I was given permission to enter the treatment rooms and lie down to wait my turn. My pain levels were high. I remember the physiotherapist was kind and caring. She was clearly concerned about my levels of pain, and I know she discussed me with her seniors. She gave me some general ergonomic advice and advised me to buy a lumbar roll and a wedge cushion. Both proved ineffective and made my pain worse. She performed some manual therapy and gave me some simple home exercises. I remember these as core stability exercises. We both knew the therapy wasn't proving effective enough, and I was discharged to wait for an epidural injection.

Around a year later, I had a second, GP-based, course of physiotherapy. I was seen for three sessions. I was given some simple advice and some simple home exercises. I remember these as neural glides and core exercises. I was conscientious about practicing the exercises between sessions. Once more, it was recognised that these routine exercises weren't improving my pain or function; in fact, they were probably making my situation worse. I was discharged to wait for an epidural injection.

I underwent back surgery 17 months after the original injury, and 6 weeks following surgery, I received a third episode of physiotherapy care as a hospital outpatient. I was assessed and given advice regarding medications, and, as far as I remember, some simple core exercises. Unfortunately, my spinal surgery did not resolve either my neuropathic or back pain, and my physiotherapist expressed concern about my condition. I was referred back to my spinal surgeons for review and was discharged from physiotherapy to await the outcome.

My surgeons arranged for an MRI with contrast, which showed nerve root scarring. They told me there was nothing more surgically they could do to help and referred me back for further outpatient physiotherapy. Their referral letter said, 'we feel that she should have an intensive course of physiotherapy to improve her core stability'. 'Core exercises' and 'core stability' had been strong themes throughout my healthcare treatment. The resultant episode of therapy included a component of core exercises but also included some general advice and manual therapy. I was also referred into the hospital's Active Back Classes, which were group exercise classes aimed at improving the function of those with back difficulties. I found these helpful.

Although I don't think I gained any benefit from the 'core' exercises, and probably only limited short term benefit in the manual therapy, overall this was a more successful episode of care for me. The therapist discussed with me my concerns about the physical nature of my work and gave me advice that proved to be profoundly important to me. Following these discussions, I decided to change my career, which has resulted in positive long-term improvements in my pain condition and ability to enjoy life whilst living with pain.

Despite the limited success in this last episode of therapy care, these four episodes were just not effective enough for me. In my view, these episodes of care were 'routine' and weren't sufficiently person centred. The approaches used may have worked well for others, but overall, they didn't work well enough for me. It appears to me that how 'most people' should be treated was of primary importance, and clinical judgement was of less importance. Figure 11.1 shows how I view those

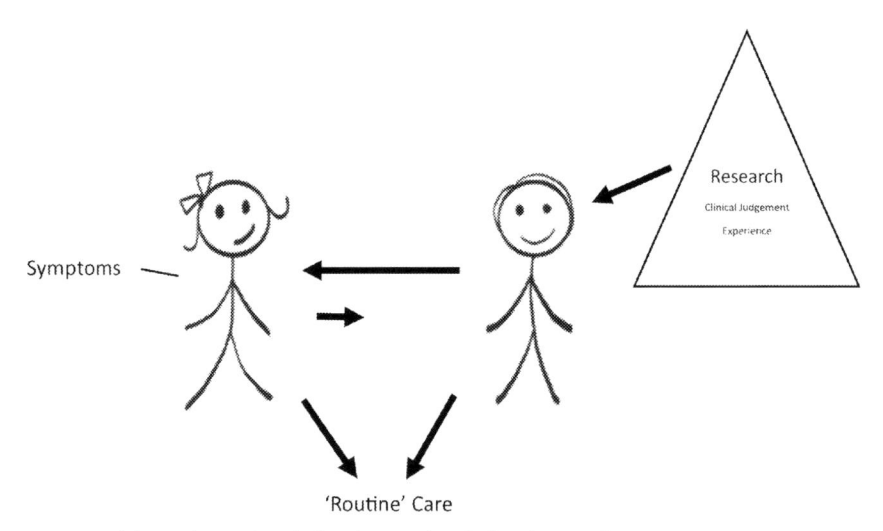

*Figure 11.1* My first four years of healthcare.

first four years of healthcare. Although my symptoms and experiences were considered, I think they were 'filtered' by the sometimes narrow questions I was asked. I believe the physiotherapists had an idea what type of 'evidence' they wanted from me and probably inadvertently led me to describe a narrow focus of my condition rather than the wider focus I lived with and the particular circumstances I was living within, which inevitably forms part of my overall condition and presentation.

Although I had experienced four years of physiotherapy care, I didn't really understand why my body was constantly in pain. I hadn't been given much, if any, help to improve my day-to-day physical function, and I hadn't been taught pain self-management. I wasn't helped to walk or to sit, despite these being huge difficulties for me. My 'lop-sidedness', and the maladaptive way I was holding and using my body, was noted but ignored. Despite my pain being predominantly neuropathic, I wasn't taught much, if anything, about neuropathic pain. Nobody taught me about the complexity of pain.

I can honestly say that there was little about those episodes of physiotherapy care that I have taken forward in dealing with my life with persistent pain. I don't look back and think about those sessions, reflect on what I was taught in them, or apply them to my everyday life. They haven't helped me cope day to day with my emotions around living with persistent pain. I didn't leave them with a better, or in fact any, understanding of the complexity of pain. I didn't gain any transferable skills, and I wasn't shown how to adapt or extend any exercises I was taught.

## *A clinical perspective on evidence-based practice*

From the perspective of evidence-based practice, the interventions described previously were typical (Hodges & Richardson, 1996; O'Sullivan, 2000; Hides et al., 2019), and the treatments were in keeping with the recommended guidelines at the time. The key guidelines that were being referenced were the National Institute of Clinical Excellence (NICE) low back pain in adults: Early management guidelines (CG88). They were drawn from a group of experts in the field of low back pain and included multiple stakeholders who painstakingly evaluated the clinical research evidence and applied their best judgement toward their aims. The aims of the guidelines were to 'systematically develop statements to assist practitioner and patient decisions about appropriate healthcare for specific clinical circumstances' (NICE 2009). The clinical research that was selected came from population studies that prioritised randomised controlled trials and systematic reviews, as they represented the best methodological way in which to reduce bias. These guidelines listed their goals to achieve a 'high impact on patient outcomes in pain, disability or psychological distress' in 'reducing variation in the treatment offered to patients leading to more efficient use of NHS resources' and to 'promote patient choice' (NICE 2009). However, CG88 was aimed at patients with low back pain but did not provide guidance with neuropathic pain. For these symptoms, the NICE guidelines that were relevant at the time were called 'Neuropathic pain in adults: Pharmacological management in non-specialist settings' CG 96 (NICE, 2010). These guidelines focused on pharmaceutical management rather than any particular guidance on physical therapy. In any case, physical therapists require clinical judgement in order to apply the clinical guidelines for the patient that most closely represent her symptoms, her situation, and her circumstances.

CG88 suggested that all patients with low back pain should be advised to exercise and that an exercise programme should be tailored to the individual. A supervised group exercise programme was recommended in preference to one-to-one supervised exercise. The caveat to the individualisation of the treatment was that the course of exercise could include a course of manual therapy (up to nine sessions over to a maximum of 12 weeks) dependent on patient preference. We saw that Christine Price received all of the previous treatments but felt isolated, not listened to, and an object of intervention. It appears that the context of 'preference' was with respect to a treatment option rather than a deliberated *choice* fostered on genuine and considered involvement. This brings us to the question of how successful the guidelines were for Christine and how she was helped, cared for, and supported.

'Core stability', or the synonym 'motor control', exercises for the lumbar spine, are intended to improve low back pain based on the original premise of segmentally stabilising the lumbar spine in its 'neutral zone' (Panjabi, 1992). The approach initially gained traction in the mid-1990s (Hodges & Richardson, 1996) and early 2000s (O'Sullivan, 2000), until one of its early pioneers, O'Sullivan (2012), and others (Lederman, 2010), began to favour multidimensional and person-centred approaches instead. The 'core stability' or 'motor control' treatment approaches are still prevalent today (Hides et al., 2019), but they maintain a reductionistic lens on a complex, multilayered problem that involves the whole person and their situation in the world (Osborn & Smith, 1998; O'Sullivan, 2012).

As multidimensional and person-centred approaches to patient care are gathering momentum, the clinician still has to consider how best to apply knowledge gained from clinical research and make sense of it in practice with the individual case. Clinical research alone does not provide us with the type of knowledge we need to make decisions about the care of individuals, nor is it appropriate without an understanding of the social, situational, relational, and professional as well as personal goals, values, and preferences of the people we serve. The clinician requires more tools than evidence-based practice has provided in order to bridge this gap. That is not to suggest that clinical research is not useful. It is indeed essential. But an understanding of the pathophysiological rationale (based upon the underlying theories of physiology, disease, and healing), system features (resource availability; societal, personal, and professional values; legal and cultural contexts), and clinical experience (including the experience of others) alongside the patient preferences, values, and expectations, is required to be integrated into clinical decision-making (Tonelli, 2011). Drawing from Aristotle, knowledge is multifaceted and emerges from the episteme (scientific knowledge), techne (craftsmanship, skill, and tacit knowledge), and phronesis (the practical wisdom and judgement to do the right thing at the right time for the right person in the right situation) and therefore is a dynamic, evolving, and socially situated phenomenon that is intrinsically value laden. Such values require a balanced and pluralistic perspective harnessed by sound reflexivity and reflection on one's self as a clinician and the best 'evidence' used in practice.

## *A philosophical perspective on evidence-based methodology and practice*

Before moving on to a more person-centred and collaborative approach, we should take a closer look at the notion of 'evidence', and specifically 'causal evidence', used within evidence-based approaches. What counts as evidence will depend on what we think causation is (ontology) and how we think causation ought to be established (epistemology). We heard that Christine was offered the best available treatment, proven to work best for most patients within her subpopulation. Evidence-based practice is thus one where decisions about individuals are based on evidence primarily from other similar individuals. A criticism of this is that one effectively treats patients as statistical averages of their relevant subpopulations. Philosophically, the evidence-based framework sits perfectly within empiricist philosophy and the corresponding theory of causation, as we will now explain.

Empiricism is the philosophical idea that one can only trust as true knowledge what can be backed up by observation. From this empiricist starting-point, David Hume (1739) formulated his regularity theory of causation. The regularity theory defines causation as a perfect correlation, where the same type of cause is always followed by the same type of effect under sufficiently similar conditions. An epistemic advantage of this theory is that causation becomes something that can be evidenced empirically, or even statistically, if one has enough relevant correlation data. A disadvantage is that one cannot easily deal with individual variations or even marginal cases where statistical data are lacking. Christine's case is marginal insofar as her responses to the best available treatment were not normal or average. What was documented to work best for other people did not work for her.

David Hume (1739) also proposed the counterfactual definition of causation, stating that a cause should make an observable difference to the effect. This definition has motivated comparative methods for establishing causation, including randomised controlled trials (RCTs), where two sets of correlation data (test and control) are compared to see whether the intervention made a statistical difference. Note, however, that we are not here establishing whether the intervention makes a difference within an individual case but only what happens on group level. To establish that an intervention made a difference in this particular case, one would have to compare the outcome with what would have happened without the intervention.

If we accept the Humean empiricist conception of causation, statistically based approaches to causal evidence are entirely justified. From this philosophical perspective, correlation data and comparisons of these provide the best causal evidence. While this might work well for public health purposes, where one deals with whole populations, we saw an example of what might happen when basing treatment decisions for single patients primarily on statistical evidence. We have here tried to show that evidence-based methodology and practice are heavily motivated by a particular philosophical framework (for a detailed discussion on the Humean influence on scientific methodology, see Anjum & Mumford, 2018). In the next section, we propose an alternative philosophical framework that again should motivate a different methodology and practice.

## Person-centred healthcare, from theory to practice

### *Dispositionalism as an alternative philosophical framework*

The Humean conception of causation is not the only available theory, and it might not even be the most serviceable one when dealing with single patients. Hume saw observed repetition as necessary for establishing causation, namely that the same type of cause should give the same effect under similar conditions. If no same cause or condition exists, causation cannot be established or even rationally asserted. In the clinic, however, one must accept that each patient is unique and that what works for most people might not work for a particular individual. A genuinely person-centred healthcare would then not sit comfortably with the Humean framework or the evidence-based methodology.

Causal dispositionalism is a philosophical theory, developed in Mumford and Anjum (2011), which takes the opposite starting point from Hume, that causation happens in the single case and no two causal situations are plausibly identical. Here, a cause is a type of disposition. Dispositional properties typically exist without ever manifesting. A person might be fertile without ever having children. Or someone can have the causal power to run five miles, break a collarbone, or suffer from prolapse without any of these things ever happening. Whether these dispositions eventually manifest will depend on the causal situation, including the person's physiology, activity, life situation, vulnerability, general health, mental state, and so on. All factors that somehow influence the causal outcome are themselves dispositions, or causes. Any effect will thus be a result of many such dispositional properties coming together and interacting.

The vector model (Figure 11.2) represents dispositional causation. It can be used to illustrate some of its essential features, such as direction and intensity of disposition, causal complexity, tipping points or threshold effects, context-sensitivity, and linear and non-linear composition, as well as additive and subtractive intervention (for details, see Mumford & Anjum, 2011).

In Christine's case, relevant threshold effects $F$ and $G$ would be chronic pain and absence of pain. From the dispositionalist theory of causation, a treatment would only be effective insofar as it is an appropriate 'mutual manifestation partner' for the individual receiving treatment, meaning that the treatment and the individual can interact to produce a joint effect. That many other people have experienced an effect from a treatment would not mean that this person will, for instance, if this person lacks some dispositional properties needed to interact with the treatment. If we were to model the treatments that Christine received, it is not clear whether they should be illustrated as disposing toward pain, away from pain, or as having no effect at all. That will depend on how we model her unique context but also on our

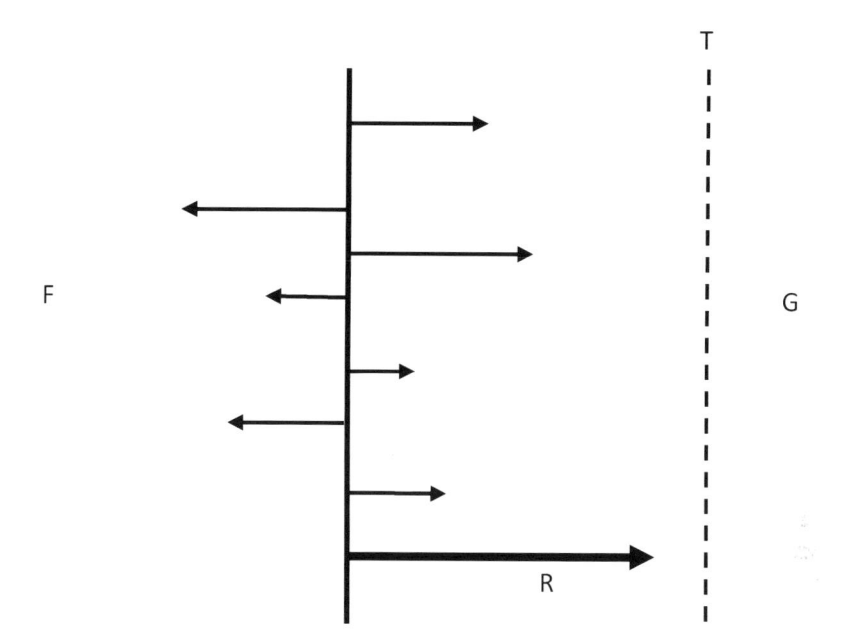

*Figure 11.2* The vector model of causation.

Source: *F* and *G* represent two opposite outcomes. The arrows illustrate causes and their lengths indicate their intensities. R is the resultant vector: the overall tendency of the dispositions combined. *T* is a threshold for a certain manifestation or effect. In this model, the overall situation is close to reaching the threshold effect.

knowledge about the intervention and how that intervention interacts with Christine. To be informed by the best available evidence here means to consider evidence primarily from the patient's context but also with a mechanistic understanding about how the intervention works. Only then can one evaluate whether the treatment is an appropriate mutual manifestation partner for the patient in their specific situation.

### *Dispositionalism as a clinical tool for person-centred healthcare*

Physiotherapists have traditionally been trained to compartmentalise their clinical observations into subjective and objective phenomena in order to form a critical analysis and create a substantive plan. As much as this approach may be considered a useful heuristic of practice, it does suggest a touch of hubris in signifying that the practitioner's interpretations are objective and that their clinical tests are definitive of a greater truth status than the subjective experience of the patient. It is, after all, the patient's experiences of pain, function, or (dis)ability that physiotherapeutic interventions are directed at. Often, patients look for support and understanding regarding the predicament that they are in beyond the subject/object divide, particularly in the context of pain.

Pain is inherently complex, and its understanding continues to be a rich area of research, opinion, and debate, from the metaphysics of theory to the empiricism and pragmatism of clinical praxis. People in pain usually seek diagnosis for more than a treatment or management plan. They are often also looking for justice, validity, and social acceptance that steer away from the stigma of psychological or psychosomatic illness. Understanding causation is central to everything that is sought from both the practitioner and the person suffering with pain. Key questions that are asked include: What is causing the pain? What treatments might be effective? And what might the future hold for a person with persistent pain? These questions require both clinicians and patients to make sense of the situation, reflecting on past experiences, current circumstances, and future possibilities. This co-constructed narrative is an important feature of the therapeutic alliance and reasoning process. This 'inter-subjectivity', or the understanding of each party's lifeworld (Osborn & Smith, 1998; Øberg, Normann, & Gallagher, 2015), is an essential aspect of drawing together the multiple sources of 'evidence' that start and end with the patient at their centre.

The sensitive and considered use of cautious conversations allows a coherent, mutual understanding to develop and is of the utmost importance. Physiotherapists are privileged in that they, within an accepted social context, have permission to touch, hold, and physically assist people through movement in both assessment and treatment. Both forms of verbal and body communication create a tacit form of interaction and are an additional method of therapeutic intervention.

A multidimensional approach that includes physical, relational, psychological, social, environmental, and lifestyle domains are considered during both the narrative and normative evaluations (Launer, 2018). Elements that are felt to have causal interactions are drawn into a mind-map which attempts to develop a written account, initially from the perspective of the clinician. The patient is given the opportunity, either at the time or at a later point, to adjust, reframe, and correct the mind-map so that it makes intelligible sense for them. Often, recounting a patient's story through the writing of a timeline with relevant causal inferences can be a helpful sense-making strategy in itself. Perhaps using this approach can act as a bridge between the first- and third-person perspective, that of the person's lived experience and that of the clinician-respective viewpoints.

In Low (2017, 2018), I describe how I used the vector model as a clinical tool to explore a person's individual circumstances and personalise a treatment plan. The patient was given explicit permission to evaluate or change the strength and direction of the dispositions as they felt their situation and circumstances evolved. Every patient is different and has varying levels of autonomy and confidence in using the mind-map and vector model. As a clinician, I ascertain this during the interaction and adjust my approach accordingly. At times, I lead the direction of the session, including planning, while at others, the patient leads. It is entirely context dependent.

It is important that the model should reflect a reflexive and evolving situation which may result in unpredictable or non-linear manifestations. The vector model is not a representation of the sum of causal factors that stack up and result in an effect. It is a means by which the interactions between causal factors can be accessed but at the same time recognises the inherent complex nature of causation. The causal dispositions may interact in ways that may at times be unseen, or, indeed, not all may be accounted for. This reflects the inherent uncertainty of the reality of clinical practice without being so relative that the model collapses upon itself. Thinking in this way facilitates epistemic humility and fosters a healthy perspective on supporting patients who are experiencing complex and often uncertain symptoms. Modelling the clinical encounter in this way provides a platform to focus or concentrate on discrete aspects that may have an effect but can also explain why, even if positive improvements have been made, there has been no overall improvement in the pain experience. The model may also describe how even small changes that may not seem important can have a large effect.

The vector model can be used to discuss how potential treatments may have a positive, stabilising, or negative effect. An example might be how non-steroidal anti-inflammatories (NSAIDs) may reduce a person's pain through their action on COX-1 and/or COX-2 enzymes but may, at the same time, inhibit bone healing following a fracture or after surgery. However, the pain relief may allow improved sleep patterns, enhanced adherence to rehabilitation strategies, and activities that enhance bone healing. Through thoughtful discussion, the patient may disclose that they have previously responded well to NSAIDs in the past and have had no negative side effects. However, in Christine's account, the use of medication had significant side effects and inhibited general function and activities of daily living. On the one hand, it might have reduced her pain, but on the other, the medication had a deleterious effect, not only on Christine but on how she interacted with the people and situations around her.

### *An experience of being treated as a unique individual*

Approximately four years after my injury, I received an episode of physiotherapy care from Matthew Low, which took a much more individualised and personalised healthcare format. With his help, I became better able to manage and deal with my pain situation. I became better able to live life well with persistent pain. For several years after, I self-managed my pain reasonably well. I stopped taking regular medications and declined the offer of a spinal cord stimulator. However, eventually my success at self-managing my pain began to decline, and nearly ten years after my injury, I was re-referred back for physiotherapy with Matthew.

At the time of my first referral to Matthew, I continued to experience high levels of pain, distress, and disability. I could walk a reasonable distance, but sitting remained very painful and problematic. My sleep remained poor, and my distress levels remained high. I had become very sensitive to pain medications and had been placed on a spinal cord stimulator pathway. On the surface, I was managing to live a reasonably independent life, and I continued to work part time. However, below the surface, I was struggling with the emotions involved in living with a long-term pain condition, both in terms of managing day to day and of being fearful of the future. I had remarkably little understanding of pain and few strategies to manage it.

150  *Christine Price* et al.

These physiotherapy sessions were very different to those I'd experienced before. Everything was tailored much more to me as a person and to my individual presentation of my condition. As we went through the first episode of care, I was gradually, and increasingly, encouraged and empowered to take a much more active part in discussions and decisions and a much more active part in managing my pain condition. I was skilfully supported to become a more equal and active partner in my care. Figure 11.3 shows how I view this more person-centred, but still evidence based, care.

In terms of 'treatment', as with other physiotherapists, I was given a range of exercises to undertake. However, unlike the exercises given by other physiotherapists, I felt these were more personalised to me and less 'routine'. For example, I was given exercises to correct my 'lop-sideness', which had not been addressed before. I was taught to ignore conventional advice about posture and sitting, and instead to find positions, chairs, and cushions that work for me.

An important element of my physiotherapy care was the widening of my understanding that the experience of pain evolves from more things than just a single body part in isolation to everything else. Before entering these physiotherapy sessions, I had no understanding about the complexity of pain. I was helped to understand, in a way I hadn't before, how everything about me as a person, my genetics, my emotions, my past experiences, my day-to-day experiences, and my 'physical' condition, all contribute to my experience of pain. In Figure 11.4, I explore the many different causal and dispositional factors contributing to my experience of pain. I learnt to understand how these elements constantly change and interact with each other, impacting my experience of pain, and how unique my experience of pain is.

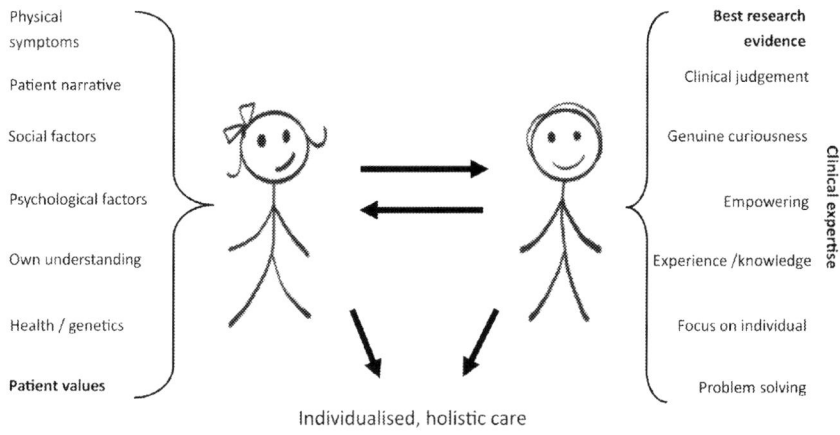

Physical symptoms

Patient narrative

Social factors

Psychological factors

Own understanding

Health / genetics

**Patient values**

**Best research evidence**

Clinical judgement

Genuine curiousness

Empowering

Experience /knowledge

Focus on individual

Problem solving

Clinical expertise

Individualised, holistic care

Genuine shared decision making, individualised explanation of pain and condition, focus on function and independence, focus on self-management, carefully considered treatments.

Condition improves beyond clinic door, including better able to self-manage and live well, with less distress.

*Figure 11.3* My experience of good, person-centred, evidence-based practice.

*Understanding chronic pain* 151

```
                    Get up and go attitude

         Experiencing distress    Past trauma    Good self-insight

         Poor pain understanding   INTJ personality   Partner and children

   Financial concerns   Disabilities            Severe pain      Poor sleep

   Fear of future in pain                              Very sensitive to meds

   Highly logical   Working part-time           Good coping skills   Asthmatic

   High IQ   Neuropathic pain                  Back pain      Shoulder pain

   Resilient   Relatively sedentary            Homeowner      Anxious

   Optimistic   Cup half full                  Fiercely independent
```

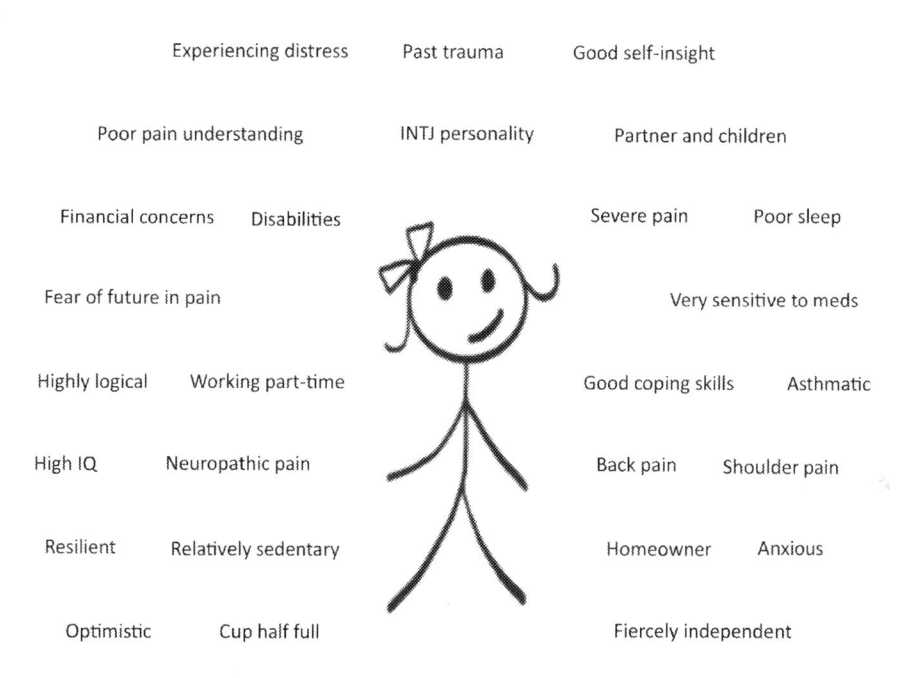

*Figure 11.4* Causal and dispositional factors contributing to my experience of pain.

Although understanding the complexity of pain has been hugely important for me in terms of living a life at peace with persistent pain, understanding pain isn't enough to successfully manage my pain on a day-to-day basis. With my physiotherapist's help, I developed a range of pain self-management skills and techniques.

I was helped to understand that there are elements of me and my life that are likely to make my pain experience worse, which I call 'pain contributors', and that there are elements of me and my life that are likely to improve my pain situation, which I call 'pain improvers'. Whilst working with Matthew, I selected a number of my pain contributors and pain improvers to work on and change. I also adapted and personalised the vector diagram to create a visual support that worked particularly well for me, shown in Figure 11.5.

In my vector diagrams, the thicker long vectors at the bottom give an indication of the overall 'level', or 'size', of either the pain contributors or pain improvers. My aim over time is to decrease the size of each of the pain contributors and increase the size of each of the pain improvers, thereby hopefully reducing my overall experience of pain. For example, if I reduce some of my work commitments, thereby reducing my workload and need to sit, and increase my understanding of pain, thereby improving my ability to manage my pain, then the associated vector lengths will change, and hopefully my overall experience of pain might improve.

## Pain contributors | Pain improvers

- Pain contributors (left, arrows pointing left):
  - Anxiety
  - Family stressors
  - Co-morbid shoulder pain
  - Poor sleep
  - Need to sit
  - Workload
  - Overall pain contributors

- Pain improvers (right, arrows pointing right):
  - Physical activity
  - Aids and adaptations
  - Understand pain
  - Relaxation
  - Pain management
  - Resilience
  - Overall pain improvers

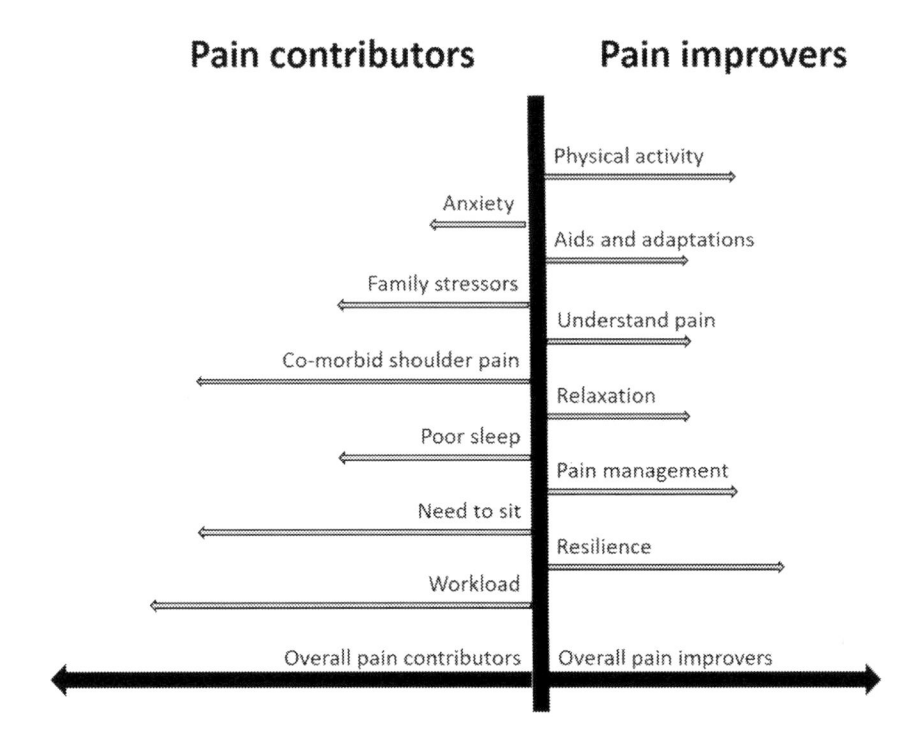

*Figure 11.5* The main contributors and improvers of my pain.

I have found this visual approach to identifying which causal factors I need to work on, and then tracking my progress over time, very helpful. As well as supporting focused improvement, the use of these vector diagrams supports discussion, shared decision-making, self-awareness, insight, and an understanding of the complexity of pain. Utilising vector diagrams, in conjunction with a range of other pain management techniques, has meant that my overall experience of pain has in reality reduced over time.

Reflecting back on my healthcare experience, there is no doubt in my mind that it was the more person-centred, but still evidence-based, care that has facilitated and enabled me to live an active and fulfilled life with pain. I cannot express how important this ability to live well with pain is to me. Although skilful, there was nothing 'magic' about this physiotherapy care. I believe it could easily have been delivered by any of the physiotherapists that I had seen in the four years before.

## Concluding remarks

According to evidence-based practice, clinicians' experience and judgement are devalued because they carry the increased likelihood of bias. However, research evidence is not without its own forms of bias. The philosophical assumptions that underpin clinical research derive, in part, from a Humean empiricist concept of causation, and the idealisation of causation favours statistical accounts over narrative ones. We have shown here how this can create a challenge for the care of individual patients.

A singularist philosophical account of causation, such as causal dispositionalism, may provide far-reaching benefits, particularly for individual cases. This is because it allows for consideration of complexity, context sensitivity, reflexivity, and individuality. Using the described framework, the patient can be given the opportunity for a fuller understanding and shared meaning of their current situation, and they are actively involved in the clinical reasoning process. This approach may foster closer shared decision-making that not only allows patients to use a variety of self-care approaches and opportunities but also provides a platform for the therapist to offer a variety of treatments in the full knowledge that the patient has greater control and informed choice. This is because the framework moves beyond the assessment, diagnosis, and reconciliation of research evidence. Attention is drawn, instead, towards the person's story, which supersedes that of a descriptive and categorical diagnosis. What lies beneath this is a person who has hopes, fears, relationships, and lifestyle considerations, as well as a lifetime of historical experiences that may have had a significant influence on them.

Statistical data are often used to determine the prognosis and management of a patient. However, a dispositionalist framework encourages the context-sensitive use of propensities that have been carefully considered in light of each individual patient. Instead of predicting effect based upon a research population, the individuality of the patient is also considered within the context of how that person relates to the research population. A genuinely person-centred approach honours and respects the person at the centre of clinical decision-making, with population data, clinical research, policy, and guidelines used to support care rather than to dictate it. All of these considerations foster a deeper person-centred approach that we consider enhances clinical care for both the therapist and patient in practice.

## References

Anjum, R. L., & Mumford, S. (2018). *Causation in science and the methods of scientific discovery*. Oxford: Oxford University Press.

David Hume (1739). *A Treatise of Human Nature by David Hume, reprinted from the Original Edition in three volumes and edited, with an analytical index, by L.A. Selby-Bigge, M.A.* (Oxford: Clarendon Press, 1896). Retrieved from https://oll.libertyfund.org/titles/342

Hides, J. A., Murphy, M., Jang, E., Blackwell, L., Sexton, M., Sexton, C., & Mendis, M. D. (2019). Predicting a beneficial response to motor control training in patients with low back pain: A longitudinal cohort study. *European Spine Journal*, 28(11), 2462–2469.

Hodges, P. W., & Richardson, C. A. (1996). Inefficient muscular stabilization of the lumbar spine associated with low back pain: A motor control evaluation of transversus abdominis. *Spine*, 21(22), 2640–2650.

Launer, J. (2018). *Narrative based practice in health and social care: Conversations inviting change*. London: Routledge.

Lederman, E. (2010). The myth of core stability. *Journal of Bodywork and Movement Therapies*, *14*(1), 84–98.

Low, M. (2017). A novel clinical framework: The use of dispositions in clinical practice: A person centred approach. *Journal of Evaluation in Clinical Practice*, *23*(5), 1062–1070.

Low, M. (2018). Managing complexity in musculoskeletal conditions: Reflections from a physiotherapist. *In Touch*, *164*, 22–28.

Mumford, S., & Anjum, R. L. (2011). *Getting causes from powers*. Oxford: Oxford University Press.

National Institute for Health and Clinical Excellence. (2009). *Low back pain: early management of persistent non-specific low back pain* (Clinical guideline 88.) www.nice.org.uk/CG88.

National Institute for Health and Clinical Excellence. (2010). *Neuropathic pain in adults: pharmacological management in non-specialist settings* (Clinical guideline 96). www.nice.org.uk/CG96.

Øberg, G., Normann, B., & Gallagher, S. (2015). Embodied-enactive clinical reasoning in physical therapy. *Physiotherapy Theory and Practice*, *21*(4), 244–252.

Osborn, M., & Smith, J. A. (1998). The personal experience of chronic benign lower back pain: An interpretative phenomenological analysis. *British Journal of Health Psychology*, *3*(1), 65–83.

O'Sullivan, P. (2000). Lumbar segmental "instability": Clinical presentation and specific stabilizing exercise management. *Manual Therapy*, *5*(1), 2–12.

O'Sullivan, P. (2012). It's time for change with the management of non-specific chronic low back pain. *British Journal of Sports Medicine*, *46*(4), 224–227.

Panjabi, M. M. (1992). The stabilizing system of the spine: Part I: Function, dysfunction, adaptation, and enhancement. *Journal of Spinal Disorders*, *5*, 383–389.

Tonelli, M. R. (2011). Integrating clinical research into clinical decision making. *Annali dell'Istituto Superiore di Sanità*, *47*(1), 26–30.

# 12 Finding the right track

Embodied reflecting teams for generous physiotherapy

*Patricia Thille, Arthur W. Frank, and Tobba T. Sudmann*

## Introduction

Emilly Munguía Marshall (2015), hereafter Emilly, wants us to remember that patients are more than their presenting complaints: 'they have a story'. And Emilly has shared one of her own.

During her first clinical rotation while studying for her physical therapy degree, Emilly encountered Mrs. B, 'an 89-year-old cute white-haired lady who was diagnosed with dementia and bipolar disorder many years ago' (para. 2). Mrs. B had accidentally overdosed on her medications, forgetting she had already taken them one day. This mistake was unlike Mrs. B, but her life was in upheaval because her husband was in hospital, dying from pancreatic cancer. Now Mrs. B was recovering in the room across the hall from him.

Physical therapy services were set up to help get Mrs. B walking and gain strength, after her body was temporarily incapacitated from the medication overdose. Before Emilly and her supervising physical therapist entered the room, the supervisor recommended that Emilly not ask Mrs. B about the assisted living facility where she lives, or about her husband, until they had a better sense of her mood and current strength.

> To my surprise, she was oriented and calm, cooperative and motivated, but teary eyed, which is never a good sign. I did a gross evaluation and we made small talk about where she was from and where she got her hair done, but all the small talk in the world couldn't keep her from mentioning that her husband was across the hall and she had just seen him. She told us how he said 'I love you,' but then she said, 'I think he's mad at me.' We somehow managed to get back on track with our session and went for a walk down the hall and back. She glanced over at his room every once in a while, but otherwise just looked down at her feet while she walked.
>
> (Munguía Marshall, 2015, para. 4)

When Emilly and Mrs. B returned from the walk, her husband's oncologist entered the room. He spoke directly, telling Mrs. B that everything medically possible for her husband had been done, and now they were giving him medication for pain to improve his comfort. Mrs. B responded by asking the physician if he thought her husband was mad at her. 'I think he's just feeling really sick, and may be needing some rest this morning'.

'Is he going to die'? Mrs. B asked.

Emily, the observer and storyteller, described her rush of emotions when Mrs. B asked this question. As Emily worked to collect herself, the oncologist replied:

> I think he's going to die, yes. He has been through a lot, so I think it will happen this week or the beginning of next week. He is very sick, and yes, I think it's almost his time to rest from being so sick.
>
> (para. 7)

The oncologist reassured Mrs. B that her husband was upset with the length of his sickness and the limitations it imposed. The clinicians, Emily included, then said their goodbyes.

Emily looked to her supervisor for support, asking how to handle 'tough situations like that', as they moved on to the next patient. The supervisor replied that it takes years of experience to build up one's ability to witness hard situations, and 'sometimes patients will stay on your mind and will affect your life a little bit' (para. 8).

Emily's stated moral of her story is that a patient is not merely a diagnosis but a human being with 'a story', actually, many years of stories. This realization was not self evident. When Emily began working with Mrs. B, she found her patient's displays of emotion 'not a good sign' and worried about getting 'back on track' after talk about Mrs. B's husband. But in Mrs. B's story, concern for her husband was the track. We, the authors, wonder how this lesson has stayed with Emily and affected her practice.

## Mindlines and the limits of clinical perception

The sense that Emily has acquired of what it is to be 'on track' can be understood using the metaphor of mindlines, as proposed by Gabbay and le May (2011). They observe that what clinicians know to do, in a particular moment of practice, depends not on articulated knowledge but rather on embodied practical knowledge, or 'mindlines'. Mindlines are internalized, in contrast to 'guidelines' which are imposed externally. Mindlines comprise integrated information from various sources, including formal training, clinical experiences with patients, stories told by esteemed colleagues, past experiences in multiple professional roles, scientific sources, understanding of local resources and context, and personal insights. Mindlines are more than personal. They are a metaphor for a collective process by which clinicians become capable of 'personalized, flexible syntheses of all the different types of theoretical and experiential knowledge that they need to be able to call upon instantaneously' (Gabbay & le May, 2011, p. 44). Flexibility means continuous modification of action responsive to the situation. Mindlines reflect a person's biography, enacted in response to a setting that calls for action. Their flexibility of response distinguishes them from protocols and guidelines.

In Emilly's story, we hear a student's discomfort and lack of embodied knowledge of how to be in such a situation with Mrs. B. Emilly appreciates the oncologist's approach, which she describes as 'direct, comforting, and honest' (para. 7). She seeks feedback and support from her supervisor about how to manage her own emotions as a therapist in the face of sadness *that is beyond intervention*. Her supervisor responds from her own embodied ability to know how to be, especially how to sustain a personal and professional self in the face of sad situations such as their encounter with Mrs. B. The story shows an active, dialogical process of learning and integrating new experiences and emotions. Hearing the story, we witness the student expanding her mindlines, as her supervisor may also be doing.

Mindlines, too, often develop by a series of contingencies: Having this or that supervisor, meeting particular patients in particular supervisory contexts, and the therapist's mood and vulnerabilities on a day of a memorable experience. This chapter proposes more systematic attention to how mindlines develop in clinical education and how they are sustained or changed in ongoing practice. Specifically, we want to offer tools to physical therapists to support a more generous physiotherapy practice. Our understanding of being *generous*, as a practice, relies on Frank's (2004) description, where generosity begins in welcome – a welcoming of the sick and the suffering without qualification. Generosity involves being in a relation of care where the host offers what the guest needs. The host can never completely provide what the guest needs, so the relation of care is one that starts with an implicit plea for forgiveness (Frank, 2004).

What we call moral life is enacted in the micro-moments of service delivery: 'Moral moments are frequently ones we would like to "escape" . . . because we sense that how we act will declare who we are. . . . But . . . the moral moment cannot be evaded' (Frank, 2004, p. 19). Emilly and her supervisor initially wanted to evade the emotional context of Mrs. B's clinical needs. Their generosity was their willingness to realize that non-recognition of this context would evade professional duty. But generosity is not easy to enact in many contemporary healthcare institutions that focus on repair or prevention of bodily vulnerability (Frank, 2004). Healthcare workers learn to stay 'on track'; they internalize limits to the scope of their professional work. Physical therapy, as it specifies and addresses bodily breakdowns, resists overtly recognizing power relations and patients' vulnerability (Nicholls & Gibson, 2010; Trede, 2012). Yet, for the patient, this vulnerability is what most needs to be addressed. When faced with sadness that is beyond intervention, such as that Emilly describes as occurring in her encounter with Mrs. B, we are confronted with part of what it means to be human. While we cannot meet all our guests' needs, we can build a relation of care that speaks person to person, recognizing the shared experiences of uncertainty, loneliness, and fear, rather than the therapist primarily relaying institutional demands (Frank, 2004).

In moments where clinicians and patients face sadness, loss, and fear – and other emotionally charged moments – 'they have a story' is a necessary but insufficient guide for a generous practice of physiotherapy. Everyone may have a story, but many stories are dangerous, destructive to the self and to others (Frank, 2009, 2010). Other stories are bland and without much significance. Stories require *discrimination* by the clinician; generosity does not mean uncritical acceptance of any story. To practice this discrimination, we propose a second metaphor, that of the reflecting team. In some clinical practices, reflecting teams are colleagues observing, commenting on, and perhaps intervening in clinical work. Complementary to that usage, we follow Frank (2004) in proposing a reflecting team of theorists offering ideas that both support and critique clinical practice. Our argument is that mindlines need a reflecting team. Rather than argue this point abstractly, we prefer to show how our own reflecting teams have affected our own mindlines.

## Methods

Instead of presenting a unified authorial 'we', for the rest of this chapter, we the co-authors write in our distinct voices, in dialogue with each other. Such writing recognizes the different positions we each occupy – how we are distinctively *situated* – in our professional histories and current concerns.

We intend to preserve the months of conversations in which we shared our own stories, sometimes finding ourselves recalling forgotten stories, as well as how our respective readings have affected what we take as the point of these stories. Those conversations and readings have shaped us, and specifically, they shape what stories we remember and how we remember them. We present stories because professional careers are the accumulation of stories. Stories are arguably humans' first and most enduring way to make sense of what happens in the world of which we find ourselves a part (Frank, 2010). Stories are not simple reflections of experience. How stories are told is shaped by prior stories. Past narrations are the resource and the limit of future narrations, and narration is a significant limit of what can be experienced. Stories *go with us* in life. Frank (2010) talks about stories as companions. The companion stories we each live with influence what we see as real, possible, and important; they are guides to action, both what is worth doing and what is best avoided (Frank, 2010). Stories can guide us to think seriously about what we seek and the values we aim to preserve (Frank, 2004).

To make the development of clinicians' mindlines less dependent on contingent interactions with patients, supervisors, and colleagues, we integrate each of our stories with an introduction to a theorist who has helped us reflect on our own experiences. The net effect is to propose at least one version of a 'theoretical reflecting team' to support physiotherapy mindlines that orient to generous practice. We advocate that critically reflective mindlines, as opposed to pre-conscious ones, are based on experiencing clinical work in companionship with theorists who exemplify values we seek to integrate into our work.

## Struggling to face sadness beyond intervention (Patty's story)

The first story we presented was about training. I opt to respond with a training story of my own. This story starts with an event over 23 years ago, though like all stories, I tell it anew here.

I was 22 when my mother died. Suddenly.

She didn't feel well after an afternoon of bowling and lay down to rest. Within hours, she had died from a heart attack. She was 60.

I was halfway through my physiotherapy program. There's much that I could say, but the story I want to tell about me as a physiotherapist starts with her death. Like anyone narrating the death of a loved one, death creates a rupture in time, a before and after.

Within a week of my mother's death, I returned to physiotherapy classes. In the month after her death, I admitted to my neurology physiotherapy professor that I did not plan to specialize as a neuro physiotherapist. She wondered why, and I answered honestly: 'Because patients and their families in need of neurology services were going through loss issues'. In little over a year's time, at the age of 23, I knew I would not be in a position to handle that confrontation with acute, charged moments with others. 'That is an excellent reason', she replied.

'They have a story' was not something I needed to be reminded of in the same way as Emily. It was my patients' stories that I could not face, not then, at least. I could not handle the immediacy of sadness that is beyond intervention. It brought my own human vulnerability and suffering to the fore. It touched on my own sadness, limiting my ability to be a generous host. I could not cope with that vulnerability in a professional setting, so I opted to work in fields with fewer of what I thought were 'loss issues'. Admittedly, I later learned that I had failed to appreciate how people dealing with 'loss issues' were ubiquitous among those I saw. The question was whether care was organized in a way that allowed me, as a physiotherapist, to join my patients in confronting these issues.

## *Inviting Bakhtin as a response*

Mikhail Bakhtin (1895–1975) was a Russian scholar during the period of Stalinism, writing literary theory that doubled as social theory and, depending on how one reads it, masked a critique of authoritarianism. Bakhtin's (1984 [1963]) book, *Problems in Dostoevsky's Poetics*, argues for a *dialogical* literary and social form. He starts from the assumption that language is social, in the specific sense that language is permeated with many voices. We are all polyglot, learning a variety of social dialects (Booth, 1984). There is no single authoritative voice. Instead, there is constant translation among voices (Emerson, 1984). We speak to each other in dialects of particular places and membership groups, including professional groups. The speech of those outside our group – for example, patients to clinicians – requires translation. If we translate well, we do no violence to the other voices; we do not betray the essence of the other speakers' intentions (Emerson, 1984).

But in what Bakhtin (1984 [1963]) calls authoritative, *monological* literature, there is an authority that is established that finalizes the story and the characters. Much of the speech in professional healthcare, from textbooks to grand rounds, is monological. The monological story assumes the validity of only one perspective rather than being committed to the unfinished quality, the *unfinalizability* of selves interacting. Monologue seeks completion; dialogue posits the perpetual incompleteness of anyone's story and of any relationship. Dialogical speech appreciates the interaction of voices and resists the authority speaking with a final word. Having Bahktin on our reflecting team also keeps us aware of the gap that always exists between people in interaction, their irresolvable otherness to each other. Mistranslation of a social dialect is always possible, requiring the humble recognition that we are always working with incomplete knowledge of the other. Bakhtin offers an ethics of generous communicative relatedness – of doing no violence to another by pretending to know all that needs to be known about that other.

Emilly's story foregrounds the movement from a monological to a dialogical way of thinking. In 'They Have a Story', Emily came to appreciate the incompleteness of her knowledge, the gap that exists in her understanding of her patient within the clinical context, and how such a gap can create trouble. A clinical session that began based as a monological performance certain of what is and is not 'on track' became what may be Emilly's first movement toward conscious clinical work as dialogue with the patient. Her story is an opening to a generous practice.

In contrast, I (Patty) didn't struggle to remember 'they have a story'. I was not in a monological mindset. Instead, I struggled with what was, at that time in my professional life, a raw grief so overwhelming that it could not admit space for my patients' stories. The trouble I faced was coping with patients' and families' emotions and vulnerability. At that time in my professional life, my grief was too raw for me to engage the stories of those with acute neurological injuries. I could not be a generous host, because my inner dialogue was too noisy for external dialogue to be possible. I had not yet developed the capacity to be deeply attuned to their suffering and sadness without being overwhelmed by them.

How to develop mindlines that enact generosity, that strive for a dialogical type of care? Here, we invite another story to think with – and another theorist.

## Facing sadness beyond intervention (Tobba's story)

The story I want to share is about a couple that I met almost weekly in 2018–2019, Elliot and Louise. Elliot participated in a three-armed RCT study of neuro plasticity and cognitive decline. The three arms in the RCT were physical activity (I was project leader), music therapy, and one-year delayed intervention (either physical activity or music therapy). The team responsible for the physical activity intervention (physical therapist [PI], sports teachers, and students at the BA program in public health) did physical tests on all participants in the project and were responsible for a weekly physical activity session, indoors or outdoors, depending on weather and season. Activities were organized to be fun and playful and to facilitate physical, cognitive, and social engagement in the group, for example, using circuit training or physical education stations. Whenever possible, we tried to utilize the participants' previous experiences or knowledge in physical education or sports.

Elliot and Louise always came together to the sessions, often hand in hand. Louise was obviously very fond of her husband, and Elliot of her, so it was quite moving to see them together. I also observed how much fun and support both got from the group of study participants and from the group of students and teachers.

During springtime, Elliot came to one session wearing a Lakers basketball T-shirt, and Louise told us he used to be a keen player and a serious fan of several basketball teams. From the start of the project, Elliot had moved slowly, struggling to understand and follow the group's activities, even if he had two students guiding him. Yet when we gave him an American basketball, he started moving with grace, bouncing the ball to the perfect position to be able to jump and put the ball right into the basket. We were all so happy, and the smile on his face, to us and his wife, was unforgettable. Alas, we did not capture that magic moment on video.

Basketball was not a magical cure. Elliot became increasingly affected by his dementia, and his problems following the group's activities increasingly bothered him. As dementia progressed, it became harder to motivate him to take part in activities that he found difficult to master and follow. Not many months later, Elliot and Louise had to withdraw from the project due to a rapid deterioration of his health.

Losing function and health is part of living. But losing health and days to incurable disease is very hard for everyone involved, whatever the cause. My encounter with this couple is an example of the 'love and sadness beyond intervention' that I have encountered several times in my professional and private life. But for me, Elliot finding himself in basketball brought together a few pivotal professional experiences where I have discovered both generosity and hospitality, or the lack thereof. I learned a lesson about how to meet, greet, and create an ephemeral communitas with people in grief and distress (Sudmann, 2018a, 2018b). The short-lived and transitory sense of community, or sense of shared experiences, may create a stirring moment with a healing potential.

### *Story meets story*

To gain permission to publish their story in this chapter, I sent the account by email to Louise, explaining our writing focus for this chapter. She answered the next day, not only granting us permission to print the story but adding that she found it touching and beautiful. She went on to tell me that her husband had passed away just a few days earlier; I had not yet seen the death notice or the obituary that were in the local newspaper the same day. Louise's comments on my story are included subsequently, again with permission, as she touches directly upon the topic of this chapter – hospitality and generosity.

It was hard and very sad to watch how my husband deteriorated and withered away. He struggled a lot with eating and swallowing, and lost weight very quickly. He died peacefully at home, with me holding his hand.

It was two things that made our life a bit better, after my husband was diagnosed with Alzheimer's disease. First and foremost, it was the project with you and your colleagues and students, these weekly group session at your university. He was always happy after these sessions. We appreciated these sessions with you very much – both the physical activity as such and being together with all of you. The second activity was a monthly arts session for persons living with dementia at an art gallery in the city, arranged by The Dignity Centre. The coordinators from the centre had chosen three different paintings to prompt conversation. My husband was very knowledgeable and skilled, and he always commented upon features in the painting that others did not notice, or facts or comments about the painter not known to the presenters. A year ago, one of the coordinators played music while showing a picture, a song well known to many adults in Norway, and my husband got up and sang 12 verses (most of us never knew there was so many verses) – no false note, no false lyric. I was so impressed, and proud. The coordinators were completely overwhelmed. I'll never forget that!

### Beyond reflection

My story has one final loop. When I was working with Elliot and Louise, I was mourning the loss of my husband, after a long and strenuous five years of cancer that included brain metastasis. I encountered in Elliot and Louise a reflection of my own experiences; they mirrored my acquired knowledge of what it is to await decline and eventual death. When Patty lost her mother, her experience turned her inward. When I met Elliot and Louise, I turned outward, recognizing their pain through my guts. This recognition was not cognitive; it came not through *reflection* or *reflective practice*, though writing about it now is an act of reflection. At the time, I felt a bodily recognition of love, loss, and fear of what tomorrow might bring. I wanted consolation and even fun – a pause or break in my day as much as in my patients' days. Those sessions created an oasis where the heavy burden of loss became more bearable.

### Practicing with Gadamer

Since my graduation as a physical therapist several decades ago, I have been struggling to understand how clinical encounters can be created and enacted to add value to our patients' recuperation or reconciliation with what cannot be healed. In *The Enigma of Health* (Gadamer, 1996 [1993]) and in many of his later writings and interviews (Gadamer, 2007 [1997]), Hans-Georg Gadamer (1900–2002) dwelled on his own experiences with longevity and bodily changes, as well as pondering how understanding is possible and how healthcare is an art that is based on communication and understanding. After immersing myself in Gadamer's texts and dialogues (Gadamer, 2006 [1960]), and in particular feminist re-interpretations of his masterpiece *Truth and Method* (Code, 2003), Gadamer became a companion for my reflections on how I can create, sustain, and end fruitful dialogues and recuperative encounters with my patients and their next of kin.

For Gadamer, health is a bodily experience to which people pay no particular attention; the body is 'forgotten' until one experiences a loss of the usual equilibrium. When equilibrium is lost, a sense of uncanniness or homelessness in the body may be experienced, a disturbance in the sense of wellbeing. What Gadamer means by the *enigma* of health is that being healthy – a state of life he calls wellbeing – is a state of not noticing health, of being ready for and open to everything. Gadamer dwells upon the miraculous existence of health and how suffering or pain has a profound power of 'inwardization'. When we are drawn into ourselves, we lose contact with the external experience of the world (Gadamer, 1996 [1993]).

For Gadamer, everything that can be understood is language, which includes not only spoken language but also signs and gestures. Human understanding evolves as an 'event of play': The interactants must let themselves be played hitherto and thitherto, back and forth, by the evolving dialogues and social interaction. Diversity between us is productive and opens up creativity – which we need in our quest for re-establishing an equilibrium in our bodies. By playing and being played, we can always be open to new possibilities (Gadamer, 2007 [1997]; Vilhauer, 2013). When loss of previously unnoticed equilibrium turns our attention inwards, our ability to understand, explore, or exploit what can be offered in the form of treatment from healthcare services is reduced. If understanding evolves as an event of play, inwardization will hamper understanding and healing, as Gadamer sees it.

Gadamer's way of thinking enables us to see how Elliot entered our project in a state of disequilibrium, inwardly focused and not at rest or home in his own body. Louise tried to facilitate Elliot's outward attention through touch, movement, and spoken words. In those sessions, Elliot eventually found a way to *play* once again. That moment was transitory, but Louise's email is testimony to its importance.

For me as a physical therapist and researcher, Gadamer offers a reminder of the primacy of being at home in one's body and how creativity and curiosity may affect our patients' inward or outward attention. I think of Gadamer's description of health as mysterious and enigmatic, and his description of understanding as an event of play, as a parallel to Frank's descriptions of generosity in healthcare encounters. The two serve as guides for finding a way of welcoming patients to my world, and inviting myself into their world, by looking for ways to increase bodily well-being and equilibrium.

## Conclusion (Arthur's commentary)

We offer three stories – Emilly's, Patty's, and Tobba's – not in order to find themes that are common to all three, much less to abstract practice guidelines from them. The stories should remain distinct, yet when placed in dialogue with each other, each signifies more than any one story by itself. Emilly's story shows a student being surprised by what she can recognize in the life of her patient. She discovers in Mrs. B not a patient requiring rehabilitation but a person who has a story, and for Emilly, Mrs. B then becomes not a *case*, denoting physical problems and therapeutic interventions, but a *story*, which includes relationships, losses, and, for the clinical professional, a dual acknowledgement of professional limits and expansive personal demand for response. That story becomes part of Emilly's mindline as a physiotherapist. It will work as a companion for Emilly in future practice, affecting what she is able to see and experience in her later patients. Mrs. B's story will shape Emilly's practice. In the future, as Emilly retells this story – certainly to herself, possibly in her own teaching and writing – she will change it, shaping the story according to other stories that the initial story attracts. It's a reasonable guess that the story of Mrs. B was not *initial* but rather that Emilly experienced what happened as narratable because of earlier stories that preceded her training in physiotherapy.

Among the three physiotherapists in these stories, Patty is living through the saddest time in her own life. Her personal sadness made engagement with certain patients too difficult for her. But what may be most interesting is how Patty, at this young age, had such reflective awareness of her contingent limitations, and she had the good luck to have a clinical instructor who respected Patty's ability to speak those limitations, which not everyone can articulate. A crucial part of Patty's mindline, so early in her career, was an awareness of *where she was* and how that affected what she could offer her patients. The sadness of that moment is, for those hearing her story, redeemed by the promise of how this self-awareness will develop and what it will eventually make possible in her career.

Patty's story helps us understand a physiotherapy session as a shared space, and whatever success is in the session depends on how much of themselves each, the professional and the patient, can bring to that space. Tobba's story is about how professionals can enable patients to bring more of themselves, by offering patients the resources they need but cannot ask for.

Tobba, also, is living through one of her saddest times, but, for multiple reasons, including their respective ages and experience, she is able to channel her sadness into her practice. Tobba's story takes us back to Emilly's phrase and the question it poses: What is it for a physiotherapy session to be 'on track'? Whatever benefit Elliot and Louise find in their participation in the project's group is physical only in the most transitory sense. Tobba's story makes us want to hyphenate the *physio* in physiotherapy. Tobba observes a clue – the Lakers t-shirt – and translates that into a clinical act, giving Elliot a basketball. That ball enables a moment of recovering a self that, Louise's email encourages us to believe, will not be lost as Elliot's abilities decline. That last moment of fluid movement will inform *how* he experiences the inevitable decline. As Louise writes, it was a time when they could still be happy. How that happiness could be measured in the evaluation of effectiveness – compared with the other two arms of this study – highlights the limits of measurement and of studies that only count what can be measured.

Tobba also offers us an opening to what may lie beyond reflective practice as it is often understood. She suggests it might be useful to distinguish between cognitive reflection and embodied reflection. The word *reflection* implies a cognition: It implies seeing and then thinking about one's own actions as if they were those of another. *Embodied reflection* may be an oxymoron, because to know from and within the body is not to stand outside and look upon that body and its situation. In Tobba's coda about how her work with Elliot and Louise was affected by her bereavement, she shows either the limits of reflection, or another form of reflection, or both.

Finally, how important are Bakhtin and Gadamer, respectively, in Patty's and Tobba's ability to tell their stories and to integrate those stories into their clinical mindlines? Bakhtin and Gadamer offer ideals of interpersonal relationships and a vocabulary that enables measuring a current, lived situation against those ideals. But beyond that, with their authority as *philosophers*, Bakhtin and Gadamer help Patty and Tobba *take their experiences seriously*, and that may be our most important point in this chapter. Professional practice is all about what physiotherapists take seriously and consider on or off track, narratable to whom, measurable for what purposes, and an appropriate use of institutional resources. Emily gives no indication of having any such reflecting team, but our point is that for more developing professionals to be able to tell a story as Emily does, it can help to add a theoretical reflecting team to whatever other teams are available to enable reflection. Emilly's story is a start; a purposeful integration of theory could deepen her appreciation of patients' stories and lives. Again, for a generous physiotherapy, we advocate supporting the development of reflective, perhaps *mindful*, mindlines, based on experiencing clinical work in companionship with theorists who exemplify values we seek to integrate into practice.

Put another way, professional practice takes place in the reciprocity between the professionals' inner dialogue – and for us, a *mindline* is a dialogue between multiple competing voices – and their external dialogues with patients, colleagues, supervisors, and whomever else. What counts as speakable and what can be heard in those internal and external dialogues is crucial. If any of the voices in these inner and external dialogues is not responded to with recognition, and, preferably, generosity, humans withdraw and dialogue ends. Stories both are companions, and they need companions. Bakhtin and Gadamer help, but so can many other theorists. For those who want to tell the kind of stories that Emily, Patty, and Tobba tell, we hope this chapter can be one companion in their ongoing dialogues.

# References

Bakhtin, M. (1984 [1963]). *Problems of Dostoevsky's poetics* (C. Emerson, Trans.). Minneapolis, MN: University of Minnesota Press.
Booth, W. C. (1984). Introduction. In C. Emerson (Ed.), *Problems of Dostoevsky's poetics* (pp. xiii–xxvii). Minneapolis, MN: University of Minnesota Press.
Code, L. (2003). *Feminist interpretations of Hans-Georg Gadamer*. University Park, PA: Pennsylvania State University Press.
Emerson, C. (1984). Editor's preface. In C. Emerson (Ed.), *Problems of Dostoevsky's poetics* (pp. xxix–xliii). Minneapolis, MN: University of Minnesota Press.
Frank, A. W. (2004). *The renewal of generosity: Illness, medicine, and how to live*. Chicago, IL: The University of Chicago Press.
Frank, A. W. (2009). The necessity and dangers of illness narratives, especially at the end of life. In Y. Gunaratnum & D. Oliviere (Eds.), *Narrative and stories in health care: Illness, dying, and bereavement* (pp. 161–175). New York, NY: Oxford University Press.
Frank, A. W. (2010). *Letting stories breathe: A socio-narratology*. Chicago, IL: The University of Chicago Press.
Gabbay, J., & le May, A. (2011). *Practice-based evidence for healthcare: Clinical mindlines*. Abingdon, UK: Routledge.
Gadamer, H. G. (1996 [1993]). *The enigma of health: The art of healing in a scientific age* (J. Gaiger & N. Walker, Trans.). Cambridge, UK: Polity Press.
Gadamer, H. G. (2006 [1960]). *Truth and method* (J. Weinsheimer & D. G. Marshall, Trans.). London, UK: Continuum International Publishing Group.

Gadamer, H. G. (2007 [1997]). *The Gadamer reader: A bouquet of the later writings* (R. E. Palmer, Trans.). Evanston, IL: Northwestern University Press.

Munguía Marshall, E. (2015). They have a story. *The Journal of Humanities in Rehabilitation.* Retrieved from www.jhrehab.org/2015/07/08/they-have-a-story/

Nicholls, D. A., & Gibson, B. E. (2010). The body and physiotherapy. *Physiotherapy Theory and Practice, 26*(8), 497–509. https://doi.org/10.3109/09593981003710316

Sudmann, T. T. (2018a). Equine-facilitated physiotherapy: Devised encounters with daring and compassion. In D. A. Nicholls, B. E. Gibson, K. S. Groven, & J. Setchell (Eds.), *Manipulating practice: A critical physiotherapy reader* (pp. 194–218). Oslo, NO: Cappelen Damm Akademisk.

Sudmann, T. T. (2018b). Communitas and Friluftsliv: Equine-facilitated activities for drug users. *Community Development Journal, 53*(3), 556–573. https://doi.org/10.1093/cdj/bsy026

Trede, F. (2012). Emancipatory physiotherapy practice. *Physiotherapy Theory and Practice, 28*(6), 466–573. https://doi.org/10.3109/09593985.2012.676942

Vilhauer, M. (2013). Gadamer and the game of understanding: Dialogue-play and opening to the other. In E. Ryall, W. Russell, & M. MacLean (Eds.), *The philosophy of play* (pp. 89–100). Abington, UK: Routledge.

# 13 Why care about culture? Encountering diversity in a paediatric rehabilitation context

Reflections on epiphanies and transformative processes

*Runa Kalleson, Linn Julie Skagestad, and Sosan Asgari Mollestad*

**Introduction**

The world today is characterized by widespread migration and increased interconnectedness. This global displacement is at a record high, with approximately 244 million international migrants (International Organization of Migration, 2018). This implies concrete changes to the environments where physiotherapists operate and increases the likelihood of encounters with cultures that contrast with a Western rehabilitation mindset.

Even though cultural competence among service providers in rehabilitation is a topic quite extensively addressed in the literature, there is still a scarcity of research that explicitly examines professional cultures and a lack of texts that bridge experiential, empirical, and theoretical perspectives from related fields. With this chapter, we aim to contribute to the literature by drawing on reflection-based insights that emerged through an innovative partnership between a physiotherapist working with minority families, a social worker with an immigrant background, and a psychologist who draws upon perspectives from the fields of sociocultural psychology, rehabilitation, and philosophy. We consider the chapter relevant to practitioners and researchers who encounter diversity in professional contexts in general and within the field of paediatric rehabilitation in particular.

The overall purpose is to sensitize readers to issues of diversity. We aim to highlight some of the challenges service providers may face encountering families of different backgrounds and illuminate the need for critical self-reflection upon one's culture, assumptions, and positionality in society. Based on these aims, we invite readers to follow a paediatric physiotherapist's path towards increased cultural awareness and personal and professional growth through encounters with a minority family, collaboration with a cultural liaison, and subsequent reflections with a psychologist.

The text presents a series of autoethnographic reflections, an approach seeking to describe and systematically analyze personal experiences in order to understand aspects of culture (Ellis, Adams, & Bochner, 2011). The culture in focus is a part of the municipal rehabilitation services directed to children with disabilities and their families in Norway. The chosen approach is in line with the recommendations to study systems and cultures of healthcare delivery in order to promote more culturally competent services (Napier et al., 2014).

We present epiphanies based on critical incidents perceived to have had a significant impact on the first author's development as a physiotherapist working with families of different cultures and background experiences. The text is composed of two parts: The first part provides a close-up, retrospective reflection on the experiences of the first author, which is analyzed in conversation with literature concerning cultural competence in healthcare services. The latter part provides a theoretical meta-perspective based on reflective discussions with a psychologist, and further delineates collaboration challenges and processes of reflection that draw on theories from a broader professional field.

Due to ethical considerations, the minority family discussed in the text is a construction of different families encountered by the main author during an overlapping period. It is the authors' reflections, rather than the family, that constitute the focal point of the story. No names are exposed except for those of the three authors. The first-person voice woven throughout the chapter constitutes the perspective of the physiotherapist and first author, Runa Kalleson, in dialogue with insights arising through collaborative reflection with the second and third authors.

## Encountering diversity

> More than ten years of experience working with children with disabilities and their families, additional education in paediatric physiotherapy, and predominantly positive feedback from patients and collaborative partners had made me both confident and perhaps at times a little complacent in my work at the well-baby clinic. However, a special encounter was about to turn this view of my own competence upside down. The turning point appeared the day a father entered the clinic carrying his daughter about the age of four over his shoulder. 'The girl is obviously severely disabled', was my first thought. My second thought was: 'This girl is in need of physiotherapy, and an adapted stroller or a wheelchair for transportation'. Finally I was thinking: 'Why is the father smiling, seeming more or less untouched by the serious condition of the child?'

In retrospect, reflecting on what happened when I first glimpsed this family, it is striking how the child's medical condition and needs for physiotherapy interventions dominated my thoughts. In the next couple of weeks, I learned that the young girl and her mother were refugees recently arriving in Norway for a family reunion with the father. The father's smile could easily be explained by joy and the relief of being reunited with his family after years apart, as well as pride in presenting his own child. However, I was more concerned about the disability being undiagnosed and the lack of documentation of previous medical intervention and follow-up.

These thoughts and concerns reflect how biomedical approaches perpetuate our consciousness and practices in rehabilitation contexts (Gibson, 2016).

> I felt great compassion for this family, obviously having lived under conditions that would be challenging for caretaking of a child with a severe disability. Now, being safely settled in Norway, they could access appropriate services fitting their needs, I was thinking. I was very happy to present available services directed to children with disabilities and their families: physiotherapy and technical aids free of charge, economic benefits, adapted daycare, respite care services, and means of service coordination, like having a service coordinator, an individual service plan, and a multidisciplinary support team. I was simply quite proud being a part of this impressive service system!

Encountering people from another country of origin provides an opportunity to compare the two countries and their healthcare systems. A comparison of Norway and Afghanistan, where the current family originated from, shows quite different socioeconomic conditions for health service delivery. Since the start of oil production in the early 1970s, Norway has enjoyed several decades of high growth and is now considered one of the richest countries per capita in the world. Afghanistan, on the other hand, is affected by decades of conflict and is among the lowest-ranked countries for several health indicators (Trani, Bakhshi, Noor, Lopez, & Mashkoor, 2010). Norway is characterized as a welfare state, with most health and social services being publicly financed based on an overarching principle of equal access to services for all inhabitants regardless of their social or economic status (Ringard, Sagan, Sperre Saunes, Lindahl, & Ringard, 2013). In Afghanistan, efforts to improve health services seem to be unevenly applied, with availability of health services being considerably better for more privileged groups. Disabilities in Afghanistan are shown to negatively affect people's access to healthcare, partly due to the stigma associated with disability (Trani et al., 2010). In Norway, the situation is quite different, with services provided based on documentation of illness and disability and people's need for health and social care. A large number of acts and secondary legislation regulate the systems, and efforts are made to include the entire family in rehabilitation processes and to coordinate the different services provided (Ringard et al., 2013). In this regard, Norway would appear to be the country of preference in which to care for a family member with disability. However, the comparison also shows how the Norwegian healthcare system may appear unfamiliar to families with experiences from completely different societies. The navigation of unfamiliar healthcare systems has previously been identified as an additional challenge for immigrants and refugees arriving to Western countries (Grandpierre et al., 2018).

> Convinced of the superiority of the Norwegian healthcare system, we expected the parents to be satisfied and grateful for all the services we were offering. Instead, the family rejected several of the services offered and questioned the

way some services were provided. For instance, they showed little interest in the processes of developing an individual service plan and establishing a multidisciplinary support team for their child, and they declined the opportunity to send their child to daycare and respite care. I was surprised and confused: Why did they reject our services? Do they not trust us? Do they not understand that this was the best way to support their child's development and well-being? The encounters between the family and service providers seemed to be dominated by mistrust: The family lacked confidence in our services, and service providers considered the family's behavior non-compliant with the recommended follow-up for children with disabilities. Some service providers even started to mutter about involving child protection services because the parents were making bad decisions on behalf of their child. The atmosphere for collaboration was far from optimal, and I experienced being involved in the rehabilitation follow-up as extraordinarily demanding. I was frustrated with all of the time and energy being directed to what appeared to be a struggle between the family and the service providers. Why were we unable to work together to uphold the child's best interests?

What I had until now considered a well-functioning healthcare system seemed to fail in the encounter with this family. Similar challenges for service providers who work with immigrant families raising a child with disability have been identified in previous literature, with lack of training in providing culturally sensitive care as one of the main obstacles to efficient collaboration (Lindsay, King, Klassen, Esses, & Stachel, 2012). In retrospect, it is apparent that we made few attempts to adapt our services to the specific situation of the family before we began to carry out our tasks. We based our services on the child's disability, without considering how the family's culture and experiences with healthcare in their former country may have affected the context for service delivery. We were also unaware of how our own culture and background influenced the services we were offering. This failure to consider culture, as exemplified in this critical incident, has in recent years been recognized as the single greatest barrier to the advancement of higher standards of health worldwide (Napier et al., 2014) and has given rise to a call for more culturally competent services (Fellin, Desmarais, & Lindsay, 2015; Lindsay et al., 2012). Recommended steps towards increasing cultural competence include raising awareness of how culture affects service delivery, gaining knowledge of cultural differences, and engaging in reflection on how we carry out our professional practices when we encounter diversity (Balcazar, Suarez-Balcazar, & Taylor-Ritzler, 2009). Involving a cultural liaison, to serve as a bridge between service providers and minority families, is presented as one way to facilitate greater cultural competence among professionals and to promote the delivery of more culturally competent services.

## Involving a cultural liaison

> I felt that we were in a cul-de-sac, with no road leading forward. We obviously needed new strategies to navigate this situation. In my quest for a new approach, I turned to Sosan Asgari Mollestad, a social worker employed in a project at my

workplace, whom I eventually invited to join as co-author of this book chapter. Sosan was not included in rehabilitation work at the well-baby clinic at that time; however, she agreed to assist in this situation. As an immigrant from Iran, she was uniquely positioned with knowledge relevant to the challenges that had arisen. Based on her knowledge and background experiences, she was not at all surprised that our offer of services turned into an unsuccessful encounter with the Afghan family. 'Misunderstandings are likely to appear when such different cultures collide', she stated. She further elaborated: 'When leaving a homeland, migrating into a new territory with a very different everyday life, you leave behind a lot of your habitual roles. However, being a parent ensures that you at least keep the significant caregiver role. Being offered help and support with caregiver tasks may be perceived as a threat to a central part of your identity. It may also be interpreted as authorities' doubts about the family's ability to take care of their child. Sosan also asked some thought-provoking questions: How could we expect the parents to be involved in services so unfamiliar to them? How could we expect engagement in written plans they probably could not read? And did we really expect them to expose their vulnerability by outlining their needs and inadequacies in meetings dominated by professionals they hardly knew?

The involvement of a co-worker representing another cultural and experiential background forced me into more explicit reflection upon culture and its influence on the interpretation of services. As exemplified by Sosan, the services we provided could be perceived quite differently based on family culture and background experiences (Grandpierre et al., 2018; Napier et al., 2014). Previous experiences of discrimination and marginalization may, for instance, lead to a scepticism of governmental services in general (Grandpierre et al., 2018). By being unfamiliar with the underlying reasons for the provision of family-directed services, these services may wrongly be interpreted by parents as a threat: as authorities' lack of trust in the family's resources and capabilities. This may contribute to shifts in self-perceptions from parents of a child in need of assistance to seeing themselves as people whose capabilities to care for their child are being questioned. This exemplifies how practitioners hold an authority not only to influence services but also to shape how recipients of care understand themselves (Gibson, 2016). Being inattentive to the possibilities of such misunderstandings may lead to disempowering practices instead of the intended capacity-building supports.

A crucial and transformative point made by Sosan was that the challenges that had arisen occurred in encounters *between cultures*, such that the family's culture could no longer be viewed as the scapegoat for the collaborative breakdown. Culture is not merely related to specific ethnic groups; we all hold certain systems of values, Sosan emphasized. This implies that services developed in a specific cultural context are influenced by the service providers' own cultural background, meaning that practices are not universal but rather particular to the context where they are developed (Napier et al., 2014). In most cases, rehabilitation services are developed by and for the majority group in a society, such that they may fail to serve the needs of minority groups (Grandpierre et al., 2018).

Language is identified as a prominent obstacle in service provision by both minority families and service providers (Grandpierre et al., 2018). In most Western societies, there are taken-for-granted skills such as the ability to read and write in the language of the majority, that underpin an optimal utilization of rehabilitation services. Without such skills, written service plans, application forms, and notices about appointments appear inappropriate for families who speak different languages. In a country like Norway, where high rates of literacy prevail, there is little recognition of the potential language needs of minority groups, and effective responses to various language needs within services are still deficient.

In addition to these practical barriers, there are also some underlying assumptions and expectations that are usually covert in the delivery of healthcare with the potential to complicate collaborative processes. The *logic of rehabilitation*, including priorities, services, and organizational structures, is commonly underpinned by the majority's views on rehabilitation and disability in a society (Gibson, 2016). With service providers representing a majority population, most of the underlying assumptions in the healthcare system are taken for granted and therefore not made explicit or openly discussed. These covert underlying expectations and assumptions may be difficult for someone from outside the culture to discern, such that misunderstandings are likely to occur. For instance, when families are not aware of the expectation of active involvement in rehabilitation processes, like those taking place in multidisciplinary support team meetings, their behaviour may be interpreted by service providers as a lack of interest in follow-up about their child. Such misunderstandings about the healthcare system, and divergent beliefs about the role of parents in rehabilitation processes, have been identified as having negative effects on the engagement of immigrant parents in the follow-up of children with disabilities (Brassart, Prévost, Bétrisey, Lemieux, & Desmarais, 2017). To avoid misunderstandings and enhance active participation in rehabilitation processes, alternative ways of delivering services may be warranted. Active use of a cultural liaison and home-based services are some adjustments suggested in the literature (Balcazar et al., 2009; Brassart et al., 2017; Fellin et al., 2015; Grandpierre et al., 2018).

## Balancing power dynamics: a home visit

> Sosan suggested that we should visit the family together in their home in order to get to know them better. My first reaction was to think that this would be unnecessarily time consuming. However, recognizing that my previous encounters with the family in my office had not been effective for moving the rehabilitation process further, I had to admit that a home visit was worth trying. What really made me hesitate was the feeling of being uncomfortable leaving the safety of my office, entering an unfamiliar environment to practice my profession. I was unsure of what was expected of me and how I should behave in these circumstances. As if in fulfillment to my concerns, visiting the family made me feel like a cultural stranger. The family had prepared a meal for us, and I didn't know how to eat it! Luckily, my obvious lack of knowledge worked as a humorous icebreaker, creating an opportunity for the family to teach me something after weeks of being exposed to my attempts to teach them physiotherapy techniques. Sosan and the

family were speaking a common language, and all of a sudden, I became the one who did not understand what was said. Sosan was translating most of their conversation, but I was still aware that I most likely missed some of the informal talk. It struck me that this is what commonly happens in multidisciplinary team meetings. An interpreter translates the professional content, while the informal talk between service providers is left untranslated. I now felt that what was easily missed by this practice had the potential to create a distance between native and non-native speakers. However, with Sosan bridging the cultural and linguistic diversities, the situation was less uncomfortable than I feared. I was very happy to notice that the atmosphere was considerably more relaxed compared with previous encounters with other service providers, and the mother was far more involved in the conversation than ever before. The topics included in the conversation were more comprehensive than I had experienced in a more traditional clinical setting. We learned about the family's social network, their ability to communicate in four different languages, and how the mother had been able to care for her seriously ill child under difficult conditions while moving between different refugee camps over years. This was not at all compatible with previous descriptions of the family as weak in resources! Further, by looking at family pictures and short cellphone videos, we gained more information about the child's previous development than we had ever before been able to capture in the medical records.

Flexibility of services, including increased length of appointment time, is highlighted as essential for gaining more contextual knowledge and for establishing an efficient relationship between service providers and minority families (Grandpierre et al., 2018). Home visits appear to be advantageous in different ways. First, they offer a unique opportunity for service providers to gain insight into the family's resources, home environment, day-to-day practices, and family roles. Such knowledge is considered an important step towards the delivery of more culturally competent services (Balcazar et al., 2009). Second, from the perspective of families, their home is likely to constitute a more familiar environment for service provision than majority-dominated public spaces like hospitals and well-baby clinics. Being an immigrant implies having experienced a loss of a known place, which may make people more vulnerable to the physical and geographical frames of service delivery (Ahlberg & Duckert, 2006). Previous research has highlighted the provision of home-based services as a way to build alliances between service providers and families and to remove some of the practical barriers for attendance (Brassart et al., 2017). Further, home visits are associated with more positive experiences of care among immigrant families raising a child with disability (Fellin et al., 2015). In short, home visits may facilitate increased engagement in the provision of services, not least when it comes to involvement of mothers in families where the father usually serves as the spokesperson in public encounters with service providers.

A striking consequence of the home visit appeared to be the altered power dynamics between the human beings involved, with both resources and inadequacies being more apparent and more evenly distributed than in a more traditional clinical setting. Such a disruption of the usual power imbalance is also noted in previous research (Brassart et al., 2017; Fellin et al., 2015). A further mitigation of power resulted from the involvement of Sosan serving as a cultural liaison. She was present to help and support both the family and me and provided a two-way explanation of how the services were delivered and understood. She mitigated language and cultural codes as barriers to communication and cleared up misunderstandings that had resulted from previous encounters. That formed the basis of a greater understanding of each other's position in the collaborative process and facilitated the establishment of a relationship more strongly based on trust and confidence.

## Altering the practice

> After this first home visit, the scene was set for a more fruitful collaboration between the family and me as a service provider. The relationship now established made it easier to communicate and reflect upon wishes, needs, and expectations, and the family became more engaged in the rehabilitation process. The acquired knowledge of the family and the awareness raised about how the services were developed and for whom, formed the basis for a discussion about customization of services to better fit the family's needs. Sosan was only occasionally involved in our further encounters however, she was still available when needed. Based on the positive experience of our collaboration, she was increasingly becoming involved when new service providers were introduced to the family. This turned out to be an effective approach to get the rehabilitation process back on track for the family and service providers involved.

This last epiphany illuminates how the process of becoming more culturally competent altered healthcare practice. The process included several steps, from becoming attentive to the need to encompass cultural aspects in service provision, to raising critical awareness of how culture affects how services are delivered and perceived, to gaining knowledge of the particular family, to developing skills and strategies for communication and collaboration. The lessons learned further influenced other co-workers and subsequent encounters with families.

Central to the processes of change was Sosan serving as a cultural liaison. Involving a liaison has been highlighted as a strategy to foster more culturally competent work environments, with particular importance when explaining healthcare processes to minority groups (Grandpierre et al., 2018). This is in line with research by Brassart et al. (2017), who identify the preparation of immigrant parents for therapeutic processes as an important feature in the follow-up of a child with disability. Based on our experiences, we suggest that service providers could benefit from being prepared before encountering minority families. This is supported by previous research that highlights the important role a social worker can have in informing service providers about the needs of the family (Fellin et al., 2015). The liaison role involves a two-way perspective that bridges knowledge between families and service providers. In addition, the liaison offers the potential to facilitate relational practices and mitigate some of the power imbalances in service provision. Based on our experiences, we propose that this represents a strategy to improve physiotherapy practices in the years to come.

## Expanding the horizon: engaging sociocultural perspectives

As time passed, I could not completely let the encounters go. My thoughts orbited around how Sosan's involvement turned the severe collaborative challenges into a process of improved services and contributed to my own personal and professional growth. I was still eager to explore perspectives from other professional fields that could illuminate and elaborate both the challenges we faced and the collaborative processes we went through. In order to deepen my understanding, I turned to my colleague, PhD candidate and psychologist Linn Julie Skagestad, who has a particular interest in sociocultural, interpersonal, and power relations in client-professional collaborations, and who subsequently joined as second author of this chapter. This collaboration resulted in a reflection-based dialogue where Linn, drawing on theoretical perspectives from the fields of sociocultural psychology, rehabilitation, and philosophy, helped identify three main collaborative challenges based on my experiences. To make our reflections more tangible, Linn put her theoretical reflections and suggestions into written text. These collaborative challenges are discussed subsequently.

### *Collaborative challenges*

Sociocultural approaches to human interaction depict reality as 'multifaceted' and 'partly shared', implying that people's interpretive positions differ and thus require attention (Hundeide, 2003; Rommetveit, 1992). This perspective could be useful when exploring challenges to genuine dialogue and the establishment of viable partnerships when facing diversity within the field of rehabilitation. Karsten Hundeide (1992, 2003), a central scholar within the sociocultural approach to human development and interaction, distinguishes what constitutes the 'foreground' and 'background' in our daily encounters. The foreground encompasses explicit utterances and is always interpreted against a tacit background composed of what is 'assumed to be known' (Hundeide, 1992, p. 139). Often, a shared interpretive background is taken for granted; however, in encounters where there is 'little sharing of background premises', for instance, due to cultural differences, assumptions must be *explicated* in order to establish shared understandings and viable working relationships (Hundeide, 1992, p. 140).

Transposed to the encounters outlined previously, one could argue that the service approach seemed to be mainly directed by a biomedical rather than a sociocultural stance. According to Gibson (2016, p. 16), a biomedical approach emphasizes 'biology, pathology and scientific method' and contrasts more holistic and interpretive approaches to rehabilitation, concerned with treating and understanding the entire person. In the first stages of the rehabilitation process, the child's medical condition and needs for interventions predominated the concerns of the service providers involved. Less effort was invested to explore the personal or interpretive background of the family, such as their personal resources and autobiographical story (i.e. previous experiences with public services or governments) or cultural meanings of the caregiver role or of disability (i.e. associated with stigma), or their roles as service receivers. Nor were the Westernized logics of rehabilitation that underpinned the service providers' perceptions of high-quality service provision subjected to explanation or exploration.

Returning to Hundeide (1992), by overlooking the interpretive background of the collaborators, it turned out to be difficult to establish mutual understandings regarding what constituted the foreground, such as the aetiology of the disease, beneficial interventions, and productive forms of collaboration. Dialogical challenges occurred when both service providers and family members interpreted the foreground matters against profoundly different cultural and experiential backgrounds – due to inattentiveness to their divergent background premises. In turn, unnecessary misunderstandings emerged, such as the parents' uncertainty about whether receiving public services represented distrust of their capabilities to care for their child, along with tendencies of mutual annoyance, distrust, and resignation. Within these arrangements, the dialogue and working relationships were deeply compromised.

## *Recognition of the family's competencies and concerns*

A second main challenge that seemed to hamper genuine dialogue and a viable working relationship was insufficient recognition of the family's competencies and concerns. A better understanding of this challenge could be provided based on a relationally oriented, cultural-historical approach to collaboration, as discussed by Anne Edwards (Edwards, 2017). Edwards is concerned with how professionals' capacity to interpret problems *with* their clients and co-workers may promote *inclusive* and *accurate* professional practices where the complexity of the clients' situation and concerns are better voiced, interpreted, and responded to. This capacity is referred to as *relational expertise* and involves recognizing, engaging with, and complementing the motives and competencies of others. Prior to the involvement of Sosan, the service providers did not appear to include or recognize the central motives or competencies of the family – such as their need for flexible services, their sense of caregiver responsibility, or their linguistic skills. Rather than engaging the family in a *joint* exploration, where meanings and solutions were co-constructed, a one-way sharing of information and assumptions about competence characterized the initial phase of the collaboration. Medical knowledge and bureaucratic procedures fitting Western societies appeared to dominate the service providers' perceptions, camouflaging the family's total resources. French and Swain (2001) suggest that recognition of clients' experiential knowledge is essential if relations between service providers and their clients are to be balanced. This occurred in later stages of the process, during the home visit, when the competencies of the family became more evident. It should be noted that some level of relational expertise was demonstrated when the physiotherapist involved Sosan in the first place and when she opened herself to being informed and transformed by new perspectives and competencies.

## *'The participant's attitude'*

Finally, drawing upon the Norwegian philosopher Hans Skjervheim (1996), it seemed that the dialogue and working relationship suffered from an inadequate display of what he refers to as 'the participant's attitude'. Skjervheim postulates that in order to establish equal relations between two interlocutors, it is critical that both hold 'the participant's attitude', meaning that they actively *engage* in the concerns raised by the other. This allows for a balanced, triangular relationship between the two subjects and the concern(s) in question. If one interlocutor simply *registers* the other's concerns, without further engaging with the problem itself, Skjervheim suggests that there is a risk of objectification of the person. In the encounters outlined previously, rather than actively engaging in whether the questions raised and choices made by the family could be reasonable and productive given the circumstances, the practitioners appeared to limit their response to registering these matters as the family's concerns and not necessarily relevant to service provision. This may relate to the service providers' focus on the child's disability and their view of the family as representing a 'different' culture. However, based on this approach, the service providers were positioned as the actors and appraisers and the family as 'acted upon' and 'appraised'. Consequently, asymmetrical power dynamics and unbalanced relations seemed to be further reinforced.

## Collaborative reflection and dialogue

In this final section, I summarize my reflections on the collaborative processes and personal growth developed through collaborative reflection and dialogue with Sosan and Linn.

Throughout the outlined period, the collaborative processes between the family and me as a service provider seemed to change, with dialogical and relational challenges becoming less evident. Simultaneously, I was taking important steps towards a deeper understanding of cultural differences, recognizing the relevance for practice and for cultivating new skills. These processes were facilitated through the involvement of the social worker Sosan, serving as a cultural liaison. Prior to her involvement, my approach might have been characterized as ethnocentric – implying an inclination towards believing that one's own values and perspectives could serve as a universal standard suitable for judging others (Hammell, 2013). This was illustrated by my questions about whether the father was minimizing his child's medical condition in our encounters. Looking back, a Western perspective on disability as being a concern for the healthcare system to diagnose and intervene with (Gibson, 2016; Goodley, 2011) seemed to serve as a 'standard' informing my initial concerns. This is opposed to taking other 'standards' into consideration that may have resonated more accurately with the perspectives of the family, such as the potential for disability to be regarded as a private issue – for instance, due to stigma or social organization (Ingstad & Whyte, 1995). In this regard, my approach seemed to be underpinned by both ethnocentric and biomedical assumptions. However, when I realized that this approach appeared to be inadequate and acquired more cultural awareness, I suggest that steps were taken towards developing what Hammell (2013) refers to as cultural competence in its early iteration. This approach to cultural competence emphasizes the importance of acquiring knowledge on the values, customs, and traditions of particular cultural groups.

Facilitated by Sosan's critical questions, reflections, and collaborative approaches which drew attention to social privilege and biases, my awareness further advanced toward what Hammell (2013) conceptualizes as 'cultural humility'. This entails a move away from seeing clients from cultural minorities as culturally different and toward a more relational understanding of cultural difference as residing within the practitioner–client relationship and occurring in encounters between cultures. To bridge differences and redress power imbalances, it is thus essential that practitioners commit to critical reflexivity regarding their own assumptions, biases, values, positions, and privileges and how these differ from those of the client (Hammell, 2013). A more critical form of self-reflection was seen when I reflected upon my privilege as a native speaker and considered how dependence on a translator created a distance that could compromise the establishment of more trusting working relationships. Deeper critical reflection was also evident in contemplations about the unreasonableness of expecting the family to understand and comply with the 'logics of rehabilitation', taking into consideration their lack of familiarity with the culture of the rehabilitation team, such as expectations of active parental engagement in interventions and services directed to the child.

Hammel (2013) suggests that cultural humility involves a recognition of how different members within a cultural group interpret and express this particular culture differently, as well as the changing nature of culture. This implies that our approach when encountering diversity is more important than learning about specific cultures. It also alludes to the fruitfulness of fostering practitioner and team reflexivity through the use of liaisons as 'cultural experts' or 'cultural interpreters' (Ahlberg & Duckert, 2006). Thus, practitioners and healthcare teams could beneficially invite liaisons into joint and explicit considerations of power, responsibility, and interpretations of culture when working with minority families. In the specific encounters outlined in this chapter, Sosan served as a facilitator of increased awareness and bridged understanding between me as a service provider and the family. To advance this cultural competence even more, the previously mentioned perspectives could in the future be given more explicit attention and discussions about increased use of liaisons in healthcare contexts and the transferability to other professional settings could be further discussed.

Further, it is suggested that the outlined reflective processes regarding the nature and interplay of cultures formed the basis for more advanced communication and interpersonal skills enhancing the quality and customization of the services provided to the family. The encounters described demonstrate how relational understandings of cultural difference encouraged by Sosan and further developed through the home visit enabled more effective interpersonal strategies that moved away from a pure medical focus and understandings of the practitioners as 'value neutral'. Instead, more advanced communicative and collaborative approaches were now found necessary, which involved the family more closely and with more flexibility in joint interpretations of their situation and needs, as well as offering opportunities to explore and reflect upon divergences in assumptions and privileges. Through my subsequent encounters with sociocultural perspectives, introduced by Linn, my insights and reflections upon the collaboration process, beneficial relational competencies, and diversity developed further. First, my awareness was raised regarding how approaches that failed to consider relationships, divergent interpretive perspectives, and motives and background assumptions of collaborators could represent communicative challenges in a rehabilitation context. These challenges include difficulties in establishing a trusting and reciprocal working relationship and common ground from which more unified and accurate understandings of the family's situation and needs could be built and more customized services provided. Through engagement with sociocultural theories, perspectives were introduced that enabled deeper reflections upon the specific encounters outlined previously, including further reflections upon my personal growth and the contributions of Sosan. Finally, an understanding of diversity as something which extends beyond differences in ethnicity, and which could fruitfully be considered in any rehabilitation or professional context, emerged.

In summary, the process of becoming more culturally competent and aware can be achieved in different and supplementary ways: by engaging in encounters with different groups of people, by raising one's critical awareness and knowledge of cultures coming to meet, by analyzing and reflecting on one's own practice, and by considering the implications for broader systems and practices (Balcazar, Suarez-Balcazar & Taylor-Ritzler, 2009). The first two approaches were facilitated in physiotherapy practice working with the minority family and through the involvement of the social worker Sosan, while the latter approach evolved to a great extent through dialogue and shared reflection with the psychologist Linn. My dialogically based collaboration with Sosan and Linn represented an innovative and potent form of practice reflection, transcending previous experiences of self-reflection in terms of facilitating a deeper understanding of myself as a physiotherapist and fellow human in a diverse world and in terms of recognizing tacit, relational, and systemic presuppositions as they relate to the practice of cultural sensitivity, humility, and competence.

## Conclusions

In this chapter, we aimed to show how service providers are embedded in a cultural context by telling the story of a physiotherapist encountering a minority family. Different characteristics of the cultural context were identified, including taken-for-granted assumptions about shared understandings of service delivery, biomedical perspectives that permeate the healthcare system, and insufficient reflection upon the influence of cultural diversity in healthcare contexts. Innovations of practice included the involvement of a liaison, raising awareness of the significance of context for delivering and receiving services, bridging and 'interpreting' diverse understandings, and facilitating effective communication and beneficial working alliances. Further discussions drawing upon sociocultural and philosophical theories contributed to an enhanced awareness of challenges related to encountering differences in general, as well as approaches to moving from ethnocentric to more relational practices. By adding insights about recognizing that there are two cultures coming to meet, cultural humility appears as a key approach to the development of both individual professional and personal competencies and in quality improvement of services at a systemic level.

However, rather than presenting one 'universal truth' or providing a prescription for practice, the intention here is to initiate further thinking, reflection, and dialogue among physiotherapists and other people and systems who shape the lives of their fellow human beings. In this regard, the baton is now passed on to those who wish to more thoughtfully respond to diversity in professional practices or other human interactions.

## References

Ahlberg, N., & Duckert, F. (2006). Minoritetsklienter som helsefaglig utfordring [Minority clients as a health care challenge]. *Tidsskrift for Norsk Psykologforening*, *43*(12), 1276–1281.

Balcazar, F. E., Suarez-Balcazar, Y., & Taylor-Ritzler, T. (2009). Cultural competence: Development of a conceptual framework. *Disability and Rehabilitation*, *31*(14), 1153–1160. doi:10.1080/09638280902773752

Brassart, E., Prévost, C., Bétrisey, C., Lemieux, M., & Desmarais, C. (2017). Strategies developed by service providers to enhance treatment engagement by immigrant parents raising a child with a disability. *Journal of Child and Family Studies*, *26*(4), 1230–1244. doi:10.1007/s10826-016-0646-8

Edwards, A. (2017). Revealing relational work. In A. Edwards (Eds.), *Working relationally in and across practices: A cultural-historical approach to collaboration* (pp. 1–22). Cambridge: Cambridge University Press.

Ellis, C., Adams, T., & Bochner, A. (2011). Autoethnography: An overview. *Forum: Qualitative Social Research*, *12*(1).

Fellin, M., Desmarais, C., & Lindsay, S. (2015). An examination of clinicians' experiences of collaborative culturally competent service delivery to immigrant families raising a child with a physical disability. *Disability and Rehabilitation*, *37*(21), 1961–1969. doi:10.3109/09638288.2014.993434

French, S., & Swain, J. (2001). The relationship between disabled people and health and welfare professionals. In G. L. Albrecht, K. D. Seelman, & M. Bury (Eds.), *Handbook of disability studies* (pp. 734–753). Thousand Oaks, CA: Sage Publications.

Gibson, B. E. (2016). *Rehabilitation: A post-critical approach*. Boca Raton, FL: CRC Press, an imprint of the Taylor & Francis Group.

Goodley, D. (2011). *Disability studies: An interdisciplinary introduction*. Los Angeles: Sage Publications.

Grandpierre, V., Milloy, V., Sikora, L., Fitzpatrick, E., Thomas, R., & Potter, B. (2018). Barriers and facilitators to cultural competence in rehabilitation services: A scoping review. *BMC Health Services Research*, *18*(1). doi:10.1186/s12913-017-2811-1

Hammell, K. R. W. (2013). Occupation, well-being, and culture: Theory and cultural humility/Occupation, bien-être et culture: La théorie et l'humilité culturelle. *Canadian Journal of Occupational Therapy*, *80*(4), 224–234. doi:10.1177/0008417413500465

Hundeide, K. (1992). The message structure of some Piagetian experiments. In A. Heen Wold (Eds.), *The dialogue alternative: Towards a theory of language and mind* (pp. 139–156). Oslo, NO: Scandinavian University Press.

Hundeide, K. (2003). *Barns livsverden: Sosiokulturelle rammer for barns utvikling* [Children's lifeworlds: Sociocultural frames for children's development]. Oslo, NO: Cappelen Akademisk Forlag.

Ingstad, B., & Whyte, S. R. (1995). *Disability and culture*. Berkeley, CA: University of California Press.

International Organization for Migration. (2018). *World migration report 2018*. IOM: The UN Migration Agency. Retrieved December 19, 2019, from https://publications.iom.int/system/files/pdf/wmr_2018_en.pdf. 2. Castelli F. Drivers of migration.

Lindsay, S., King, G., Klassen, A. F., Esses, V., & Stachel, M. (2012). Working with immigrant families raising a child with a disability: Challenges and recommendations for healthcare and community service providers. *Disability and Rehabilitation*, *34*(23), 2007–2017. doi:10.3109/09638288.2012.667192

Napier, A. D., Ancarno, C., Butler, B., Calabrese, J., Chater, A., Chatterjee, H., Guesnet, F., . . . Woolf, K. (2014). Culture and health. *The Lancet*, *384*(9954), 1607–1639. doi:10.1016/S0140-6736(14)61603-2

Ringard, Å., Sagan, A., Sperre Saunes, I., Lindahl, A. K., & Ringard, Å. (2013). Norway: Health system review. *Health Systems in Transition*, *15*(8), 1–162.

Rommetveit, R. (1992). Outline of a dialogically based social-cognitive approach to human cognition and communication. In A. Heen Wold (Eds.), *The dialogue alternative: Towards a theory of language and mind* (pp. 19–44). Oslo, NO: Scandinavian University Press.

Skjervheim, H. (1996). *Selected essays: In honour of Hans Skjervheim's 70th birthday* (Vol. 12). Bergen: The Department of Philosophy.

Trani, J.-F., Bakhshi, P., Noor, A. A., Lopez, D., & Mashkoor, A. (2010). Poverty, vulnerability, and provision of healthcare in Afghanistan. *Social Science & Medicine*, *70*(11), 1745–1755. doi:10.1016/j.socscimed.2010.02.007

# 14 Using Deleuze

## Language, dysphasia, and physiotherapy

*Michael Gard, Rebekah Dewberry, and Jenny Setchell*

> Forming grammatically correct sentences is for the normal individual the prerequisite for any submission to social laws. No one is supposed to be ignorant of grammaticality; those who are belong in special institutions. The unity of language is fundamentally political.
>
> Deleuze and Guattari, A Thousand Plateaus (1987, p. 112)

As always, society changes, and relationships evolve. This is particularly important for this chapter because we, as the authors, have been involved in different and changing dynamics, including but not limited to friendship, supervision, therapy, coffee partners, and academic colleagues. Therefore, while we do not explain these relationships in depth, there are some important details that may help the reader to understand these arguments.

First, this chapter is about different ways of approaching people with dysphasia using qualitative data, post-structural theory, music, and poetry. There will be, potentially, dead ends and promising strategies. For example, this chapter may be 'old news' or intriguing ideas, depending on the reader's personality, discipline, professional experience, or views on the use of theory in the caring professions.

Second, this text is a team effort. Although throughout this chapter we use the term 'I' rather than 'we', and each section is written by one author, we have discussed each section with each author in mind.[1] In other words, this chapter is a collection of single-author narratives, but we see something useful in bringing academic, therapist, and patient experience together.

Third, I (Michael Gard) had an accident. For me at least, at that moment, the world became different, and it would never go back. I was riding my bike in a small town in Australia and was knocked over by a car. I woke up on the road with a serious head injury and, two days later, I had a major stroke. Technically speaking, I had a middle cerebral artery territory ischemic infarct, a secondary traumatic internal carotid artery (ICA) dissection and fractured facial bones. Although I have permanent numbness on my face, I was fortunate that my body was mostly uninjured. My problem was communication, and three days after the accident, I could not talk, read, or write. Part of my brain injury included an acquired dysphasia disability, although there will be more information about this condition later in this chapter. For now, I spent three months in the hospital and the next nine months at home before eventually going back to work on limited duties.

Fortunately, my bike accident was in an area in Australia in which the insurance system paid for my various types of therapy to help to re-develop my communication skills. Through recovery processes, I had many supportive family, friends, and colleagues, including co-author Jenny Setchell. I was also lucky enough to be cared for by hospital and community professionals, including co-author Rebekah Dewberry, who was and is a private practice speech therapist. Rebekah and I have worked together for over two years. Of course, over this time, our discussions ranged across professional and personal issues, including my experience of hospital speech, occupation and physiotherapy, and private services once I left the hospital.

Fourth, as we have already mentioned, relationships are crucial but changing. My relationship with Jenny began with my co-supervision of her PhD thesis (Setchell, 2016), but soon it morphed into academic colleague and collaborator, and, following my accident, I changed from teacher to beginning student. My relationship with Rebekah Dewberry was also shifting, including a fairly conventional 'patient–doctor' dynamic and using 'talk' as a way of approaching dysphasia but also time spent between individuals who are interested in overlapping problems.

Against this background, the issue we want to focus on in this chapter is the care of stroke patients and, in particular, dysphasia patients. There can be absolutely no doubt about the professional care that I received over the last four years. My relationships with therapists gave me a completely new knowledge about the complexities of practice, and I would defend them against any questions about their level of professional service. But experience often produces new questions. For example, during the later years of my recovery, my carers and I tried to find a specific program for people who have had a brain injury but who also want to return to a professional job. Most of the programs that we found, including software or internet-delivered platforms, are for people to improve their domestic skills, including buying food in shops and talking with family members. In the end, we stopped searching. As I improved my communication skills, repetition, including paper-based speech exercises, was absolutely crucial, but there was still a 'gap'.

Over time, including talking with both Jenny Setchell and Rebekah Dewberry, the gap emerged as an important practical and theoretical issue. This gap can be exploited in intriguing ways. During my own recovery phase, for example, I had a chance to talk with a fellow stroke survivor. Reflecting on his experience with serious dysphasia only 20 years ago, he received only one month of treatment in hospital, and then the doctors told him simply to go home.[2] This situation has changed somewhat, particularly if a person with a brain injury is covered by a health or an accident insurance policy. But for many people, including dysphasia patients, there can be the daunting prospect of life without professional programs.

In summary, then, this chapter will be written by individual authors. Following this introduction (written by Michael), Jenny will add more detail about the potential new ways of seeing physiotherapy from our discussions, using Deleuze as a starting point for writing for the chapter. Rebekah will then describe her career, from public hospital care as a young speech therapist to becoming an experienced private practitioner. In the next section, Michael will sketch the interactions between clinical practice, experiencing dysphasia as a patient, and academic theory. In the concluding theory section, Jenny considers some new directions for physiotherapists and researchers to consider.

Of course, with the quote from *A Thousand Plateaus* with which we began this chapter, there is no destination in mind. There are only diverse, potentially uncomfortable, and stimulating ways of travelling.

## New directions for physiotherapists – part 1

As multiple chapters in this book suggest, I (Jenny, a physiotherapist) believe it is important to find ways to think/do physiotherapy differently. Despite seeming sociopolitically agnostic to many of those within it, physiotherapy, in its contemporary, 'professionalised' Western sense, has many dominant cultural norms of practice and thinking which limit our ability to adapt. The profession favours measurement and order (Gibson, 2016; Setchell, Nicholls, & Gibson, 2017), categorisation and diagnosis (Gibson, 2018), and normal and typical function (Setchell, 2017; Setchell, Gard, Jones, & Watson, 2017). As Setchell, Nicholls, et al. (2017, p. 16) put it, physiotherapy textbooks:

> show bodies that could be any body, their therapeutic spaces bring the body under the biomedical gaze (Armstrong, 1995) and their practices focus on the ways the body can be measured and known. Education is one point where this way of practicing becomes biomedical, but it is reified throughout the career – in the focus of physiotherapy journals, conferences, professional development opportunities, conversations in lunchrooms and procedures in workplaces.

The profession seeks tools to measure dysfunction and compare against norms (Nicholls & Gibson, 2010), with normal bodies (or those that approximate normal) as the ideal to be strived for. The medicalised bodies these foci produce are ones that become a pliable '*machinic* structure in which "components" can be altered, adjusted, removed or replaced' (Grosz, 1995, p. 35). These discursive and material underpinnings of physiotherapy are lasting impressions of the profession's strategic alignment with biomedicine and, increasingly, with positivist science. As Nicholls and Gibson (2010, p. 500) argue, '[v]iewing the body-as-machine was a supremely important and highly effective strategy for the founders of modern physiotherapy practice, since it played a large part in establishing the profession's legitimacy'. These alignments are understandable, as they were likely considered beneficial for patients, and come with significant gains in status and power for the profession. However, there has been growing concern that these cultural norms come at a cost for those who seek care.

What are the costs of biomedical perspectives and positivist science in the context of physiotherapy and healthcare more broadly? This is, of course, a large question with multiple complex answers that have been explored elsewhere in detail. However, I will attend briefly to a few key concepts related to physiotherapy in the literature to date. Reductionist approaches to physiotherapy come at the cost of creativity due to narrowed parameters and options (Abrams & Gibson, 2016;

Setchell, Nicholls, et al., 2017). There is a loss of attention to things that cannot easily be quantified – such as considerations of emotions and social, cultural, and embodied experiences (Bjorbaekmo & Mengshoel, 2016; Setchell, Abrams, McAdam, & Gibson, 2019; Trede, 2012) – and the cost of devaluing difference – with resultant 'othering' and stigmatisation (Thomas Abrams, 2014; Bjorbaekmo & Engelsrud, 2011; Setchell, 2017; Setchell, Watson, Gard, & Jones, 2016; Synnott et al., 2015).

How might we work differently to avoid such costs? There are a number of suggestions, including moving away from striving for independence and attending to the complexities of patients' human and non-human connections (Gibson, 2006; Nicholls et al., 2016), resisting reductionism by attending to the multiple effects of any physiotherapy enactment (Setchell, Nicholls, et al., 2017), and a move towards embodiment (Bjorbaekmo & Mengshoel, 2016; Nicholls & Gibson, 2010). An additional approach that has been little considered is to work *with* disability itself to find some ways to think again about what we value and strive for.

Working *with* disability offers physiotherapy a different way of thinking through its practices but also a different way to attend to patients (French, 1994; French & Sim, 2008). Thinking through disability provokes questions such as: What can I learn from the different ways of moving through the world offered by my patient? How might these differences be enjoyed, celebrated, worked with rather than against? Of course, there are many values to striving for 'normal' function: we don't want to discount that this focus is important to many. However, we would like to suggest that striving for normality should not be the default, that we should consider difference and at times promote it over normality. Who wants to be normal, anyway?

In this chapter, we explore dysphasia – not usually the realm of physiotherapy but certainly the realm of what we are doing right now – in writing. We use writing and dysphasia and speech therapy as a way to think physiotherapy through disability. As I sit here and write this chapter, it feels pertinent right now: writing is an embodiment of dysphasia. Together, we will use our *dysphasianalysis* to consider, through our academic writing/speaking – our articulations – how disability can be worked with and link this to how we think/do disability and physiotherapy. In this chapter, we will attempt to work with disability in order to articulate ourselves. By working across our disciplines of speech therapy, sociology, and physiotherapy – as well as one author's lived experiences with dysphasia – we will conduct a dysphasanalysis (which is a play on Deleuze and Guattari's 1987 'schizoanalysis' where these philosophers drew from different ways of thinking conceptualised via 'mental illness' to reconceptualise how to think about the world) to look at what biomedicine in allied health does to disability – and move to other possibilities of what else it can do.

Deleuze and Guattari are, in some ways, an obvious choice. Their writing has been taken up across the social science disciplines but particularly in psychology, psychiatry, mental health, and its various of care professions. For example, one advantage of their 'open' style of writing and thinking is that they give the reader 'permission' to experiment, to look *again* at supposedly 'true' statements, and to listen *carefully* to the narratives of patients and for other ways of working. We must not necessarily view treatments as a rational process leading to a 'cure' ($x + y = z$) but rather consider emotions and tangential thinking pedagogical tools, teaching us in their own somewhat non-rational ways. 'Rational' thinking can be useful and damaging, depending on the situation and one's attitude. We are also using a series of 'single' but connected narratives; we are building – like all conversations – 'gigantic memory' (Roberts, 2005).

The stories in the final section of this chapter evoke the *multiple* possibilities of data interpretations. Yes, one can play a 'role' between a 'patient and doctor' for capital (money, prestige, fun, etc.), but this is only the beginning. One's relationships with others can be framed through multiple lenses; our conversations/narratives can offer us different positions, both by writing these narratives (as authors) and by reading them (as readers). As we (authors) re-call and re-make these clinical and relationship experiences, we hope to entice physiotherapists into new ways of working with patients. In other words, we do not want to *build* on Deleuze theory but rather use it to look again at dysphasia/physiotherapy. Dysphasia is a new – some readers might say novel – condition for physiotherapy to consider. But following a group of physiotherapist researchers, this chapter uses narrative and patient-centred strategies, not because they are better but because they could 'work in harmony with more traditional biomedical approaches' (Nicholls et al., 2016, p. 167).

## New approaches in speech therapy

The hospital environment is an alluring option for new graduates in the various health professions. It is a fast and exciting place, with a plethora of clinical presentations and learning opportunities. As a new graduate, I took to my role as a hospital speech pathologist like a duck to water. Mixing my metaphors, I was also a sponge, and the learning curve in the first 12 months was very steep indeed. Learning to work with the medical, nursing, and allied health teams gave me a deep appreciation for the complexities of the human body and the mind, as well as a considered appreciation for disability and what it means for the individual person.

Working with people who have suffered a stroke is a core business for adult speech pathology. Dysphasia is an acquired neurogenic language disorder that can occur after an injury to the brain and usually affects the left hemisphere, which is responsible for language. Dysphasia is typically described through verbal language expression, auditory language comprehension, written expression, and reading comprehension. A person with dysphasia will often have relatively intact non-linguistic cognitive skills (memory and executive function); however, they are not mutually exclusive. The treatment and care protocols for a person who has suffered a stroke are clearly documented. The Australian Clinical Guidelines for Stroke Management (2007) recommend rehabilitation to commence the first day after a stroke in order to maximise the participation of the individual back into the community through interventions focused on impairment, activity, and participation (Stroke Foundation, 2017; see Chapter 5 especially).

A typical pathway from hospital to home may begin with an acute hospital admission and subsequent transfer to a stroke or neurosurgery ward. On these wards, the speech pathologist is focused on checking for safe swallowing, and they will perhaps conduct a communication screen to identify if any dysphasia is present. There is little scope at this early stage for functional, formal therapy that is focused on rehabilitation of language/communication due to limited time, resources, the environment, and the acute health status of the patient.

Once the patient is stable, they then move on to a brain injury or stroke rehabilitation ward. The patient will typically see daily speech therapy, focusing on structure- and impairment-based therapy. Impairment-based therapy for dysphasia may include naming, semantic therapy, conversational language therapy, and work on reading speed.

On discharge, follow up is often through outpatient day hospital, a transitional rehabilitation program (where available), and then home. Before the introduction of the National Disability Insurance Scheme (NDIS) in Australia, health services would typically cease after discharge. The person may have been entitled to a disability pension, but typically, accessing private services was often the only form of formal ongoing therapy. Even today, an online search of private speech pathologists will yield a majority of paediatric clinicians, with perhaps some practices providing a mix of adult and paediatric work.

Having worked across all stages of the recovery process within the public health system, I quickly found myself in a state of frustration. The nature of the hospital and health system is to treat, achieve a level of function that is suitable for discharge, and then encourage staff to move on to the next patient. I felt that I was not able to make a meaningful impact or affect change in people's recovery, often due to the lack of time and resources.

I eventually 'burned out' of what felt like a fairly formulaic hospital model in this acute setting. I found the impairment-based models of therapy to be limiting; they did not address the immediate functional goals of the patient, nor did they meet the needs of the individual when they returned home to a bustling family, accessing their community, re-engaging with their friends, or returning to study or work.

The medical and allied health worlds strive to be robustly evidence based. This is driven by quantitative data that often compares people against a set of controls or norms. Of course, this is necessary to ensure a deeper understanding of how our brains and our bodies work, but there has recently been a push towards more qualitative research in healthcare. An individual, experiential body of work that provides insights into the workings of each individual is emerging, and when considered alongside quantitative data, it can provide powerful information that is meaningful to the individual.

Michael is one such individual with dysphasia that I have worked with. During his hospital admission, Michael was seen by a speech pathologist. Michael was described as having:

> very severe impairment for aphasia and severe impairment for language. Michael reportedly completed a course of speech therapy (rehabilitation) focusing on core semantics, phonological skills and naming, functional

conversational language, and IPAD therapy apps. At the conclusion of that treatment, Michael was considered to have severe expressive and moderate to severe receptive aphasia that impacted all aspects of language function.

On discharge from hospital and accessing insurance-funded private speech therapy, it was noted that he had 'significantly improved in several areas of language function by mid-2016. Improved areas included reading, writing and sentence construction. He was noted to have improved discourse and importantly the ability to self-correct grammatical errors.'

When I met Michael in 2017, he identified his goals in a more functional framework, wanting to increase his hours and duties of work at the university, to be able to write research grants, and to present at conferences. To achieve these goals, he needed to be able to write, research, publish, supervise, teach, and speak publicly at an exceptionally high academic level.

These goals can be hard to achieve while recovering on a stroke ward, although, of course, it depends on the patient. The transition from impairment-based therapy to activity- and participation-based therapy often correlates with the transition from hospital to home and in relationship with the trajectory of recovery being made.

By building awareness and understanding of his own thought processes, analysing and testing different strategies, and reflecting and generating possible solutions in tangible situations that were important to him, Michael has directed his therapy. This means we have been able to utilise metacognitive strategies to achieve his goals. Problem solving, identifying cause and effect, remembering to use strategies, and reflecting on strengths and weaknesses are all ways Michael used to improve his skills. Spoken and written discourses are discussed in relation to fluency, planning, organisation, content, coherence, and quantity but also in utility and satisfaction.

Dysphasia recovery is not a one-dimensional trajectory. It is a unique journey for each person recovering from dysphasia. There are no right or wrong goals. There is no right or wrong time frame. There is, however, an inherent need for a distinctive, person-centred, customised approach to rehabilitating dysphasia, tapping into the person's personality, environment, and personal circumstances. Although much of this seems like standard approaches to healthcare, subsequently Michael draws out some of the moments where the therapy was able to diverge in a way that is consistent with a dysphasanalysis – thinking *with* disability, not against it.

## Poetic language, musical behaviour, and language

In my experience, most books about surviving a stroke mention the personal freedom of being without language. In some senses, I understand this. Being let free in a world of fluid connection, rather than operating in a structured language, can be, they say, astounding. In her book *My Stroke of Insight*, Jill Bolte Taylor (2017) describes her career as neuroanatomist and then her long recovery journey after having a major stroke. Throughout the book, she writes touchingly about the 'deterioration of my cognitive abilities' and the moment when – having lost her connection with language – she was 'at *one* with the universe', and she experienced her capacity to touch the '"mystical" or "metaphysical"' (p. 3)'. Later in her book, she describes this experience more fully:

> The harder I tried to concentrate, the more fleeting my ideas seemed to be. Instead of finding answers and information, I met a growing sense of peace. In place of that constant chatter that had attached me to the details of my life, I felt enfolded by a blanket of tranquil euphoria. . . . As the language centres in my left hemisphere grew increasingly silent and I became detached from the memories of my life, I was comforted by an expanding sense of grace.
> (p. 41)

The problem for me was that, after waking up a couple days after my accident, my memory was that I could not talk, but there *were* thoughts. Of course, it is difficult to wind the clock backwards. Lying there in a hospital room without language, I remembered who I was and who was there. My lasting sense of these days was also of exhaustion and – well – blankness. I wanted to sleep, but my partner and my friends were told by doctors to use the precious moments after the event to use language. So they played games with me. They wrote the names of things on cards and glued them all around the room. Eimear, my partner, told me that this was toothpaste rather than deodorant. I did not exactly resist anyone, and, in many ways, I was fairly determined (or compliant, depending on the position you take) to improve. But, at the time, words were difficult to find. Every single word was an effort.

My life without any language at all was brief. It is said that strokes are as individual as the patient, but obviously, there are also overlaps. Defining an experience like 'blankness' – somewhat similar to, but not exactly like, living without words – depends, of course, on the use of language. And there is another important word, recollection: a small word but enormously difficult to define. It is not a memory. It is not narrative. It is not just a body experience. It is all these things, but it is different. Nonetheless, my *recollection* is that a few days later, words began to emerge. At that time, my way of explaining this to my friends was to say that there is a room full of words, but there is a blanket that has been thrown over them. I would try to 'find' a word but, most times, either I would find nothing or the 'wrong' word.

Back in the hospital in the early days of my recovery, there was also something else. I am not sure how, but at first, without spoken language, I could sing. Without spoken words in the way, some hurdles seem to dissolve. I recalled the words of 'Blackbird' by the Beatles appeared. It seems that the 'volume' of spoken word was ratcheted down to zero, so there was some space for the singing voice.

Having spent three weeks in the first phase of my recovery, I was then transferred to another hospital with a specialist ward for brain injury patients. I was always eager for anything – printed work exercises, physical activity, conversation – but that also meant constant speech, occupational, and physiotherapy. A couple of weeks into my rehabilitation program, my speech therapist had given me, as always, some printed exercises for homework. Having finished my homework, I presented myself to my next class one day later. Of course, at this moment, I did not fully understand the seriousness of my condition, and I claimed, smugly, that I was improving and that other therapists said that I would go back to work next semester.

The problem was that when my therapist looked at my answers, I received a reaction that I was not prepared for. The therapist asked me *why* did I not answer the questions correctly, rather than the unlikely poetic response that I actually gave. I tried to explain my responses to my speech therapist, and this was followed by a longer and somewhat painful discussion about my care. As minutes passed, I noticed that I was getting angry. I was so upset about this situation that I left my therapy session and returned to my hospital bed. That night, as I always did, I did my paper-based exercises, but I decided that this therapist was obviously young and probably inexperienced.

Reflecting on this encounter years later, I realised that I acted like a child. With many years of therapy ahead, I was just beginning to see that my recovery is a long journey. My heart now goes out to that young therapist. Perhaps this encounter might be interpreted as a way for the patient to build their response, word by word. The therapist kept calm throughout this discussion. The problem was that my anger became such a large hurdle that my therapist and I had to work hard to regain that relationship.

But reflections breed new interpretations. The night before this particular encounter, with my homework just finished by my bedside table, I lay there telling myself that actually therapy can be fun. I saw new words waiting to be used. Many of the words that I chose were perhaps not the obvious option, but there was some poetic pleasure here as well. For example, in one exercise, I used the word 'goannas' rather than 'cows'; the speech therapist looked at me as if I was mad.

In school many years ago, I saw poetry as difficult or, worse, just a foreign land that I did not want to venture into. But the bicycle accident somehow let me be free of rational discourse and opened new ways of expressing myself. Certainly, I will not say that a poetic genius was born in that hospital, but I enjoyed creating poetic phrases. Once I began to locate particular words, there were many 'errors', but sometimes poetic 'shoots' emerged, too. Once I said to Eimear, 'the sky is full of inscription'. In one sense, it makes no sense in this conversation. Like poetry, though, it lets one's mind be free to make new connections. Is the sky *written*? Is the sky a monument? Of history? Of the past? Is the sky a poem? The stroke was, in some senses, a gift, at least for me.

If I could return to that encounter, perhaps the therapist could have taken this conversation in a completely new different direction. For example, rather than correcting these 'errors', the therapist could have let me make 'errors' and led us 'forward'. First, they may have let me go, understanding that I was a 'child' who needed not a teacher but a listener. Second, the therapist might have asked me different questions about the words that I *had* used rather than the missing words that I had not used.

Furthermore, one way of approaching speech therapy exercises is to slow the patient down and practice 'error-free' patterns of speech. Simplifying this concept, there is a conversation between the brain and the mouth. The mouth of the patient is looking for words that are there, but the brain needs extra time to find those words. Therefore, the purpose is for the patient to speak very slowly without errors. I understand the logic, but it was difficult to have a normal conversation or even say 'good morning' without qualifying my answer with an apology for the errors I had made. For a couple of years, I just worked hard to avoid these interactions. I am pretty sure that was much harder for me than the people that I talked with. In other words, this encounter between my speech therapy and me has many potential outcomes; are we correcting the speech errors, or are we providing circumstances for poetic shoots to flourish? There is no magic here, but in this encounter, poetic language gave me some pleasure in *talking*, and pleasure in therapy was very rare.

My accident actually happened in a different state of Australia to the one I live in. I will not bore the reader with Australian state politics, just to say that the importance of state-based accident policies can have a profound effect on your life course. As an example, in the week before I was released from the hospital, I met the representative from *Icare*, the state government disability program delivering insurance and care services. This person managed my post-hospital program and, via *Icare*, paid for all future my speech and occupation therapy. Having been a (very) amateur musician, I raised the possibility of music therapy. As it turned out, the *Icare* representative said that there might be some local music specialists focusing on brain injuries. A few weeks later, a music therapist was there in my lounge room.

I might be accused of saying the obvious, but personalities make relationships work, and this was extremely important for someone like me, who was creating themselves as well as working with another therapist. This person worked. They listened. They thought about what I had said, and the next time we met, we tried different strategies, some of which were dismal failures, at least from my perspective. But there were also successes. I was prepared to try anything, so we tried singing together. For example, we launched into sing-around techniques. This involved singing often medieval and renaissance songs which the therapist and I would take turns in singing. My therapist also recorded themselves singing a series of sentences that I would listen to and then sing. In these exercises, there were brief moments when I could recognise my old 'self', rising above the 'water line', only then to disappear from view.

The music therapist and I often talked about these successes. I remember telling them about waking up from sleep next to my partner when, in that brief instance, I am 'free' from the stroke and I can talk. An instant later, I remember the stroke is there again, and normality returns. For me, there is an important point about the patient 'forgetting' the stroke and, by extension, their dysphasia. In those moments, the words are *there*. The old voice returns. Furthermore, stroke and dysphasia are not only biological and mechanical. In those micro-moments, the brain 'forgets' the dysphasia. For me, my ability to locate words greatly depends on, for example, fatigue, ambient noise, the size of the audience, people's familiarity, and the time of day. There is, in other words, a part of this condition that moves beyond the materiality of the body to the discursive and the environmental. The point here is not that the condition is partly discursive – which is well understood – but, at least in Queensland, there seems to be a dearth of new (or old) discursive approaches to dysphasia or, particularly, specialists who do not use cognitive behavioural therapy.

Which brings me back to poetry and music. Or, closer to this point, poetic language and musical behaviour can be one way of using the *irrational* strategies. I am absolutely *for* 'repetition', but there is still a gap there. Of all my reflections over the past four years of my recovery, the absence of pleasure from my treatment is still apparent for me.

When I began my recovery phase, I had a large amount of time in hospital to wonder and reflect. As I said, my body was basically uninjured, so I walked everywhere, including a café some distance outside hospital grounds. I am not sure, but I think the staff were comfortable for me to walk wherever I wanted. Staff are always busy, and getting me away from hospital unattended, breathing the air and having random conversations with the public, was always going to be beneficial. When I was not absconding, I was meandering around various hospital wards. As a curious patient, I would ask random questions (I was always practicing locating words) to staff, including the absence of poetry and music from brain injury rehabilitation. Some nurses and doctors were actually quite interested in new ways of doing care, and they said there were some interesting findings in the literature, particularly around music therapy. Of course, I imagine that hospital practice has to be led by both the weight of 'science', the day-to-day health economics, and pragmatic considerations of how to see many patients in only so many minutes.

Once I left the hospital, I became a day patient. This meant that I had to catch a weekly cab from home to the hospital. I was told that I was seeing another speech therapist. The therapist was somewhat older than the other therapists that I had seen previously. My experience was similar, but it was also different. I understood that I was now seeing a more senior therapist and, therefore, I had moved into a different phase of my recovery process. The therapist I was seeing was more relaxed. Of course, they also gave me endless supply of printed paper-exercises to do and gave the therapist extra time to complete other administration duties which, of course, I understood.

Some two years later, having worked with many therapists, I asked my *Icare* representative to look for a different approach. As always, I was patient with my therapist, and, over time, I had improved my talking skills appreciably. But there were also times when I thought the exercises were somewhat debatable. One therapist gave me a lengthy questionnaire to do for homework. The problem for me was I still had severe difficulties locating the written and spoken words and phrases for answers. In the end, I had to retreat from this encounter and start the search again.

Was I searching for a relationship somewhat like my music therapist? Perhaps. Many experts would say that having a stroke changes your outlook on your whole life, and so the therapist becomes more like a friend, in much the same way that my stroke became a constant companion.

Once I met Rebekah Dewberry, she realised that paper or computer exercises were, for many reasons, fairly useless for me. Many paper exercises are focused on re-building a patient's grammatical skills, but I had no difficulties completing these. My struggles were locating, in that instant, particularly words and phrases. But she did other things which distinguished her from other therapists. She listened *carefully* to my voice. She saw the pleasure I experienced when my 'old voice' emerged, albeit briefly. And Rebekah never corrected me. Of course, she had to test me periodically, similarly to other therapists, but while she might have used the results in her reports to *Icare*, the tests were wide open to many interpretations.

I was engaged in a test to show whether I could build sentences, construct ideas, and talk slowly. I am not sure how this test was useful and, certainly, I have forgotten these various scores. What I do remember was, in the middle of this verbal exercise, I tried to make the sound of 'rolling hills' but it came out '*reow*ling hills', a bit like a cat making the sound 'meow'. Some therapists might have marked me down on that error. With Rebekah, this 'error' was not a mistake and, instead, we looked at it as a normal variation in speech, and we chatted about the words that rhymed with 'reowling'.

There were also a series of bodily behaviours that were, at least for me, interesting but were not raised throughout my treatment. We would watch some videos of me talking where I would brush my mouth with my hand as if I wanted to remove 'errors' from my face. There was some sagging of skin on the left side of my face that had somewhat of a random effect on my word production. I lost some use of salivary gland function on the left side of my mouth, and I often needed more hydration to help me talk. I had three fractured facial bones, which affected the shape of my face, but they also altered my sense of myself as a 'talker'. But, rather than Rebekah choosing these for correcting, my behaviours emerged and become more obvious to *me*. These behaviours became links for further conversation and reflection.

At this moment of writing this section of this chapter, the stroke and dysphasia are still intimate companions for me. If you had to ask me, I would say that these practices that I have described here probably helped me, for better or worse, to 'cure' my disabled self. But they also gave me the chance to take magical pleasure in the use of language, poetry, and music. There is only one of me, and it is difficult to know whether *this* therapy worked better rather than *that* therapy. This is not a science. If Deleuze were here, he might have said that a narrative, although non-rational, can be useful to us now. Poetry and music *can* be effective in the hospital and private practice, but perhaps they just need a slightly different perspective.

## New directions for physiotherapists – part 2

So, what happens to physiotherapy when we think through Michael and Rebekah's discussions previously? In some ways, not much. Overall, their discussion does not suggest a dramatic shift in how we might understand or approach physiotherapy practice. Many aspects of the approach to working with Michael's dysphasia were very similar to customary physiotherapy practice – testing function, setting patient goals, shifting goals as the patient's needs change, preparing patients to return to work – all this is standard physiotherapy fodder. But there were some key moments which I (Jenny, a physiotherapist) believe present some quite radical ways to think differently about physiotherapy. These were the times when Michael and Rebekah (and his other therapists) were thinking *with* disability, not against it. The moments of dysphasanalysis – *using the dysphasia*. When dysphasia was celebrated and enjoyed – or at least embodied and experienced – rather than quantified and judged against a norm or pushed aside as 'incorrect'.

A key moment that we might consider in our dysphasanalysis was the use of pleasure and creativity – be it what Michael termed the 'poetic pleasure' of speaking differently or the use of music as a creative way to articulate. Applying these practices to the context of the work physiotherapists might do with 'physical' disabilities, it is possible to consider that this enjoyment/celebration might be played out through creative movement and/or dance. As Michael said – sometimes therapy was fun! This idea is not new – see, for example, the work of physiotherapists Molinaro, Kleinfield, and Lebed (1986), who discussed how, after breast cancer surgery, patients might adjust to their changed bodies through 'the freedom of total body movement'. However, such creative approaches are rare in physiotherapy, where movement is normally constrained to a very functional focus (Nicholls, Fadyll, & Gibson, 2015). Creativity and pleasure are rarely prioritised in physiotherapy.

Another key opportunity for dysphasanalysis is in Michael's description of Rebekah's lack of correction of his 'errors'. How would it be if physios reconceptualised their lists of 'errors' (e.g., abnormal gait, decreased range of movement, abnormal patterns of breathing, poor core stability) as poetic pleasures or creative moments rather than mistakes? Might we be able to play a little more by letting go of the measuring devices, the checklists, the numbers, and the pre-determined outcomes that create 'errors' in the first place? Deleuze and Guatarri would say so: there is much to be gained by being less teleological and 'remaining in the fray'. After all, there are so many different ways to work with our different ways of being in the world. As Michael said to his partner, 'the sky is full of inscription'.

> [Forming correct movement] is for the normal individual the prerequisite for any submission to social laws. No one is supposed to be ignorant of [normal movement patterns]; those who are belong in special institutions. The unity of [movement] is fundamentally political.
> Adapted from Deleuze and Guattari (1987, p. 112)

## Notes

1 Having said this, there are some points where we break our rules about 'I' and 'we'. In the end, we have used 'I' or 'we' intentionally. There is no error here, at least from our perspective.
2 It is interesting when two stroke survivors talk. They might 'understand' each other without explaining the symptoms and effects of strokes. That is, they already know what each other is talking about. From my memories of hospital and home care, we rarely talked directly to *other* stroke patients in a semi-formal, structured way. But the understanding is not so important but, rather, the physical relief that somebody else *knows*.

## References

Abrams, T. (2014). Is everyone upright? Erwin Straus' "the upright posture" and disabled phenomenology. *Human Affairs*, *24*(4). doi:10.2478/s13374-014-0249-2

Abrams, T., & Gibson, B. E. (2016). Putting Gino's lesson to work: Actor-network theory, enacted humanity, and rehabilitation. *Health* (London). doi:10.1177/1363459315628039

Armstrong, D. (1995). The rise of surveillance medicine. *Sociology of Health & Illness*, *17*(3), 393–404. https://doi.org/10.1111/1467-9566.ep10933329

Bjorbaekmo, W. S., & Engelsrud, G. H. (2011). Experiences of being tested: A critical discussion of the knowledge involved and produced in the practice of testing in children's rehabilitation. *Medicine Health Care and Philosophy*, *14*(2), 123–131. doi:10.1007/s11019-010-9254-3

Bjorbaekmo, W. S., & Mengshoel, A. M. (2016). "A touch of physiotherapy": The significance and meaning of touch in the practice of physiotherapy. *Physiotherapy Theory & Practice*, *32*(1), 10–19. doi:10.3109/09593985.2015.1071449

Deleuze, G., & Guattari, F. (1987). *A thousand plateaus: Capitalism and schizophrenia*. Minneapolis: University of Minnesota Press.

French, S. (1994). Attitudes of health professionals towards disabled people: A discussion and review of the literature. *Physiotherapy*, *80*(10), 687–693.

French, S., & Sim, J. (2008). *Physiotherapy: A psychosocial approach* (3rd ed.). London, UK: Elsevier.

Gibson, B. E. (2006). Disability, connectivity and transgressing the autonomous body. *Journal of Medical Humanities*, *27*(3), 187–196. doi:10.1007/s10912-006-9017-6

Gibson, B. E. (2016). *Rehabilitation: A post-critical approach*. Boca Raton, FL: CRC Press.

Gibson, B. E. (2018). A post-critical physiotherapy ethics: A commitment to openness. In B. E. Gibson, D. Nicholls, J. Setchell, & K. Synne-Groven (Eds.), *Manipulating practices: A critical physiotherapy reader* (pp. 35–54). Oslo, NO: Cappelen Damm.

Grosz, E. (1995). *Space, time, and perversion: Essays on the politics of bodies*. Abingdon, Oxon: Routledge.

Molinaro, J., Kleinfield, M., & Lebed, S. (1986). Physical therapy and dance in the surgical management of breast cancer: A clinical report. *Physical Therapy Journal*, *66*(6), 967–969.

Nicholls, D. A., Atkinson, K., Bjorbaekmo, W. S., Gibson, B. E., Latchem, J., Oleson, J., . . . Setchell, J. (2016). Connectivity an emerging concept for physiotherapy practice. *Physiotherapy Theory & Practice*, *32*(3), 159–170. doi:10.3109/09593985.2015.1137665

Nicholls, D. A., Fadyll, J., & Gibson, B. E. (2015). Rethinking movement: Postmodern reflections on a dominant rehabilitation discourse. In K. McPherson, B. E. Gibson, & A. Leplege (Eds.), *Rethinking rehabilitation: Theory and practice* (pp. 97–116). Boca Raton, FL: CRC Press.

Nicholls, D. A., & Gibson, B. E. (2010). The body and physiotherapy. *Physiotherapy Theory & Practice*, *26*(8), 497–509. doi:10.3109/09593981003710316

Roberts, M. (2005). Time, human being and mental health care: An introduction to Gilles Deleuze. *Nursing Philosophy*, *6*(3), 161–173. https://doi.org/10.1111/j.1466-769X.2005.00221.x

Setchell, J. (2016). *Weight stigma in health: (Re)thinking weight in a physiotherapy context* (PhD thesis). School of Psychology, The University of Queensland. doi:10.14264/uql.2016.466

Setchell, J. (2017). What has stigma got to do with physiotherapy? *Physiotherapy Canada*, *69*(1), 1–4.

Setchell, J., Abrams, T., McAdam, L., & Gibson, B. E. (2019). Cheer* in healthcare practice: What it excludes and why it matters. *Qualitative Health Research*, *29*(13), 1890–1903. doi:10.1177/1049732319838235

Setchell, J., Gard, M., Jones, L., & Watson, B. (2017). Addressing weight stigma in physiotherapy: Development of a theory driven approach to (re)thinking weight related interactions. *Physiotherapy Theory & Practice*, *33*(8), 597–610.

Setchell, J., Nicholls, D. A., & Gibson, B. E. (2017). Objecting: Multiplicity and the practice of physiotherapy. *Health: An Interdisciplinary Journal for the Social Study of Health, Illness and Medicine*, 1–20. doi:10.1177/1363459316688519

Setchell, J., Watson, B., Gard, M., & Jones, L. (2016). Physical therapists' ways of talking about weight: Clinical implications. *Physical Therapy Journal*, *96*(6), 865–875. doi:10.2522/ptj.20150286

Stroke Foundation. (2017). *Clinical guidelines for stroke management*. Melbourne, Australia.

Synnott, A., O'Keeffe, M., Bunzli, S., Dankaerts, W., O'Sullivan, P., & O'Sullivan, K. (2015). Physiotherapists may stigmatise or feel unprepared to treat people with low back pain and psychosocial factors that influence recovery: A systematic review. *Journal of Physiotherapy*, *61*(2), 68–76. doi:10.1016/j.jphys.2015.02.016

Taylor, J. T. (2017). *My stroke of insight: A brain scientist's personal journey*. London, UK: Hodder & Stoughton.

Trede, F. (2012). Emancipatory physiotherapy practice. *Physiotherapy Theory & Practice*, *28*(6), 466–473. doi:10.3109/09593985.2012.676942

# 15 How are we doing? Placing human relationships at the centre of physiotherapy

*Jean Braithwaite, Tone Dahl-Michelsen, and Karen Synne Groven*

**Introduction**

As this anthology itself attests, an urgent spirit of reform and self-critical reflection is now widespread at the cutting edge of physiotherapy research. Three recent approaches are the 'tinkering' recommended by Gibson and colleagues (2019) in pursuit of person-centred care, Buetow (2019)'s proposal to rebrand the aims of therapeutic intervention as 'ultrabilitation' rather than 'rehabilitation', and Groven, Braithwaite, and Dahl-Michelsen (2019)'s exposure of unintended harms of treatment in the form of 'iatrogenic dys-appearance'. This latter term refers to a variety of ways in which therapeutic interventions may make patients unpleasantly aware of their own bodies, ranging from physical pain and discomfort to embarrassment, alienation, feelings of social inferiority, stigmatization, conspicuousness, and so on, in any combination or degrees. We'll return to this concept subsequently. (See Groven et al., 2019 and references within for a fuller discussion.)

It is scarcely in dispute that it is desirable for healthcare providers involved in rehabilitation practice, including physiotherapists, always to treat their patients foremost as fellow human beings rather than as raw materials to be sculpted by us into more desirable configurations. However, in a profession dominated by biomedical metrics (of illness and health), it is very easy, even with the best of compassionate intentions, to slip into a normalizing frame of mind, to follow the script of 'best practices', sometimes to the detriment of the individual person. Gibson and colleagues (2019) examine in microscopic detail nine 'care events'. In one of these, a home healthcare provider, 'Ginny', unwittingly pressures 'Irene', an elderly patient recovering from a stroke, to work toward walking without an aid, at least indoors. The transcript, though, makes it quite clear that Irene strongly prefers to keep her 'stick' nearby at all times for the physical and emotional support it gives her. Ginny is attempting to follow the rules of her institutional treatment program, in which, according to Gibson, 'care is focused on the person's stated preferences to counter any paternalistic imposition of the practitioner's goals' (Gibson et al., 2019, p. 4). Yet because of the pressures Ginny's job places on her (to solicit and record individualized patient goals related to recovering prior function), Ginny ends up pushing Irene in a direction she clearly does not want to go. 'Paradoxically', Gibson notes, 'the patient *and practitioner* as persons became lost in the process' (Gibson et al., 2019, p. 4).

Part of what went wrong in the Ginny–Irene interaction is the surrounding theoretical framework which takes for granted that *recovery* of *prior* function should guide Irene's aspirations for her future. This sort of assumption is arguably etymologically inherent in the word *rehabilitation*, which is why Buetow, Kapur, and Wolbring (2019) suggest replacing it with a different term. After all, what is the ultimate goal of treatment, if one thinks about it carefully? Surely it is not recovery per se but a flourishing life. Recovery is not a realistic goal in every case, and, in particular, when a condition is present from birth, there *is* no 'prior' unimpaired state. However, *increased life satisfaction* in accordance with patients' own values and priorities is almost always available, no matter how dire the prognosis. Indeed, it is not uncommon that persons with a health challenge or disability even manage to use their atypical physical condition as a springboard to personal growth and sometimes extraordinary achievement (Solvang, 2019; Hatterud, 2018). Sometimes such individuals even end up considering themselves better off than they would have been without the disability (or health challenge) (Hatterud, 2018). Thus, Buetow Kapur, and Wolbring (2019) propose the cover term '*ultrabilitation*' to describe the pursuit of flourishing 'around, toward, and beyond recovery' (see Figure 15.1). In a similar vein, Gibson describes the 'micro-politics of caring' in which both patients and care-givers commit to a fine-grained process of mutual 'tinkering' to find the optimal interventions to maximize patient outcomes *from the patient's perspective* (rather than exclusively biomedical metrics) (Gibson et al., 2019).

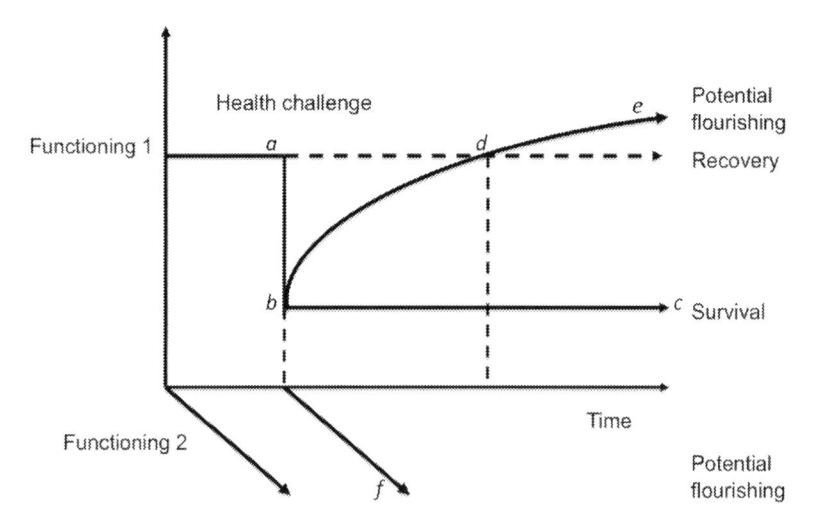

*Figure 15.1* Flourishing around, toward, and beyond recovery. A health challenge (at point *a*) may cause a type of functioning to decline (to point *b*). The person may continue to languish (point *c*), move toward recovery (at point *d*), move beyond recovery (point *e*), or strengthen another type of functioning (at point *f*).

For several years now, Groven and Braithwaite and their colleagues (Groven et al., 2013; Groven & Braithwaite, 2016; Groven et al., 2019) have focused on studying *patient* accounts of physiotherapeutic treatment in order to discover insights useful to healthcare practitioners. In Groven et al. (2019), we introduced the concept of *iatrogenic dys-appearance* into the literature, comparing the cases of two prominent Norwegian authors, both suffering from chronic muscular degenerative diseases, Jan Grue and Geir Hellemo. Grue finally decided to reject physiotherapy on the basis of his lifetime of negative experiences with dozens of physical therapists, while Hellemo, though also critical of many of his caregivers' attitudes, embraced a radically intensive program of physiotherapy going far beyond what his initial treatment team recommended. Similarly, we here present the contrasting cases of two young Scandinavians born with cerebral palsy, each of whom, in their own way, represents a success story. The two have quite different relationships to rehabilitation processes and physiotherapists, however. Maria Bjurstrøm is just 19, a competitive boccia player on the Swedish team, and has recently published a memoir *Mitt liv som CP* [My Life with CP]. Jacob Nossell is 31 and currently works as head of communications and disability consultant at Enactlab S/I, in addition to frequent public lecturing on disability, diversity, and related subjects.

In combination with our prior research, these two new cases persuade us that a key strategy in maximizing the patient's subjective benefit from treatment is that the caregiver never lose sight of two relationships important to the therapeutic context: (1) the relationship existing between the patient and the caregiver and (2) the perhaps even more crucial 'relationship' existing between the patient and their own body. As Gibson and colleagues point out, 'there is no guarantee of getting it right, no general "principle of tinkering" that can be universally applied to all situations' (Gibson et al., 2019, p. 7). But we are convinced that a therapeutic mindset which keeps specifically these relationships at the centre of attention will generally lead to better results than practices which neglect them in favour of other priorities. What counts as success, what counts as progress, cannot even be determined without taking into account the patient's own subjective experience, which requires a healthy two-way communication and shared goal-setting.

### 'Physiotherapists never say "you are good enough as you are"'

A recent issue of *Fysioterapeuten* – a Danish journal focusing on research and issues related to physiotherapy – includes an interview with Jacob Nossell, as well as describing in some detail a lecture he gave to the Danish Midlands Physiotherapists (Jensen, 2018). Nossell has had CP from birth and consequently has worked with some 25–30 physiotherapists over the course of his lifetime. By now, he has developed a fairly detailed philosophy regarding the therapeutic relationship, and he offers professional advice to physiotherapists from this position of expertise on the patient experience. Though there are serious moments when he lectures, much of Nossell's commentary is packaged in the form of a stand-up comedy routine. Extended quotes by the interviewer/journalist illustrate Nossell's light touch: his assessments of our profession, in general, express generous-minded constructive criticism, not bitterness. One such assessment is used to title the interview: 'Physiotherapists never say "You are good enough as you are".' Nossell's point comes across clearly: what healthcare providers say – and what they *don't* say – can inadvertently send messages that have a negative impact on their patients' ability to feel good about their bodies/themselves.

Similar concepts are expressed repeatedly in the course of Nossell's routine, in a variety of ways. More than once he mentions the danger of a 'myopic' focus on exercise and biometric progress. There are 'more things in life than just improving [oneself] physically'. On the one hand, he is grateful that his family and early physiotherapists had high expectations for him and were deeply invested in his progress: he felt 'privileged' to be given 'opportunities' and was able to make remarkable progress. On the other hand, he often felt pushed to 'fulfill the ambitions of others', with insufficient freedom and leisure to explore what he most wanted for himself. One of his lecture slides bears the title 'Progress-mania'. It is very easy, Nossell says, for physiotherapy to produce a 'chronically bad conscience' for the patient, because there is 'always something you can do better', such as 'lift your leg a little higher'.

'Why do we always have to do the exercises I'm worst at?' Nossell asks. 'It's like if I went home to my girlfriend and I said, "Honey, I'd really love to have sex with you, but you have to do it in just the way that's worst for you".' This remark is intended humorously, of course, but there is a great deal of emotional wisdom buried within the joke. It's worthwhile to take some time to unpack Nossell's punchline fully. The hypothetical boyfriend's romantic invitation to his partner is laughably poorly designed. If we want to coax our sexual partners to engage in an activity that *we* consider desirable, we must make it seem desirable to them as well. Insisting on precisely the positions or activities which are least comfortable for the other party, the least producing of any physical satisfaction, or pleasure, or pride, is a poor strategy for seduction or relationship-building, especially in the long term. We would consider a boyfriend who did this selfish and stupid, at best, if not outright abusive.

In a therapeutic relationship, unfortunately, because of the inherently unequal authority of the two people, it is all too easy for either the caregiver or the patient to slip into thinking that the professional generally knows best and needs to be obeyed for the patient's 'own good', despite any discomfort. Coming to the therapeutic encounter with this frame of mind establishes conditions under which what we call *iatrogenic dys-appearance* can readily emerge, despite the best of therapeutic intentions. Of course, sex and romance are not at all the same thing as a therapy relationship. However, the two have at least a few things in common. Like sex, physiotherapy is an activity that foregrounds the body, and thus it is always an opportunity for either bodily pleasure or dissatisfaction, bodily pride or shame. Also, like sex, physiotherapy involves two people, so consent and mutual respect are of paramount importance to establishing a good long-term relationship. Physiotherapists must never forget that the bodies they work with are the precious site of consciousness of another human being, and they must never forget that their actions may have the power to improve or worsen that person's long-term relationship with their own body.

## 'How are you doing?'

Nossell himself overtly stresses the importance of the physiotherapeutic relationship *as a human relationship*. During the discussion period following his talk, an audience member asks what question Nossell thinks it most desirable for a physiotherapist to ask. 'How are you doing?' is his answer. The simple, open-ended expression of interest with which most people greet one another at the beginning of a social conversation is also the best starting point for the therapeutic conversation. Of course, one must also then listen to the answer and allow it to guide the subsequent shared therapeutic projects.

Nossell stresses 'meaningful cooperation' in the therapeutic relationship. 'I know you [physiotherapy professionals] are under constant pressure', he says, generously. 'But you have to translate for me why exactly these exercises are important to me'. He tells an anecdote from his childhood: his parents were concerned about his uncontrollable drooling and consulted a number of specialists to address it. But it was only when he reached puberty and got interested in girls that Nossell himself embraced the goal of not slobbering as crucial to his social success.

As Nossell points out, the therapeutic relationship is inherently asymmetrical, with the doctor or physiotherapist presumed to be in possession of specialized knowledge of what might be good for the patient. But 'a normative assessment is not an objective truth', and the patients bring something to the table that 'you cannot read in the books', including valuable information about their own lived experience. Thus, 'an equal dialogue' is desirable.

Therapists, Nossell says 'are not used to receiving feedback or having their work questioned' by the disabled, who themselves may have difficulty resisting therapeutic authority. 'It's about finding the balance of the relationship'. In the therapeutic context, Nossell still often feels like 'a sausage in a sausage factory', but he does give credit to the profession for improvements, noting that 'in recent years you have focused on meeting the citizen where he is'.

What about children? An audience member asks. Children do not always know what is best for them. Nossell refers to his own childhood, during which his parents' 'strong attitudes and aspirations on [his] behalf' sometimes made him feel that he 'had to live up to something', not just for his own sake but to satisfy his parents and so the physiotherapist could 'note that progress had been made'. Thus, he now seeks to raise awareness among professionals about the dangers of making decisions for other people, even when those other people are children and young people. 'What interests underlie the decisions you make on our behalf? Even though we need treatment, we are first and foremost human beings'.

## Bjurstrøm's life story: a brief summary

At the time of writing her memoir, Maria Bjurstrøm had completed high school and was taking a year off before college in order to participate on the Swedish national boccia team. Boccia is a sport related to the more familiar bocce, but specifically designed for athletic competition by disabled players. Bjurstrøm has made athletics central to her life for many years, and her writing is generally enthusiastic about exercise and strenuous physical training. The overall narrative arc of her memoir follows a relatively conventional pattern in which an afflicted young person triumphs over adversity through her strength of will, with help along the way from her family and other dedicated coaches and assistants, some of whom are physiotherapists. Bjurstrøm's writing is prone to simple, affirmative slogans such as 'Nothing is impossible' and 'I never saw myself as disabled', although the details of the narrative itself reveal considerably more nuance.

Like Nossell, Bjurstrøm's connections to the world of physiotherapy began in infancy; she was diagnosed with CP and had a habilitation team before she was one year old (Bjurstrøm, 2015, pp. 11–12; all subsequent page number references in this section refer to the same text). Presumably the earliest recollections in Bjurstrøm's narrative are drawn from her parents' memories rather than directly from her own. From the age of two, she went to daycare, where her dedicated individual assistant Birgitta helped her participate fully in the other children's activities. Birgitta led Bjurstrøm through an hour of daily exercises, as well as taking her out of the school once a week to the habilitation clinic, where she did group sessions with other disabled children (p. 16). At this earliest stage of life, the little girl's experiences with physiotherapy were far from pleasant: she 'hated it when health professionals hugged me and touched me' and started to cry whenever she arrived for her weekly session at the habilitation clinic (p. 13). But the 19-year-old narrator presents this suffering as something necessary to her ultimate benefit (the team was 'forced to do it') and describes the young child's reactions with a certain amount of irony: the habilitation team was 'not popular with me' and so 'it was not easy' for them to do the tests they had to do (p. 13). By her tone, 19-year-old Bjurstrøm distances herself from the now-outgrown reactions of the child but also suggests a certain pride in the stubbornness which is a more lasting trait.

When she was approximately four years old, at her parents' insistence, Bjurstrøm was enrolled in a very intense program called Move and Walk, despite the opinion of her physiotherapist that the program was excessively 'strict'. Bjurstrøm had to live away from home for four weeks with one of her parents while the other stayed home to care for her younger sister. In Bjurstrøm's telling, the Move and Walk program was a turning point in terms of her progress: 'Even when the other children cried and were tired, I fought, because when I had decided on something I was going to make it' (p. 21). She practiced walking without support, as well as sitting with no seatbelt on a specialized wooden apparatus while moving her limbs. Her prior team of physiotherapists had advised against both of these things – clashing advice from different experts is apparent repeatedly through the narrative, although Bjurstrøm herself does not stress this theme overtly. Bjurstrøm fell many times at Move and Walk, but after a few days, she succeeded in balancing herself to sit upright without help. In addition to this functional progress, she also made a close friend, Ebba. The family was delighted with the program and resolved to attend again the following year; moreover, they kept up the pace of intense exercising at home. It was Bjurstrøm herself who set the pace, she says; her parents occasionally tried to persuade her to take it easy.

When she started public school at age 6, travel to the Move and Walk program was less feasible, so Bjurstrøm's family negotiated a place for her in a similar program, LEMO, which still required travel but not as far. She had to miss the last class of the school day when attending LEMO several times each week. In this program, she met another favourite physiotherapist, Pia. Bjurstrøm brags that she never tired of exercising, 'even when the rest of the children decided to have a break and rest' (p. 57). Her goal was to walk unsupported, and she achieved it the day before starting second grade. However, she then fell and got a concussion while demonstrating her walking skills to her family (p. 58). There were many such incidents of falls that required medical treatment. Bjurstrøm notes 'It took me many years before I could exercise without being afraid. And when my worries were gone, exercising went much better'.

Bjurstrøm's family and caregivers worked with her to make it possible for her to engage in a wide variety of sports hobbies. She could not manage soccer, but she had a tricycle and specially adapted bicycles and, like many adolescent girls, became passionate about horseback riding, which she felt improved her balance. At age 11, she and her friend Ebba enrolled in a special sports school for the disabled, 'the best thing I have ever done' (p. 72). Here, once again, she had a particularly intense and affectionate bond with a physiotherapist, Berit. Six years later, Bjurstrøm's physical strength and dexterity had improved to the point that she could operate a manual wheelchair on her own, something she claims nobody had believed possible at the outset.

The boccia playing began at age 14, and Bjurstrøm soon began entering competitions, and then winning prizes, beginning with a bronze medal at the Malmø open. 'It came as a surprise and the feeling is not possible to describe', she says (p. 113). 'How is it possible that I who had only been competing for a year could win a medal and beat more experienced players?' Four years later, she was the fourth-ranked player in Sweden, and now her goal is to win a gold medal. In an interview quoted in the promotional materials for her memoir, Bjurstrøm describes herself as 'an elite athlete' who is living her 'dream life', travelling the world for competitions. She believes that it will take a long time, but she will surely achieve her goals by investing 'a lot of sweat and tears' and with family support.

## Contrasts and discussion

On the surface, Bjurstrøm and Nossell may seem to have little in common. Her life revolves entirely around exercise and competitive sports, while he is adamant that there are 'more things in life' than striving toward greater physical fitness and that it is a mistake for the profession of physiotherapy to concentrate monomaniacally on that goal for all patients. In terms of narrative style, there are also considerable differences. Bjurstrøm tends to express emotions and attitudes in simple, black-and-white terms, while Nossell's assessments are much more complex, mixing criticism of physiotherapy with empathy toward its practitioners, for instance. Nossell tells the interviewer 'I have a hard time with my story always being the completely stereotypical sunbeam story', while Bjurstrøm appears determined to fit her story to the most basic possible pattern of achievement through willpower, even when this requires forcing a square peg into a round hole. One of her slogans – 'Nothing is impossible' (if one wants it enough and works hard enough) – really cannot be considered literally true, and, in fact, her own narrative contradicts it. For example, she practiced for a long, long time, trying to master all the movements necessary to dress herself without assistance, before she finally, reluctantly, conceded defeat (Bjurstrøm, 2015, p. 35). Of course, Bjurstrøm is still a teenager, and her mature views may likely become more nuanced, but some part of the difference in how she and Nossell portray their experiences comes down to personality.

For a person like Bjurstrøm who is highly competitive, the type of physically measurable goals and progress that serve as the foundation of evidence-based medicine may very well be the ideal motivators to engage in sustained physiotherapeutic training. For many other people, though, this type of focus will be disagreeable or even harmful, potentially damaging the patient's relationship to exercise in general, healthcare providers in general, or their own feelings of adequacy as embodied human beings. 'Why do we always have to do the exercises I'm worst at?' laments Nossell, and many people who are repeatedly put in this frustrating position will have a bad reaction. They may, as Nossell says, develop a 'chronically bad conscience', or they may rebel completely and reject everything physiotherapy has to offer.

Although Nossell and Bjurstrøm may be very differently disposed toward sports and exercise by reason of personality differences and values, it is worth pointing out that they are both influenced by living in a larger culture that valorizes exercise and physical fitness for its own sake, tending to treat physical activity as a form of virtue rather than a form of life-enhancing pleasure. It is not necessarily that medically trained health promoters generally *intend* to send the message that people's human value depends on their 'fitness' level – but this implicit message has nevertheless become widespread in our mass-culture media and is easy to internalize (Kennedy & Markula, 2011). Thus, large numbers of people in the developed world suffer from that very same 'chronically bad conscience', thinking they are not exercising enough or are not as 'fit' as some vague, socially established norm. So it is perhaps no coincidence that Bjurstrøm has relatively little to say about the pleasure she derives from her sport and much more to say about the social sacrifices she makes to pursue it and the intensity of her determination and tenacity in comparison to her peers. Presumably she *does* get physical pleasure from her current very intensive training regimen (as she once did from horseback riding and cycling), but it doesn't occur to her to emphasize that topic when telling her story. An interesting contrast here is author Geir Hellemo (Hellemo, 2017; Groven et al., 2019, who writes very eloquently about how physical exercise puts him in greater harmony with his body, giving him joy despite his degenerative illness.

Another point of similarity between the accounts of Bjurstrøm and Nossell is the common trope of outperforming medical expectations. Bjurstrøm writes, 'When I was born, the doctors told me that I would need help with everything for the rest of my life, but I like to prove the opposite, and I have done so several times'. Similarly, Nossell says that when he was first diagnosed, '[t]he doctors said: Jacob will never walk, nor will he ever speak. Fortunately, my parents didn't believe it, and they wouldn't accept it either'. True to form, Nossell then goes on to complicate his point: he is grateful for his family's support, grateful for the functional progress he has made over his lifetime, but at the same time, he also fears that other children may be under too much emotional pressure – as he was himself – to achieve those functional goals. Children may often be at risk of undervaluing their own individually chosen interests or tying their self-esteem exclusively to measures of 'progress'. Nossell warns us against these risks. By contrast, Bjurstrøm, at least if we take her writing at face value, is gleefully free from ambivalence about progress. Her self-image as an achiever is not in doubt, and she is certain that progress is inevitable in her case.

Bjurstrøm presents her life as a series of correct choices made, first by her parents and then by herself. Despite the reservations of her habilitation team, she was enrolled in Move and Walk at age four, and then LEMO, and then the sports school. Despite falls and injuries, she pressed forward with aggressive exercising and is convinced that this was for the best: she triumphed over her fears and now exercises 'much better'. Objectively, there is no way to be certain that the intensive approach chosen by Bjurstrøm's parents (and then Bjurstrøm) actually produced better results than a more cautious approach might have. Could she possibly have made similar functional breakthroughs more gently, without so much risk of injury? We have no control group to compare her to, no Bjurstrøm who stuck with the original team's recommendations, who didn't attend Move and Walk, who didn't start second grade with a concussion. We cannot be certain that she (or her parents) was right or wrong in any one decision. What does seem clear is that the general strategy her parents pursued, and that she continues to pursue now, is a good fit for her competitive, self-willed, optimistic personality and the sports interests she developed early in life. It would not be a good fit for every child or every family, though. Nor would every family have the resources and stamina to invest quite so much in travel, sports equipment, and so on.

Nossell speaks of the need for patient feedback to physiotherapists and even 'resistance' to their recommendations. Such resistance is a frequent topic in recent literature (see, for instance, Bjorbækmo & Engelsrud, 2011; Groven et al., 2019; Gibson, 2018). Bjurstrøm and her family have not waited to be given our permission to resist; they seem always to have taken it completely for granted that they had the right to make their own decisions. Her treatment team recommended that she sleep every night with braces, in order to stretch her Achilles tendons. Bjurstrøm says, 'Even though I was supposed to wear braces every night, I did not use them that often because it was uncomfortable to sleep with my legs stretched. After a few months we put them in my wardrobe and never wore them again'. This example contrasts interestingly with that of author Jan Grue (Grue, 2018; Groven et al., 2019), who faithfully wore his prescribed braces despite the pain and sleeplessness they caused. Ultimately, the Grues did resist this painful treatment, but not until the boy had first suffered with the braces for many years.

Bjurstrøm is entirely confident shopping around for second opinions until she gets the answer she wants. For example, since 'fitting in with the crowd' is deeply important to her, she wants to start high school with stylish shoes rather than specially designed orthopaedic ones. Her physiotherapist supports her in this wish and suggests a sports shoe store, where Bjurstrøm buys Reeboks. Bjurstrøm's orthopaedist, however, does not go along, so she fires him. 'What mattered the most was that the shoes were pretty and I did not care how stable they were', Bjurstrøm says. 'That was the last time I went to see the orthopedist. After all, they're my feet, right?' (Bjurstrøm, 2015, p. 65). Many healthcare providers might find a headstrong patient like Bjurstrøm challenging to deal with, but in fact an exceptionally compliant one like Grue actually poses a greater, more subtle danger in the long term. Bjurstrøm easily embraces physiotherapists – some of them, anyway – as her close friends and collaborators. She credits Pia in particular for helping to rein in her overenthusiasm and keep her on an even keel. Grue, on the other hand, once he attained maturity and confidence in his own judgment, resolved never to go to any physiotherapist ever again (Grue, 2018). Because the field and its practitioners failed him early on, he has become permanently alienated from anything we might have to offer.

Even this small handful of examples makes it very clear that there is no one-size-fits-all approach and also that patients' experiences in physiotherapy are multidimensional. On a scale measuring appetite for therapeutic exercise, Bjurstrøm and Hellemo would both score high, but not for the same reasons. Nossell would measure out somewhere in the middle and Grue very low. Bjurstrøm would score high for competitiveness and appetite for measurable 'progress', perhaps agreeing with the 'no pain, no gain' philosophy of exercise. Bjurstrøm has a strong tendency toward resistance but an equally strong drive for sociability; a physiotherapist who can establish a rapport with her secures her strong loyalty and very enthusiastic cooperation, at least with some projects. Nossell occupies a more central position in terms of resistance, but in terms of two-way communication and providing articulate feedback, he is at least Bjurstrøm's equal if not superior. By contrast, the Grue family, at least for many years, had little inclination to resist expert medical and therapeutic advice. Compliant patients like the Grue family perhaps need to have their feedback and input more actively solicited during treatment. They may not be complaining or obviously rebelling, but that doesn't mean that all is well.

Health professionals, including physiotherapists, therefore need to ask patients not only 'How are you doing?' but also 'How are *we* doing?' Therapists need to interact with patients as individuals deeply enough to discover what a flourishing life means for them and whether our treatments are promoting their perceived wellbeing more than they hamper it. Therapists can aim to work with them to promote joyous appreciation of their own bodies as part of a flourishing life, without suggesting that they aren't good enough as they are.

## Conclusion

One happy side effect of adopting a relationship-centred approach toward physiotherapy is that it can somewhat relieve the pressure on the physiotherapist. Some recent articles have called for a more self-critical, self-questioning attitude in physiotherapy as a necessary corrective to overconfidence in medical-scientific authority

(Ahlsen & Solbrække, 2018; Ahlsen, Mengshoel, Bondevik, & Engebretsen, 2018; Bjorbækmo & Engelsrud, 2011; Bjorbækmo & Mengshoel, 2016; Gibson et al., 2019; Chowdhury & Bjorbækmo, 2017; Gibson et al., 2019; Groven & Dahl-Michelsen, 2017; Groven & Dahl-Michelsen, 2018; Nicholls et al., 2016; Nicholls, 2018; Setchell, Watson, Gard, & Jones, 2016; Setchell, Nicholls, & Gibson, 2018). To some, this drive toward increasing self-examination and doubt may seem undesirable, punitive toward practitioners, or even a form of self-flagellation, but in fact, humility has some definite advantages. If physiotherapists solicit more patient input and a more equal balance of power, that means that they don't themselves have to carry the whole of the responsibility for the success of the relationship. Physiotherapists can admit they're only human, too, and ask their patients to cut them some slack in an atmosphere of mutual compassion, two-way communication, and jointly seeking to improve. Gibson et al. (2019)'s concept of 'tinkering' is clearly applicable here. Therapists can admit that there are differences of opinion in their field, that 'best practices' are always only provisionally established, and (in difficult cases) that shopping around for a physiotherapist who might be a better philosophical fit is always an option.

Buetow (2019)'s concept of *ultrabilitation* is another type of corrective to the unstated background assumption that physical therapy's main goal is restoring the patient to some prior, better condition of health or else striving to approach a more species-typical level of function which may or may not even be attainable. Whether physiotherapists call their work rehabilitation, habilitation, ultrabilitation, or something completely different, its ultimate goal should always be the 'flourishing' of the patient on their own terms. Therapists are there to facilitate their patients' pursuit of their best possible life, 'around, toward, and beyond recovery' (Buetow, Martínez-Martín, & McCormack., 2019). Since flourishing is a very individual matter, the goals of any particular therapeutic encounter can only be set in the context of that specific relationship.

Yet even though flourishing is very individual, some generalizations can still be made. The regular experience of bodily pleasure and pride will tend to promote flourishing, while bodily shame and feelings of bodily inadequacy will surely impair it. Elsewhere (especially in Groven et al., 2019), we have argued that physiotherapists should seek opportunities to create the former bodily situation ('eu-appearance') and avoid the latter ('dys-appearance'). Here we will put it in less technical terms: physiotherapists should remain aware of their power to influence patients' long-term good relationships with their own bodies. This relationship is crucial for wellbeing as an integral part of human flourishing, and the therapeutic relationship has the potential to have a strong impact on it, either positive or negative.

## References

Ahlsen, B., Mengshoel, A. M., Bondevik, H., & Engebretsen, E. (2018). Physiotherapists as detectives: Investigating clues and plots in the clinical encounter. *Medical Humanities*, *44*(1), 40–45.

Ahlsen, B., & Solbrække, K. N. (2018). Using narrative perspectives in the clinical setting of physiotherapy: Why and how? In B. Gibson, D. Nicholls, J. Setchell, & K. S. Groven

(Eds.), *Manipulating practices: A critical physiotherapy reader*. Oslo, NO: Cappelen Damm Akademisk.

Bjorbækmo, W. S., & Engelsrud, G. H. (2011). Experiences of being tested: A critical discussion of the knowledge involved and produced in the practice of testing in children's rehabilitation. *Medicine, Health Care and Philosophy*, *14*(2), 123–131.

Bjorbækmo, W. S., & Mengshoel, A. M. (2016). "A touch of physiotherapy": The significance and meaning of touch in the practice of physiotherapy. *Physiotherapy Theory and Practice*, *32*(1), 10–19.

Bjurstrøm, M. (2015). *Mitt liv som CP* [My life with CP]. Altermi, AB.

Buetow, S. A. (2019). Psychological preconditions for flourishing through ultrabilitation: A descriptive framework. *Disability and Rehabilitation*, *42*(11), 1503-1510. doi:10.1080/09638288.2018.1550532

Buetow, S. A., Kapur, N., & Wolbring, G. (2019). From rehabilitation to ultrabilitation: Moving forward. *Disability and Rehabilitation*. *42*(11). 1487-1489. doi:10.1080/09638288.2019.1620873

Buetow, S. A., Martínez-Martín, P., & McCormack, B. (2019). Ultrabilitation: Beyond recovery-oriented rehabilitation. *Disability and Rehabilitation*, *41*(6), 740–745.

Chowdhury, A., & Bjorbækmo, W. S. (2017). Clinical reasoning: Embodied meaning-making in physiotherapy. *Physiotherapy Theory and Practice*, *33*(7), 550–559.

Gibson, B. (2018). Post-critical physiotherapy ethics: A commitment to openness. In B. Gibson, D. Nicholls, J. Setchell, & K. Groven (Eds.), *Manipulating practices: A critical physiotherapy reader*. Oslo, NO: Cappelen Damm Akademisk.

Gibson, B., Terry, G., Setchell, J., Bright, F. A. S., Cummins, C., & Kayes, N. (2019). The micro-politics of care: Tinkering with person-centred rehabilitation. *Disability & Rehabilitation*. doi:10.1080/09638288.2019.1587793

Groven, K. S., & Braithwaite, J. (2016). Happily-ever-after: Personal narratives in weight-loss surgery advertising. *Health Care for Women International*, *37*(11), 1221–1238.

Groven, K. S., Braithwaite, J., & Dahl-Michelsen, T. (2019). Iatrogenic dys-appearance: First-person accounts of chronic neuromuscular disease reveal unintended harms of treatment. *European Journal of Physiotherapy*. doi:10.1080/21679169.2019.1598490

Groven, K. S., & Dahl-Michelsen, T. (2017). Critical physiotherapy ethics: Openness and doubt in physiotherapy encounters in lifestyle programs for children and adolescents with obesity. *Fysioterapeuten*, *9*(17), 38–43.

Groven, K. S., & Dahl-Michelsen, T. (2018). "I enjoy the treadmill very much": Moving beyond traditional understandings of self-efficacy in anti-obesity interventions. *Physiotherapy Theory and Practice*, 1–7.

Groven, K. S., Råheim, M., Braithwaite, J., & Engelsrud, G. (2013). Weight loss surgery as a tool for changing lifestyle? *Medicine, Health Care and Philosophy*, *16*(4), 699–708.

Grue, J. (2018). *Jeg lever et liv som ligner deres* [I live a life similar to yours]. Oslo, NO: Gyldendal.

Hatterud, B. (2018). *Mot Normalt* [Against normality]. Oslo, NO: Samlaget.

Hellemo, G. (2017). My body as a microcosm. *Tiddskrift for den norske legeforening*. doi:10.4045/tidsskr.17.0253

Jensen, M. B. (2018). Fysioterapeuter siger aldri du er god nok som du er (Interview with Jacob Nossell). *Fysioterapeuten*, *8*. Retrieved from www.fysio.dk/fysioterapeuten/arkiv/nr.-8-2018/fysioterapeuter-siger-aldrig-du-er-god-nok-som-du-er

Kennedy, E., & Markula, P. (2011). *Women and exercise: The body, health and consumerism*. New York: Routledge.

Nicholls, D. A. (2018). *The end of physiotherapy*. Abingdon, UK: Routledge.

Nicholls, D. A., Atkinson, K., Bjorbækmo, W. S., Gibson, B. E., Latchem, J., Olesen, J., . . . Setchell, J. (2016). Connectivity: An emerging concept for physiotherapy practice. *Physiotherapy Theory and Practice*, *32*(3), 159–170.

Setchell, J., Nicholls, D. A., & Gibson, B. E. (2018). Objecting: Multiplicity and the practice of physiotherapy. *Health*, *22*(2), 165–184.

Setchell, J., Watson, B. M., Gard, M., & Jones, L. (2016). Physical therapists' ways of talking about overweight and obesity: Clinical implications. *Physical Therapy*, *96*(6), 865–875.

Solvang, P. K. (2019). *(Re)habilitering: terapi, tilrettelegging, verdsetting* [(Re)habilitation: Therapy, adjustment, acknowledgement]. Bergen: Fagbokforlaget.

# Index

Note: Page numbers in *italic* indicate a figure on the corresponding page.

able-bodied and disabled children 128–129, 131
Abonyi, S. 6, 97
Active Back Classes 142
activities of daily living, attending to bodily happenings during 35–37
Afghanistan 169
Ahlsen, B. 5, 41
Alcoholics Anonymous (AA) 58
Amelia, P. d' 21–22, *22*
Amnesty International USA 74
Anjum, R. L. 1, 7, 140, 146
Ariès, P. 71
Armstrong, D. 73
arthritis 61
Askheim, C. 5, 41
assisted physical education (APE) classes 136
attention: habits of 33; types/modes of 31, 33, 36
Auckland Hospital Board 75
Australian Clinical Guidelines for Stroke Management (2007) 186

Bakhtin, M. 159–160, 164–165
Barker, K. 26
Beauvoir, S. de 115
*Being and Time* (Heidegger) 48
Berend, H.W. 11
best life as a goal of treatment 198, 207
Biesta, G. J. J. 90
biology 57, 83, 87–89
biomechanical/biopsychosocial approach 26, 34, 57, 106–108, *107*
biomedical model, the 44, 45, 49, 84, *107*, 131
biomedical risk management 124

biomedicine 75, 77, 106–108, 185
*Biopolitics of Disability, The* (Mitchell and Snyder) 138
biopsychosocial (BPS) model 57, 107
Bjurstrøm, M. 199, 201–203, 204–206
Boardman, J. 58
boccia 201, 203
bodily awareness 33–34, 36
bodily knowledge, in physiotherapy education 33–39
body(ies): analyzing movements 35–37; awareness 33–34, 36; ethical complexities of seeing through camera lens 11; function 58; generalized 34; impaired 130; individual/social/political 107; learning about and through 34–39; management 73; mind and 45, 73; physiotherapy and 29–31, 184, 200; tactile-kinaesthetic/bodily-emotional knowledge 37
Braden, P. 19
Braidotti, R. 78
Braithwaite, J. 8, 197
Brassart, E. 174
British Medical Journal 44
Brun-Cottan, N. 65
Buetow, S. A. 197, 198, 207
Bulley, C. 6, 83
Burrows, L. 6, 70
Bury, M. 59
Bush, K. 17
Butler, J. P. 125

camera 10–11, 19
Canada: access to healthcare 109; colonization history in 100–101; physiotherapy in 106

capitalism 74
care: 24 postural care 83, 85–86, 88–89, 90; access to 105, 109; cure and 49; ethics of 49; landscapes of 89; logic of 50–51; within nursing 42; person-centred 23, 26, 197; in physiotherapy 41–51; postural 89, 90; recovery and 44; spectre of 48; uncanniness of 46–47
Cartesianism 45
causal dispositionalism 146, 153
causation: conception of 145, 146; understanding 148; vector model of 146, *147*
cerebral palsy 72, 199
CG88 (NICE guidelines) 143–144
Cheek, J. 115
child/childhood: coming into attention 71–72; as consumer-citizen 74; as having potential 72–74; requiring protection 72; *see also* disabled children
Child Potential Unit 76–77
choice, logic of 50
chronic illnesses 61
citizens, children as 74
Clarke, B. 92
Clark, M. I. 115
clinical consequences 45–46
clinical guidelines 64, 84, 144
clinical practice: perspective of evidence-based 143–145; predictability and uncertainty in 64–65; vs. school-based physical therapy 134–136; standardization and differentiation in 62–64
colonization, truths of 100–102
community lead research 99
competition 118–119
complexity 48, 90; of 24hPC 86; of embodiment 135; of pain 150–151; of physiotherapy interventions 83, 91; reduction 91; of seeing bodies through a camera lens 11
consumer-citizen, child as 74
co-production: of knowledge 54, 55; of recovery 54, 62–65
core stability 144
corporeality 38
Corrigan, P. W. 58, 59
cripistemology 131
Crippled Children Society 75
critical disability studies 132
Critical Physiotherapy Network (CPN) 1, 2, 4
cultural competence 177

cultural humility and cultural safety 103–106, 178, 179
cultural liaison, involving 170–172
culture 98, 105, 167–180
*Cura* (goddess, care) 41
cure, and care 49
cystic fibrosis *15*

Dahl-Michelsen, T. 8, 197
Danish Midlands Physiotherapists 199
Davey, S. 15–17, *16*
Deegan, P. 59
Deleuze, G. 8, 88, 182, 185, 194
dementia 155, 161
Derrida, J. 42
Despret, V. 5, 32–33, 35
Dewberry, R. 8, 182
dialogic imagination 32, 36, 37, 157, 159–160
Dignity Centre 161
disability studies, integrating into physical therapy professionalization 128–138
disabled children: able-bodied and 128–129, 131; care for their bodies 135–136; challenges for service providers 170; construction of 70, 74–77; free and appropriate education for 128, 133; as individual citizens 74; participation in school for 137; respond to physical rehabilitation interventions 74; social identity for 74–75
discrimination 158
disease, health and 57
disease-oriented recovery outcome 55–56, 63
dispositionalism: as alternative philosophical framework 146–147; for person-centred healthcare 147–149
diversity, encountering 168–170
Donoghue, G. 12
Douglas, S. 118
Duchenne, G.-B. 11
duck-rabbit illusion 33
Dupré, J. 86–87
Durocher, L. 6, 97
dys-appearance 197, 199, 200, 207
dysphasanalysis 185, 193–194
dysphasia 185–188

*Educating the Deliberate Professional* (2016) 3
educational policy of inclusion, in US 128
Education for All Handicapped Children Act, The (1975) 128, 133

Edwards, A. 176
embodied phenomena 30
embodied reflection 164
embodiment 30, 99, 106–108, 135
empathy 14
empiricism 145
Engel, G. L. 57
*Enigma of Health, The* (Gadamer) 162
Enlightenment 48, 71, 89
epistemology 106, 145
Ermine, W. 100
ethical space 100, 103–106
ethics of care 49
E-ti-miyoyat (on a journey towards wellness) 102–103
eu-appearance 207
Eurocentric care model of service delivery 105
event of play, understanding as 163
evidence-based practice (EBP) 43, 56, 77, 91; challenge to 85–86; clinical perspective 143–145; defined 84; dominance in physiotherapy 92; paradigm of 83–85; patient's perspective 140–143; philosophical perspective 145–146; purpose of 64
Ewing, W. A. 11
exercise: physical 44, 49, 73; valorization of 204
experience-based co-design method 91

Fallacy of Misplaced Concreteness 89
Fay, D. 137
Feiring, M. 5, 54
feminism 118
Ferreira, M. L. 65
Ferreira, P. H. 65
fibromyalgia 60
FitBit, 'New Moms' community 114–126
flexibility: of response 156; of services 173
flourishing life 198, 206, 207
focal attention 31, 33, 36
Frank, A. F. 62, 63
Frank, A. W. 7, 155, 157, 158
French, S. 176
Freud, S. 46–47
funding 83, 86
*Fysioterapeuten* issue 199

Gabbay, J. 156
Gadamer, H. G. 162–163, 164–165
Gaffney, M. 6, 70
Galileo 89
Gard, M. 8, 182

Garro, L. C. 61
gaze 10, 14–17, 21, 70
generalized body 34
generosity 157–158, 161
Gesell, A. 73
Gibbons, M. 62
Gibson, B. 30, 57, 63, 131, 175, 184, 197–199, 207
Gilles, A. 75
Giugni, M. 78
Goodley, D. 78
*Great Interactions: Life with Learning Disabilities and Autism* (Braden) 19
Groven, K. S. 1, 8, 197, 199
Grue, J. 199, 205, 206
Guattari, F. 88, 182, 185, 194
Guerrero, A. V. S. 6, 113

habits 31, 33, 36
habitual movements 35
Hall, A. M. 65
Hammell, K. R. W. 57, 177–178
Hannink, E. 26
Hastings, J. 65
hauntology 42
health: defined 57; enigma of 162–163; and illness 30; inequities 98, 101; and wellness 108
healthcare: evidence-based 140–146; facilities 105; services, in Indigenous communities 108–109; visual methods emerging in 12–13; workers 157
healthy aging 99, 105, 108
Hebron, C. 25
Heidegger, M. 42, 48–49
Hellemo, G. 199, 204, 206
hierarchy of evidence 64, 83–86
home visits, and services provision 172–174
hope 59, 61
Hughes, B. 17, 130
humanism 77
human rights frameworks 74
Hume, D. 145
Hundeide, K. 175, 176
Hyginus, G. J. 41

iatrogenic dys-appearance 197, 199, 200
id 49
Illich, I. 26
illness 60; health and 30; individuals' experiences of 58, 59–60; meaning of wellness and 60; perception of 26

images: types of 13–25; use in physiotherapy practice 9, 12–13
impaired bodies 130
impairment: -based therapy, for dysphasia 187; and disability, interconnectedness of 130, 135; remediating 134
inclusion educational policy, for children in special education 128
Indigenous epistemology 101
Indigenous knowledge systems 101, 105
Indigenous worldviews 109
individual body 107
Individualized Education Program (IEP) goals 134
Individuals with Disabilities Education Act (IDEA) 133
indwelling 35
inequality 11, 85, 86, 91, 116
In Sickness and In Health conference 1
intercorporeality 38–39
intergenerational teaching 108
intergenerational trauma 105
International Classification of Diseases (ICD) 55
International Classification of Functioning, Disability, and Health (ICF) model 57, 84, 137
International Classification of Impairments, Disabilities and Handicaps (ICIDH) 57

Jacobson, N. 54, 59
James, W. 33, 37, 38
Jasanoff, S. 55

Kalleson, R. 7, 167, 168
Kapur, N. 198
Kearney, M. H. 61
kinesthetically attuned/attuned kinesthetically 32, 38
King, T. 12
Kinsella, E. A. 1
Kleinfield, M. 194
Kleinman, A. 59, 60
knowledge: co-production of 54, 55; indigenous systems 101, 105; mobilizing to improving PT practice 108–109; physiotherapy 76; scientific 144; self- 60; tacit 31, 33–39, 144; tactile-kinaesthetic/bodily-emotional 37
Kodak 10
Krieger, N. 30

landscapes of care 89
Landsman, G. H. 129–130

Langaas, A. G. 5, 29
language: biomedical 113; and cultural practices 100–102, 105, 107–108; and dysphasia 186–188; in federal education law of educating children 128, 136; poetic 188–193; in service provision 172; signs and gestures 38, 163; verbal 29, 38
Latimer, J. 65
Latour, B. 32
Law, J. 92
learning, about and through bodies 29–39
'learning to become affected' concept 35
least restrictive environment (LRE) 136–137
Lebed, S. 194
LEMO program 203
Leplège, A. 57
*levain* 87
line drawings 13
Ling, P. H. 56
Lock, M. 107
logic: of care 50–51; of choice 50; of rehabilitation 172, 178
long-term conditions (LTCs), people living with 85
looking: ethics of 15; inward/outward 1; as part of practice 1, 9; skills of 9, 13
loss issues 159
low back pain, in adults 143–144
Lowe, W. 6, 113
Low, M. 7, 140, 148, 149
lumbar spine 144
Lupton, D. 60, 63

Macdonald, H. 30
Maher, C. G. 65
Mâmawi (altogether) 97–99
Mâmawi-atoskêwin (working together in partnership) 99–100
*Manipulating Practices* (2018) 1, 3, 106
Marshall, E. M. 155
massage treatment 43–44
Mattingly, C. 60, 61
May, A. le 156
McMillian, D. 65
McRobbie, A. 118
Medical Research Council (MRC) guidance 86
Mengshoel, A. M. 5, 54
Merleau-Ponty, M. 33, 38
Métis community 6, 97–108
Michaels, M. 118
microbiology 83

micro-politics of caring 198
Middelthon, A.-L. 5, 29
Miller, E. 12
Milligan, C. 89
mind and body 45, 73
mindlines and limits of clinical perception 156–158
minority families and service providers 170, 173–174
Mitchell, D. 78, 130–131, 138
*Mitt liv som CP* [My Life with CP] (Bjurstrøm) 199
Miyo-kisinahamowat (mobilizing knowledge to improve PT practice) 108–109
Miyo-mâmti-nitsigan (thinking clearly in a good way towards wellness) 106–108
Mol, A. 42, 50–51
Molinaro, J. 194
Mollestad, S. A. 7, 167, 170–175
motherhood and mothering 115–120
motor control treatment 144
Move and Walk program 202
movements: analyzing 35; focusing on human body 107; posture and 73; primacy of 32; as sensitizing process 36, 129
multidimensional and person-centred approaches, to patient care 144, 148
Mumford, S. 146
Murris, K. 78
musical behaviour 191–193
*My Stroke of Insight* (Taylor) 188
myth of substance and fallacy of misplaced concreteness 89–91

narratives 42, 61–62, 75, 148, 186, 202
National Disability Insurance Scheme (NDIS), in Australia 187
National Institute of Clinical Excellence (NICE) guidelines 143
neoliberalism 74
Nerland, M. 3
neuropathic pain 140, 143
New York City Department of Education (NYC DOE) 129, 132
Nicholls, D. A. 1, 5, 6, 9, 30, 63, 70, 184
Nicholls, J. 5, 9
Nicholson, D. J. 86–87
nonlinear and symbiotic relationships of systems 87–89
non-steroidal anti-inflammatories (NSAIDs) 149
normality and disability 77
Norway 169

Nossell, J. 199–201, 204–205, 206
Nowotny, H. 62

observation 9, 30
online community and wearable devices, mothers engaging with 115–126
ontology 83, 86–87, 89, 145
Oosman, S. 6, 97
Oslo Metropolitan University 31
O'Sullivan, P. 144
Ottesen, A. 5, 41

paediatric physical therapy 132
paediatric rehabilitation context, encountering diversity in 167–177
pain 148; causal and dispositional factors 150, *151*; contributors/improvers 151, *152*; low back 143–144; medications 149; neuropathic 140, 143
Pallesen, E. 92
Parsons, J. 92
participants, attitude of 176–177
Paterson, K. 130
patient and physiotherapist, interaction between 38–39
patient-specific instruments 58
personal experiential recovery process: developing personal expertise 61; noticing 61–62; social movement promoting 58–59; studies on 59–60; wellness and meaning 60
person-centred care 23, 26, 84, 146–152, *150*, 197
philosophical perspective, on EBP 91, 145–146
philosophy 79, 83, 86–87, 89, 91–93, 107, 199
photography: as art form 11; feature of 15; lessons of 25–26; and physiotherapy 10–11; use in healthcare 12
phronesis 144
physical accomplishments 120
physical exercises 44, 49, 73
physical therapy education 128–133, 207
physical therapy (PT) practices 97–109; biopsychosocial (BPS) model 107; changing in partnership 109; enhancing 102–103; ethics in relation to disability 129, 131; evolving towards embodiment 106–108; in Indigenous communities 105–106; least restrictive environment and 128; mobilizing knowledge to improving 108–109; school-based 132, 134–136

physiotherapists, new directions for 184–186, 193–194
physiotherapy: adoption of biomedical paradigm 47; biomedicine and 75, 77; body and 184, 200; in Canada 106; care in 41–51; for children 70–79; creativity and pleasure in 194; developing observation skills in practices 9; development of 44; disabled child and 74–77; education in 92–93; healthcare and 90–91; images and 9, 12–13; issues related to 199; knowledge 76; learning about/through bodies 29–39; photography and 10; placing human relationships at centre of 197–207; re-centring care in 41–51; reductionist approaches to 184–185; relationship-centred approach toward 206; tacit ways of knowing in 33–39; types of image 13–25; *see also* evidence-based practice (EBP)
placebo studies 65
poetic pleasures 190, 194
Polanyi, M. 5, 31, 33, 35, 36, 38
polio epidemics 73
poliomyelitis epidemic, in 1950 56
political body 107
positioning 88
posthumanism 78
postural care 89, 90
power: dynamics, balancing 172–174; imbalances 17, 104, 105, 173, 174, 178
practice, altering 174; *see also* clinical practice; evidence-based practice (EBP); physical therapy (PT) practices
Price, C. 7, 140
*Problems in Dostoevsky's Poetics* (Bakhtin) 159
process philosophy 83, 86, 87, 91–93
process thinking 87, 90, 91
'proper treatment' images 17–19, *18*, *20*
psychoanalysis 42
PT/OT DOE Practice Guide, The (2011) 134, 136

Queen Elizabeth Hospital 75
questionnaires, disease-specific 58

radiological imaging 55
Ralph, R. O. 58, 59
randomized controlled trial (RCT) studies 64–65, 84, 143, 145
rational thinking 186
'real physiotherapy' images 19, 21–25, *21–25*

reciprocity 17, 24, 26, 105–106
*Reconstructing Motherhood and Disability in the Age of "Perfect" Babies* (Landsman) 129
recovery: as absence of disease 57; around, toward, and beyond 198, *198*; as co-production 54, 62–65; and cure 44; determined by measured treatment outcomes 58; developing personal expertise 61; disease-oriented outcome 55–56, 63; from dysphasia 188; as experience 54, 59; identified in people's storytelling 62; in medical care 54; as outcome 54; partial 57; personal experiential process 58–62; rethinking 54–65; social movement 58–59; studies on personal accounts of 59–60; wellness and meaning 60
reductionism and fallacy of misplaced concreteness 89–91
reflecting team 158, 160, 165
reflection 162, 164
reflection-in-action 35, 36
reflective practice 98, 162
*Reflective Practitioner, The* (Schon) 2
reflexivity 145, 153, 178
regularity theory of causation 145
rehabilitation services 57–58, 130–131, 149, 171–172, 175, 198
Reivonen, S. 6, 83
relational expertise 176
relationship: dynamic and dialogical 37; and kinships 108; non-linear and symbiotic 83, 87–89; practitioners and clients 104, 178; service providers and minority families 173; social 60, 61, 65; therapeutic 105, 199–201; trusting 108
researching processes 91–92
rhizoanalysis 92
rhizome 88
rights-based rehabilitation policies 130, 131
Roberts, G. 58
Rose, N. 62
Roy, TJ 6, 97
Runswick-Cole, K. 78

sadness, facing 158–163
Sakitawak Métis 99–100, 101
Sanchez, S. 134
schizophrenia 59
Schön, D. A. 2, 35, 36
school-based physical therapy 132–136
School Functional Assessment (SFA) 132

scientific knowledge 144
Scott, P. 62
Seers, K. 26
Seibt, J. 89
self-knowledge 60
self-policing 125
self-reflection 8, 104, 167, 178, 179
sensitization 32
sensitizing process 34–36
service providers: challenges for 167, 170; and minority families 170, 172–177
Setchell, J. 8, 182
Shakespeare, T. 130, 135
Sheets-Johnstone, M. 32, 36–37, 38
Shildrick, M. 78
Shubowitz, D. 7, 128
Shuttle Run (SR) 137
Sim, F. 6, 83
Skagestad, L. J. 7, 167, 175
skills of looking, developing 9, 13
Skjervheim, H. 176–177
Smith, L. 6, 97
Snyder, S. 78, 130–131, 138
social body 107
social interaction 70, 163
social movement, promoting personal recovery 58–59
sociocultural perspectives: collaborative challenges 175–176; engaging 175–177; participant's attitude 176–177; recognition of family's competencies and concerns 176
Solvang, P. K. 1
Sontag, S. 11
sourdough 87, 88, 90
spectre of care 48
speech therapy, new approaches in 186–188
standardization 137–138
'staying attuned kinesthetically' concept 32
Stewart, S. 116
story 41–51, 62, 103–105, 108, 156–165, 186
stroke and dysphasia 191, 193
structuring binaries 115
subliminal attention 31, 33, 36
substance ontology 89
Sudmann, T. T. 7, 155
Sullivan, N. 25
Swain, J. 176
symptomatic reading 42

tacit knowledge 31, 33–39, 144
Taylor, A. 78

Taylor, J. B. 188
Thille, P. 7, 155
'thinking in movement' 36–37
thinking through processes 86–87
Thirty-Second Walk Test (30sWT) 137
Thompson, H. E. 89
thoracic spine *18*
Thorpe, H. 115
Timed Floor to Stand-Normal (TFTS-N) 137
Timed Up and Down Stairs (TUDS) 137
Timed Up and Go (TUG) 137
tinkering 198, 199, 207
Törnbom, K. 12
touch 37, 43
Toye, F. 26
transcendence 118–119
*Truth and Method* (Gadamer) 162
Truth and Reconciliation Commission of Canada's Calls to Action 109
twenty-four-hour postural care (24hPC) 83, 85–86, 88–89, 90
'typical presentation' images 13–17, *14*, *15*

UK National Institute for Health and Care Excellence 84
ultrabilitation 198, 207
uncanny, the (Freud) 46–47
unconscious 47
United Nations World Health Organization 137
University of Toronto 131

Vehmas, S. 132
verbal language 29, 38
visual illusions 33
visualization 35
visual methods, use in healthcare 12–13
Vuoskoski, P. 25

Walking 77, 115, 126
Waterworth, K. 6, 70
Watson, N. 132
Weedon, F. 5, 19, 21–25, 26
wellness: health and 108; meaning of 60
Whitehead, A. 89
Wiles, J. 89
with-ness/being with, concept of 32–33
Wolbring, G. 198
Workweek Hustle 114
World Health Organization (WHO) 57

Yoshida, K. 131

Printed in the United States
By Bookmasters